# Precise Neurovascular Anatomy for Radical Hysterectomy

Shingo Fujii • Kentaro Sekiyama

# Precise Neurovascular Anatomy for Radical Hysterectomy

Springer

Shingo Fujii
Department of Gynecology and Obstetrics
Kyoto University
Kyoto
Japan

Kentaro Sekiyama
Department of Obstetrics and Gynecology
Kitano Hospital
Kita-ku
Osaka
Japan

ISBN 978-981-13-8097-6 ISBN 978-981-13-8098-3 (eBook)
https://doi.org/10.1007/978-981-13-8098-3



The illustrations were first appeared in the Japanese edition "Sanfujinka Shujutsu Series II Kohansei Fukushiki Shikyu Zentekijutsu"published in 2013 by Shindan To Chiryo Sha, Inc.



This Springer imprint is published by the registered company Springer Nature Singapore Pte Ltd.
The registered company address is: 152 Beach Road, #21-01/04 Gateway East, Singapore 189721, Singapore

# Preface

Since Ernst Wertheim reported the first systematic data on radical hysterectomy in 1911, radical hysterectomy has been considered the most interesting and challenging operation in gynecologic surgery. Naturally, many surgeons have endeavored to improve on Wertheim's radical hysterectomy. Among them, the most pioneering modifications might be by Latzko in 1919 and by Okabayashi in 1921. Okabayashi's radical hysterectomy became popular by 1930 and has been performed as a standard technique for the treatment of Stage Ib and IIb cervical cancer patients in Japan. In contrast, radical hysterectomy was not popular in Western countries until 1954, when Meigs established radical hysterectomy as a safe and effective treatment modality for the cervical cancer patient with early invasive lesion.

In order to accomplish a safe radical hysterectomy, knowledge of the precise anatomical female pelvis is essential. Many advances in our understanding of anatomy have been necessary for further development of techniques in radical hysterectomy. Until recently, the exact anatomy of the bilateral cardinal and the vesicouterine ligaments in the retroperitoneal space at the level of the uterine cervix and upper vagina was a black box for many years. Moreover, quality of life after radical hysterectomy, particularly the bladder function, has been pursued by many doctors under the name of nerve-sparing radical hysterectomy, and the precise neurovascular anatomical knowledge of the pelvic cavity has been elucidated.

This book is focused on the detailed neurovascular anatomy during the open-abdominal radical hysterectomy. Color illustrations are used as much as possible to depict each surgical step during a radical hysterectomy. For the introduction of radical hysterectomy, illustrated figures from the early twentieth century describe each original surgical step of Okabayashi's radical hysterectomy. This is followed by a step-by-step guide to radical hysterectomy without nerve-sparing, illustrating the precise neurovascular anatomy of the retroperitoneal space of the uterine cervix and upper vagina (the cardinal ligament and the vesicouterine ligament). The last chapter of the book is focused on nerve-sparing radical hysterectomy, illustrating the detailed anatomical relationship between the vascular system of the vesicouterine ligament and the nerve plane of the inferior hypogastric plexus formed by the hypogastric nerve, the pelvic splanchnic nerve, the uterine branch, and the bladder branch. Five video disks are provided, with these titles: (1) Radical Hysterectomy, performed by Okabayashi himself; (2) Nerve-Sparing Radical Hysterectomy, by Shingo Fujii; (3) Mibayashi's Original Super-radical Hysterectomy; (4)–(5) Live Surgical Videos of Step-by-Step Nerve-Sparing Radical Hysterectomy, by Shingo Fujii.

With the benefit of magnified views during laparoscopic surgery, surgeons have a greater appreciation of the clear anatomy of the blood vessels in the connective tissues in the female pelvis. Laparoscopy is now well established in the surgical management of gynecological malignancies, with laparoscopic and robotic approaches becoming commonplace in radical hysterectomy. A sound understanding of the neurovascular anatomy is a necessity for emerging gynecological oncology surgeons for open-abdominal and laparoscopic radical hysterectomy.

We hope the book will be a helpful and valuable addition for surgeons who would like to brush up their surgical skills to perform a safe and comprehensive radical hysterectomy.

Kyoto, Japan — Shingo Fujii
Osaka, Japan — Kentaro Sekiyama

# Acknowledgments

I would like to acknowledge Kenji Takakura, M.D., Noriomi Matsumura, M.D., Toshihiro Higuchi, M.D., Sigeo Yura, M.D., Masaki Mandai, M.D., Tsukasa Baba, M.D., Shinya Yoshioka, M.D., Kentaro Sekiyama, and colleagues of the Department of Gynecology and Obstetrics at Kyoto University for their sincere support during the clarification of the precise anatomy of the vesicouterine ligament and the inferior hypogastric plexus.

Kentaro Sekiyama and I would like to express our gratitude to Dr. Ranjit Manchanda, Clinical Senior Lecturer and Consultant Gynecological Oncologist, Barts Cancer Institute, Queen Mary University of London, and his associate Dr. Dhivya Chandrasekaran for editing this textbook.

Shingo Fujii

---

The original version of the book was revised: Copyright page text has been updated. The erratum to the book is available at https://doi.org/10.1007/978-981-13-8098-3_9

# Contents

# 1 Brief History of Surgical Treatment for Cervical Cancer

## 1.1 Cervical Amputation and Simple Total Hysterectomy (Figure 1.1)

Cervical cancer that was visible from the vagina enabled the vaginal resection of the lesion in the prolapsed uterus. The amputation of the cervix of the prolapsed uterus for the surgical treatment of cervical cancer started in the early seventeenth century. However, due to the poor outcomes following local excision, clinicians began to postulate that removal of the uterus may be necessary for the treatment of invasive cervical cancer. By the end of the nineteenth century, simple total hysterectomy was developed either transabdominally (Freund 1878 January) and transvaginally (Czerny 1978 August) for the treatment of cervical cancer. Nevertheless, the outcome of these surgical treatments was still very poor. Consequently, wider resection of the paracervical tissues (the uterine supportive tissues), termed the *radical* approach (extended hysterectomy) was introduced for the treatment of cervical cancer.

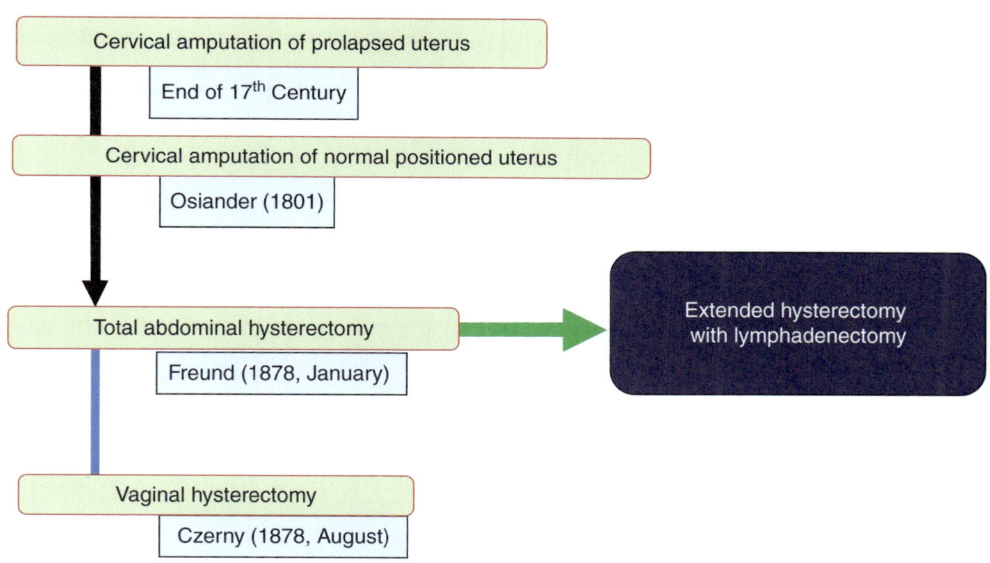


**Figure 1.1** History of surgical treatment for cervical cancer

**Electronic Supplementary Material** The online version of this chapter (https://doi.org/10.1007/978-981-13-8098-3_1) contains supplementary material, which is available to authorized users.


S. Fujii, K. Sekiyama, *Precise Neurovascular Anatomy for Radical Hysterectomy*,
https://doi.org/10.1007/978-981-13-8098-3_1

## 1.2 Extended Hysterectomy with Lymph Node Resection as a Radical Approach for Cervical Cancer Patients (Figure 1.2)

In 1895, JG Clark [1] reported the surgery of wider resection of the paracervical tissues with the uterus, (with bougie insertion into the ureters) as a novel cervical cancer surgery in Johns Hospital Bulletin (USA). Each of the 12 surgeries performed by Clark et al. differed slightly. In some cases the lymph nodes were removed, and in others the parametrium and a vaginal cuff were removed. This is considered as the first report of radical hysterectomy.

In 1898, Ernst Wertheim in Vienna developed a novel procedure of total hysterectomy; removal of the uterus with the parametrium, longer vaginal cuff, and lymph nodes. Then, he reported his improved technique and pathological findings of the removed uterus and lymph nodes with the prognosis of 500 cervical cancer patients in 1911 [2]. Since then, Wertheim's method was accepted as the "radical hysterectomy" and it became a representative method of radical hysterectomy in Western countries.

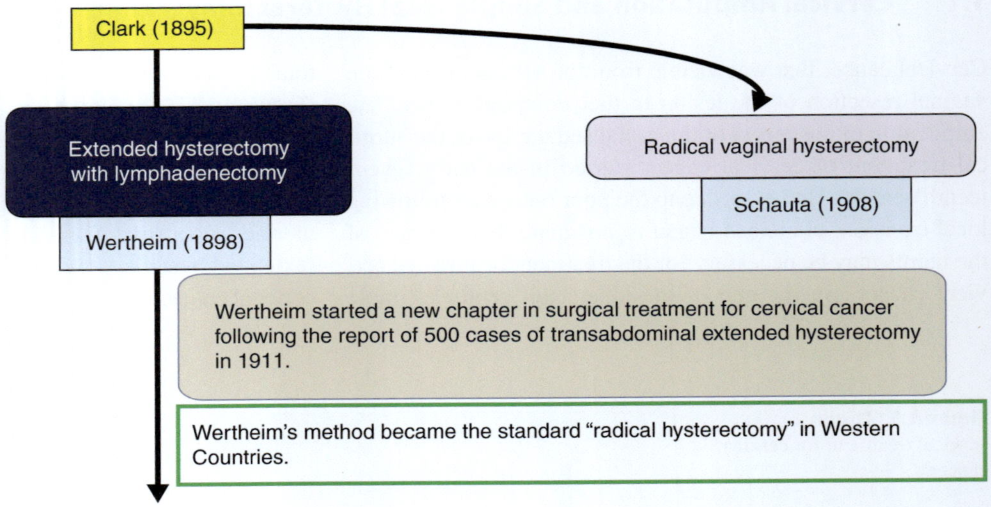


**Figure 1.2** Introduction of extended hysterectomy

## 1.3 Modification of Wertheim's Radical Hysterectomy with Pelvic Lymphadenectomy (Figure 1.3)

After the Wertheim's publication, many doctors attempted to modify the techniques of Wertheim's radical hysterectomy. Two novel surgical approaches were reported from Europe and East-Asia. In 1919, Wilhelm Latzko [3] published novel and more anatomically reasoned radical hysterectomy than that of Wertheim's. Latzko's surgery develops the paravesical space and the pararectal space and divides three ligamentous structures such as the uterosacral ligament (retinaculum posterior), cardinal ligament (retinaculum medial), and paracervical/vaginal tissues (retinaculum anterior).

In Japan, Wertheim's radical hysterectomy was introduced in Kyoto Imperial University. Shohei Takayama [4], Professor and Chairman (1906–1921) of the Department of Gynecology and Obstetrics at Kyoto Imperial University considered that Wertheim's method was not radical enough for the treatment of cervical cancers. Consequently, he endeavored to improve the technique of the Wertheim's operation to a more radical removal of the parametrial tissues, and reported his new technique at the meeting of the Japanese Gynecological Association in 1917. Moreover, Takayama's student, Hidekazu Okabayashi published the novel radical hysterectomy in 1921 [5]. Okabayashi's surgery opens the paravesical space and pararectal space and divides three ligamentous structures: the uterosacral ligament (retinaculum posterior), cardinal ligament (retinaculum medial), and paracervical/vaginal tissues (retinaculum anterior), which is line with that of Latzko's surgery. However, Okabayashi's radical hysterectomy contained novel steps on the division of the paracervical/vaginal tissues. Although the paracervical/vaginal tissues are clamped and divided as a mass in Latzko's surgery, Okabayashi's surgery separates the paracervical tissues into the vesicouterine ligament (anterior (ventral) leaf and posterior (dorsal) leaf) and the blood vessels of the vaginal wall (paracolpium), and divides independently [5, 6]. In order to get an appropriate length of the vaginal cuff, Okabayashi's surgery was much more extensive than that of Latzko's surgery.

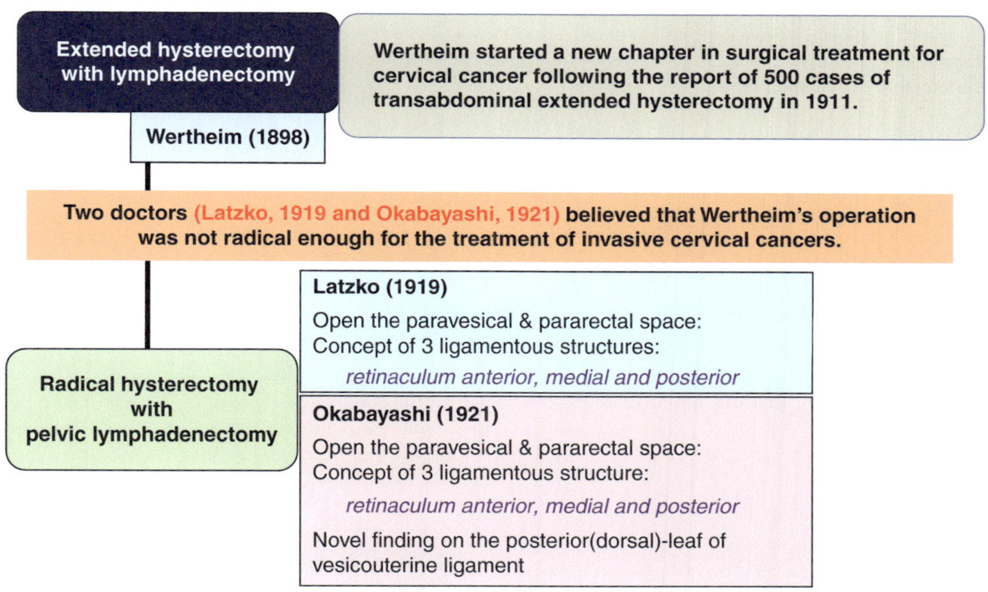


**Figure 1.3** Modification of Wertheim's radical hysterectomy

## 1.4 Situation of Radical Hysterectomy in Mid-Twentieth Century (Figures 1.4 and 1.5)

After the report of Okabayashi's radical hysterectomy in 1921 [5, 6], his surgery was undertaken by the doctors at Kyoto Imperial University, but it gradually spread across Japan. Particularly, when Kyusaku Ogino (Tokyo Imperial University) watched Okabayashi's radical hysterectomy at Kyoto Imperial University, he felt that Okabayashi's method was the most appropriate radical hysterectomy. Then, Ogino introduced Okabayashi's radical hysterectomy to Tokyo Imperial University. Moreover, Ogino started to improve Okabayashi's radical hysterectomy and his modified technique was succeeded by Takashi Kobayashi [7] at Tokyo University. Including Ogino, many doctors such as Kobayashi [7], Masanao Magara [8], Misao Natsume [9], Toshio Fujiwara [10], and Syouichi Sakamoto [11] in Japan tried to improve Okabayashi's radical hysterectomy. Among them, Fujiwara [10] was the first man to introduce liposuction for safe pelvic surgery and lymphadenectomy in 1983. In Japan, doctors of Obstetrics and Gynecology had been brushing up their surgical skills in order to understand the anatomy of the female pelvic cavity through Okabayashi's radical hysterectomy as reported. Therefore, Okabayashi's radical hysterectomy is the most esteemed procedure among the gynecologic surgeries in Japan. Consequently, Okabayashi's radical hysterectomy was accepted and became the standard technique for the treatment of cervical cancer patients in Japan.

In Western countries, Wertheim's radical hysterectomy had been employed for the treatment of cervical cancer in the early twentieth century. However, surgery was not always safe in that period and radiotherapy gradually became the first-line treatment of cervical cancer. Consequently, Wertheim's method was not so frequently undertaken until mid-twentieth century. In 1954, an American gynecologic surgeon, Joe Vincent Meigs reported a modified technique of Wertheim's radical hysterectomy with en-bloc pelvic lymphadenectomy [12]. The results achieved by Meigs were remarkable; almost 90% 5-year survival rate for Stage I disease, and more than 60% 5-year survival rate for Stage II disease. Since then, radical hysterectomy was revived for the treatment of early cervical cancer in Western countries. The radical hysterectomy performed by Meigs was very comparable to Latzko's radical hysterectomy. However, Meigs' radical hysterectomy is named as Wertheim–Meigs radical hysterectomy (later Piver Type III radical hysterectomy: Chap. 2).

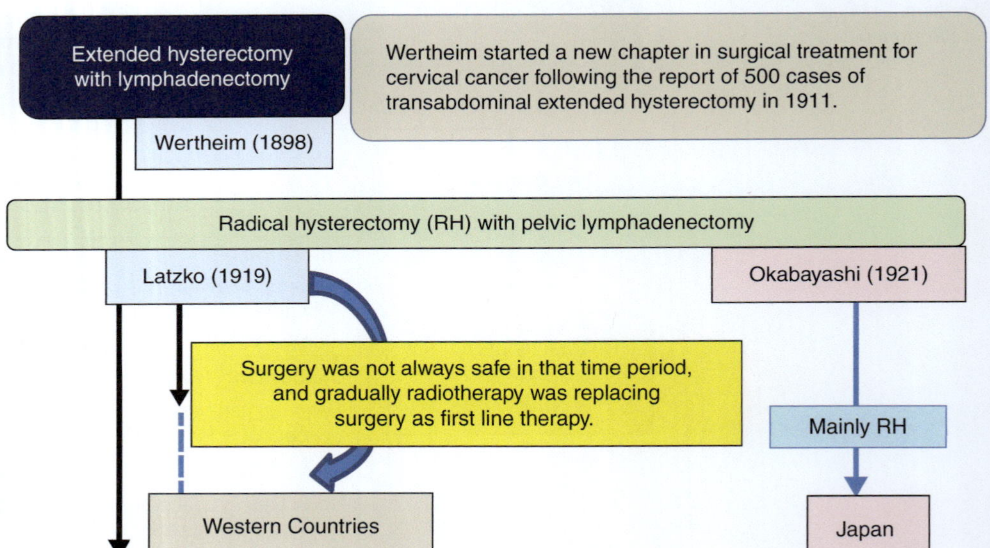


**Figure 1.4** Radical hysterectomy or radiotherapy

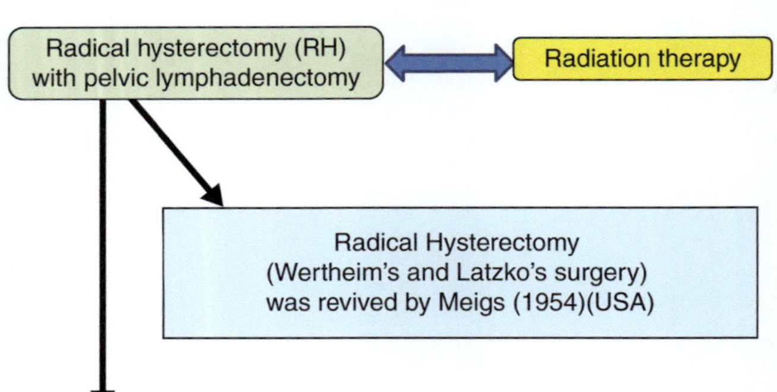


**Figure 1.5** Revival of radical hysterectomy

## 1.5 Recent Novel Findings and Methods on Radical Hysterectomy

In 1994, Daniel Dargent [13] reported a new transvaginal fertility-preserving radical surgery that amputates the cervix with parametrium for women with early invasive cervical cancer. The surgery was named as radical trachelectomy [14]. Currently, this surgery is predominantly done either transvaginally or transabdominally although a laparoscopic approach has also recently been described. For the early invasive cervical cancer patients who wish to retain their fertility, radical trachelectomy is a very important surgical technique. Recently, however, radical trachelectomy is being performed in women with larger tumor volumes than that primarily indicated. Recurrences and fatal outcomes are higher with the expansion of indications. An application of this surgery to the deeply invaded cervical cancer is still controversial.

In 2003, Hockel et al. [15] introduced a new concept on radical hysterectomy, namely: mesometrial resection (MMR) radical hysterectomy. Under the concept of embryological compartment of the mullerian mesometrium, he performs extensive dissection of the uterosacral ligament whilst maintaining the surgical body of the original Wertheim radical hysterectomy. This procedure however, appears to entail a more extensive pelvic lymphadenectomy. The surgery is conceptually new, but anatomical resection margin is very close to the original Wertheim's radical hysterectomy. The good outcome of MMR radical hysterectomy reported by Hockel et al. attracted many clinicians. The extensive lymphadenectomy performed in this surgery appears to contribute to the good surgical outcome. The concept of MMR is understandable, but the anatomy of MMR surgery stays true to the original Wertheim's surgery.

During the technique of radical hysterectomy, the surgeon usually encounters trouble during the separation of the ureter from the connective tissues between the cervix and urinary bladder. In order to remove the vaginal cuff safely, it is necessary to separate the ureter in the connective tissue that is called the vesicouterine ligament (anterior (ventral) leaf and posterior (dorsal) leaf). The vesicouterine ligament had been considered as the tissue that bled easily during surgery. Moreover, the detailed anatomy of the vesicouterine ligament was a black box for more than 90 years. In 2007 Fujii et al. reported detailed vascular anatomy of the anterior (ventral) leaf and posterior (dorsal) leaf of the vesicouterine ligament [16]. We also described the inferior hypogastric plexus hidden behind the posterior (dorsal) leaf of the vesicouterine ligament. Moreover, it becomes possible for us to isolate the uterine branch from the inferior hypogastric plexus. By isolating and dividing the uterine branch alone, well-defined anatomy for the nerve-sparing radical hysterectomy was introduced by Fujii et al. in 2007 [17].

## 1.6 Super-Radical Hysterectomy

In cases of advanced cancer with lymph node metastasis adherent to the blood vessels in the cardinal ligament, Okabayashi's radical hysterectomy is not a suitable surgery due to the risk of microscopic metastasis being left in the divided portion of the cardinal ligament. In this situation, we recommend surgery to extirpate the whole base of the cardinal ligament with internal iliac vascular bundle (Figure 1.6).

Both the internal iliac artery and vein are ligated and divided in this procedure. The internal iliac artery is ligated and divided at the obliterated umbilical artery. The obturator artery and vein are ligated and divided before they pass inferiorly to enter the pelvic side wall. The internal iliac vein is ligated and divided above the base of the pelvic wall (i.e., inferior gluteal, internal pudendal) exposing the roots of the sciatic nerve (Figure 1.7).

With these steps, the whole base of the cardinal ligament is extirpated along with the internal iliac blood vessels (Figure 1.8).

The above described surgical technique was introduced by Ryuukichi Mibayashi, a successor to Okabayashi at Kyoto University, in 1941 as super-radical Hysterectomy [18]. Current opinion suggests that such cases should be treated with radiation or chemoradiation. However, in young women with radio-chemo resistant cancer, this type of surgery can save their lives. The same kind of surgery was introduced by Palfalvi-L and Ungar-L as laterally extended parametrectomy (LEP) in 2003 [19]. Recently, this aggressive surgery is indicated in patients with lymph node positive disease, where it has shown good outcomes without adjuvant radiotherapy [18]. Because super-radical hysterectomy and LEP are extirpating the base of the cardinal ligament with internal iliac blood vessel systems, *Total Extirpation of Internal Iliac Blood Vessel System (TEIIBS) with Cardinal Ligament* seems to be a more suitable name for this surgery.

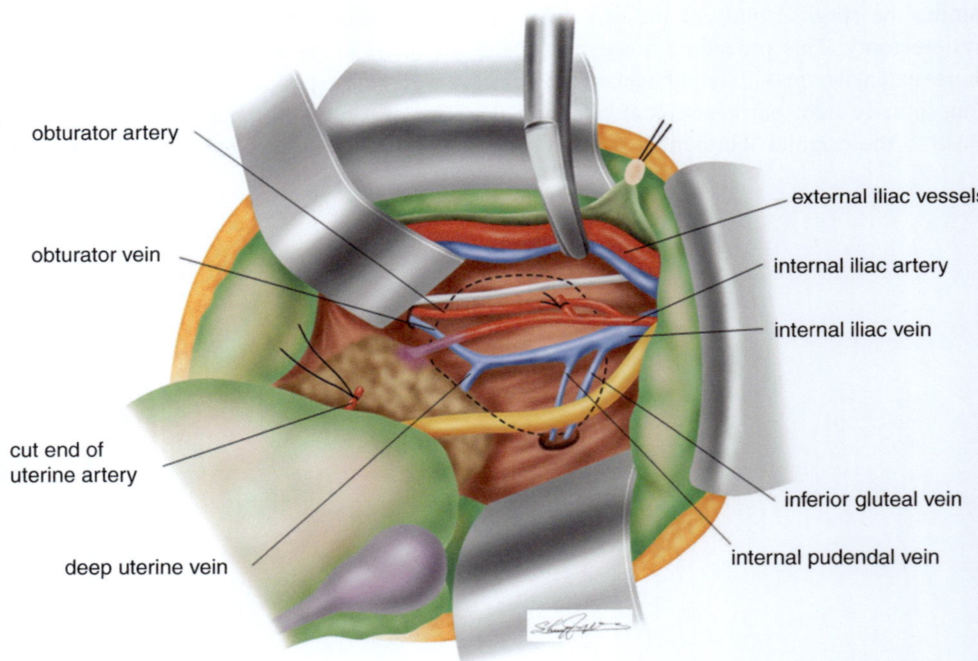


**Figure 1.6** Anatomy of the blood vessels in the pelvis focused on the location of the internal iliac blood vessel system (circle of dotted line)

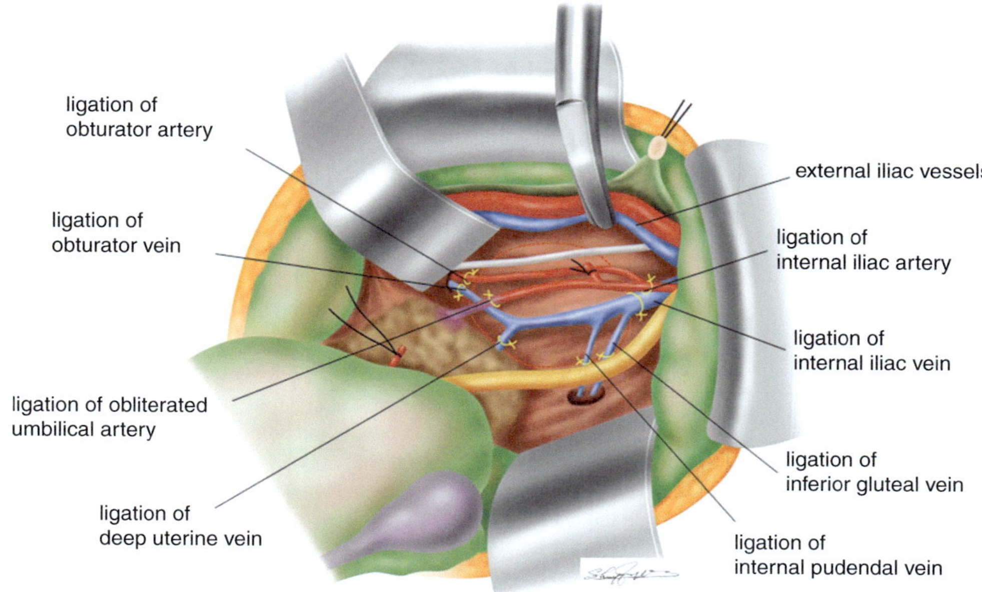


**Figure 1.7** Sites of ligation of the internal iliac vessels for the extirpation of the internal iliac vessels

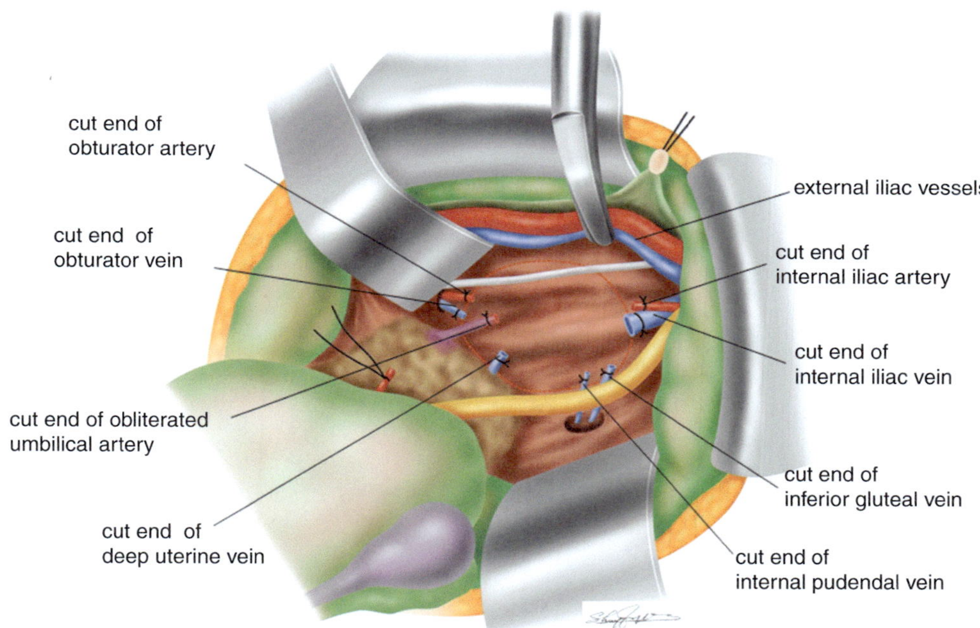


**Figure 1.8** Extirpated figure of the internal iliac blood vessel system

## 1.7 Notes

### 1.7.1 Surgical Novel Concepts and Anatomical Findings on Radical Hysterectomy

Figure 1.9 is a list of surgical novel concepts and anatomical findings on radical hysterectomy.

| | |
|---|---|
| 1895 Clark | Abdominal extended (radical) hysterectomy |
| 1898 Wertheim | Abdominal extended (radical) hysterectomy |
| 1908 **Schauta** | Vaginal extended (radical) hysterectomy without lymphadenectomy |
| 1911 **Wertheim** | Abdominal extended (radical) hysterectomy. This surgery became a standard of radical hysterectomy in Western countries |
| 1917 Takayama | Modified Wertheim method in Japan and demonstrated his live surgery at the 15th Scientific Meeting of Japan Society of Gynecology in Kyoto |
| 1919 **Latzko** | Radical hysterectomy: Lymphadenectomy at first, then developing paravesical and pararectal spaces, divide the cardinal ligament wider than that of Wertheim |
| 1921 **Okabayashi** | Radical hysterectomy: Almost the same type of Latzko's surgery, but characterized by the separation of the vesicouterine ligament independently from the paracolpium |
| 1941 **Mibayashi** | Super-radical hysterectomy is the surgery of total extirpation of internal iliac blood vessel system (TEIIBS) with the cardinal ligament. Laterally extended parametrectomy (LEP) by Palfalvi & Ungar (2003) is almost the same surgery. |
| 1951 **Meigs** | Reevaluation of Radical Hysterectomy (Wertheim, Latzko) in the USA :Meigs' radical hysterectomy is almost the same as that of Latzko's radical hysterectomy |
| 1961 **Kobayashi** | Pioneer of nerve-sparing radical hysterectomy (pelvic splanchnic nerve) |
| 1994 **Dargent** | Pioneer of fertility-preserving radical surgery: Radical vaginal trachelectomy |
| 2003 Palfalvi & Ungar | Laterally extended parametrectomy (LEP) is almost the same as that of Mibayashi's surgery |
| 2003 Hockel | Mesometrial resection (MMR) radical hysterectomy. New concept of radical hysterectomy within the area of the embryological mesometrial compartment. Surgical margin is almost the same as that of Wertheim |
| 2007 Fujii | Clarification of the detailed anatomy of the vesicouterine ligament for ideal radical hysterectomy |
| 2007 Fujii | Clarification of the detailed anatomy of the inferior hypogastric plexus for nerve-sparing radical hysterectomy |

**Figure 1.9** Surgical novel concepts and anatomical findings on radical hysterectomy

### 1.7.2 History of Radical Hysterectomy in Western Countries and in Japan

Since Wertheim reported his radical hysterectomy in 1911, the technique was modified both in Western countries and in Japan. Figure 1.10 is a chronological chart of the development of surgical technique on radical hysterectomy in Western countries and in Japan (Kyoto & Tokyo University).

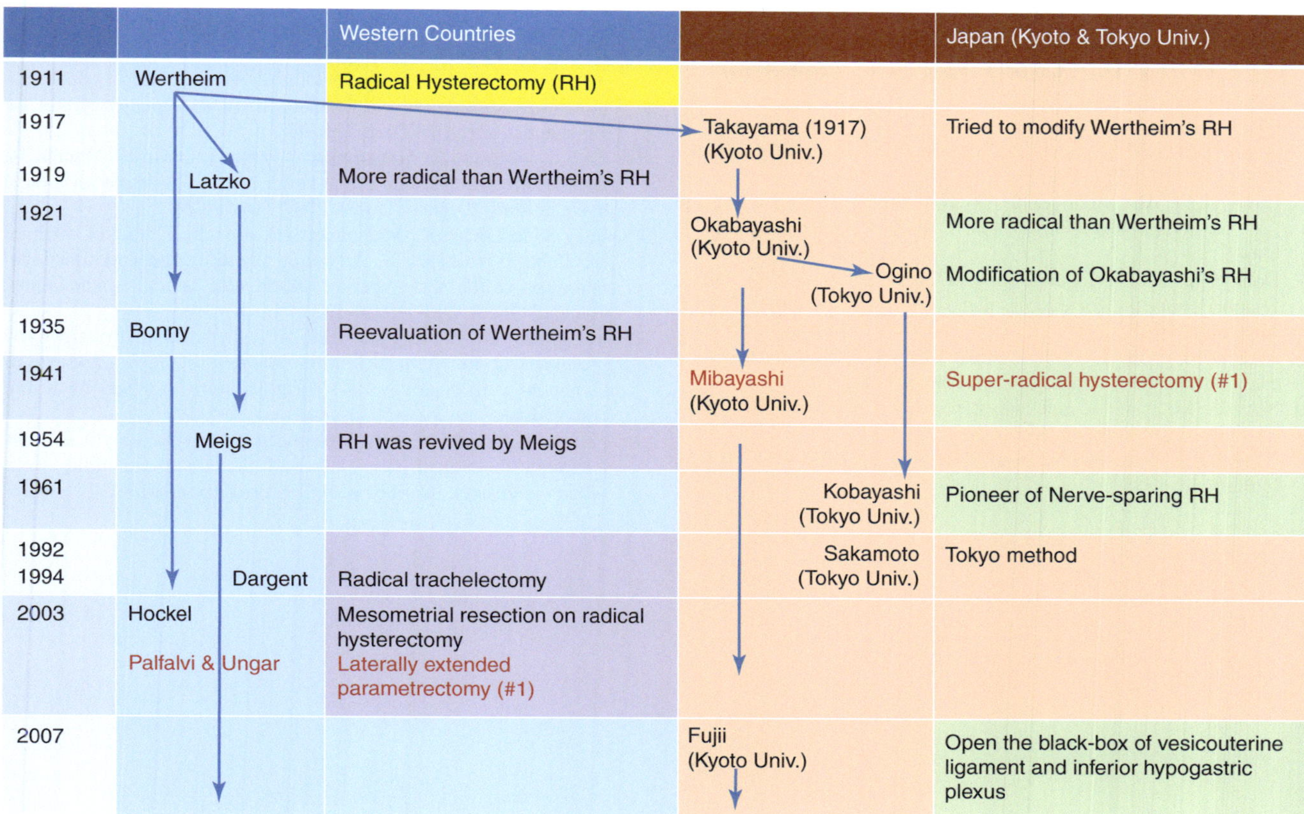


**Figure 1.10** History of radical hysterectomy in Western countries and in Japan (Kyoto & Tokyo Univ.) #1: Total extirpation of the internal iliac blood vessel system with the cardinal ligament

## References


1. Clark JG. More radical method of performing hysterectomy for cancer of the uterus. Johns Hopkins Hosp Bull. 1895;6:120–4.
2. Wertheim E. Die erweiterte abdominale Operation bei Carcinoma colli Uteri (auf Grund von 500 Fallen). Berlin: Urban & Schwarzenberg; 1911.
3. Latzko W, Schiffmann WJ. Klinisches und Anatomisches zur Radikaloperation des Gebärmutterkrebses. Zbl Gynäkol. 1919;34:689–705.
4. Takayama S. Live surgical demonstration of modified Wertheim method at the 15th Scientific Meeting of Japan Society of Gynecology in Kyoto; 1917.
5. Okabayashi H. Radical abdominal hysterectomy for cancer of the cervix uteri, modification of the Takayama operation. Surg Gynecol Obstet. 1921;33:335–41.
6. Okabayashi H. Abdominale systematische Panhysterektomie fur Karzinoma des Uterus. Jpn J Obstet Gynaecol. 1928;11:136–53.
7. Kobayashi T. Abdominal radical hysterectomy with pelvic lymphadenectomy for cancer of the cervix (in Japanese). Tokyo: Nanzando; 1961.
8. Magara M, Iwata H, Senda T. Abdominal radical hysterectomy for cancer of the cervix (in Japanese). Tokyo: Nanzando; 1964.
9. Natsume M. Systemic radical hysterectomy for cancer of the cervix (in Japanese). Tokyo: Nankodo; 1974.
10. Fujiwara T. Surgery for cervical cancer (in Japanese). Tokyo: Igakushoin; 1983.
11. Sakamoto S. Radical hysterectomy with pelvic lymphadenectomy—the Tokyo method. In: Coppleson M, editor. Gynecologic oncology. 2nd ed. Edinburg: Churchill Livingstone; 1992. p. 1257–68.
12. Meigs JV. Surgical treatment of cancer of the cervix. New York: Grune & Stration; 1954.
13. Dargent D, Brun JL, Roy M, Mathevet P. La trachelectomie élargie: uné alternative á l'hystérectomie. Radicale dansu traitment des cancers in filtrants. Jobgyn. 1994;2:285–92.
14. Dargent D, Martin X, Sacchetoni A, Mathevet P. Laparoscopic vaginal radical trachelectomy: a treatment to preserve the fertility of cervical carcinoma patients. Cancer. 2000;88:1877–82.
15. Höckel M, Horn LC, Hentschel B, Höckel S, Naumann G. Total mesometrial resection: high resolution nerve-sparing radical hysterectomy based on developmentally defined surgical anatomy. Int J Gynecol Cancer. 2003;13:791–803.
16. Fujii S, Takakura K, Matsumura N, Higuchi T, Yura S, Mandai M, Baba T. Precise anatomy of the vesico-uterine ligament for radical hysterectomy. Gynecol Oncol. 2007;104:186–91.
17. Fujii S, Takakura K, Matsumura N, Higuchi T, Yura S, Mandai M, Baba T, Yoshioka S. Anatomic identification and functional outcomes of the nerve sparing Okabayashi radical hysterectomy. Gynecol Oncol. 2007;107:4–13.
18. Mibayashi R. A surgical film of super-radical hysterectomy presented at the 39th Scientific Meeting of Japan Society of Gynecology in Nagoya; 1941 (original film is owned by Kyoto University).
19. Palfalvi L, Ungar L. Laterally extended parametrectomy (LEP), the technique for radical pelvic side wall dissection: feasibility, technique and results. Int J Gynecol Cancer. 2003;13:914–7.

# 2 Classification of Radical Hysterectomy

In Western countries, since Meigs' publication on radical hysterectomy in 1954 [1], radical hysterectomy was revived as the standard treatment for early invasive cervical cancer. The surgical technique of Meigs' radical hysterectomy contained the isolation and division of the cardinal ligament which is the same as that of Latzko's surgery or Okabayashi's surgery. In Japan, by the end of twentieth Century, surgeons met with major bleeding during Okabayashi's radical hysterectomy. Bleeding could occur at the time of dissection of the cardinal ligament at junction with the internal iliac vascular system, after the development of both pararectal and paravesical spaces. The bleeding was usually from the cut-end of the cardinal ligament of the internal iliac vascular side. Therefore, some cases could be finished without any trouble, but other cases may face heavy bleeding during Okabayashi's radical hysterectomy. The risk of hemorrhage was hidden in the separation and clamping processes of the anatomically insecure tissues. As the results of many efforts by Japanese doctors such as Yoshihiko Yabuki [2–5], recently Okabayashi's radical hysterectomy has proven safer. In order to reduce bleeding during surgery, isolation of each blood vessel in the cardinal ligament has been practiced in Japan and recently the risk of hemorrhage has reduced significantly.

In order to avoid heavy bleeding from the base of the cardinal ligament, partial division of the cardinal ligament was considered and extended hysterectomy was classified according to the resection length of the cardinal ligament, in 1974.

## 2.1 Piver–Rutledge–Smith's Classification (1974) [6]

In 1974, Piver–Rutledge–Smith [6] proposed the classification of extended hysterectomy according to the length of cardinal ligament. Class I was extrafascial simple total hysterectomy (minimum excision of the cardinal ligament and more excision of the vagina than that of simple total hysterectomy), Class II was slight resection of the cardinal ligament resembling that of Wertheim's method. Class III was resection of the cardinal ligament at the level of the pelvic side wall (Meigs' surgery was the example of Class III surgery). Class IV was characterized by the complete removal of all peri-ureteric tissue and a more extensive excision of the paravaginal tissues. The class V hysterectomy is removal of central recurrent cancer involving portions of the distal ureter or bladder.

This classification became popular, because Class III was considered as a standard radical hysterectomy for doctors in Western countries. However, it generated the chaotic state of surgical outcomes in cervical cancer treatment because the classification was used without checking the original article. In addition, many different types/extent of radical hysterectomy were termed as Class III radical hysterectomy. Gradually, majority of the published papers started to use the name of Class III radical hysterectomy for each institution's radical hysterectomy. The submitted manuscript to English journals from Japan also started to use the terminology of Class III radical hysterectomy to the radical hysterectomy done by Okabayashi's method to get better understanding from the referees of Western countries.

Differences in surgical margins, lymphadenectomy, and quality of surgery in each institution created variable surgical outcomes of Class III radical hysterectomy across the world. Consequently, the published literature accumulated considerable data on surgical outcomes on Class III radical hysterectomy of varying anatomical dissection. This therefore explains the considerable variation and differences in the data for Class III radical hysterectomy.


S. Fujii, K. Sekiyama, *Precise Neurovascular Anatomy for Radical Hysterectomy*,
https://doi.org/10.1007/978-981-13-8098-3_2

## 2.2 Querler & Morrow's Classification (2008) [7]

In 2008, Querler & Morrow [7] proposed a new classification of radical hysterectomy. The title of classification by Piver–Rutledge–Smith was "Five classes of extended hysterectomy for women with cervical cancer" but the title used by Querler & Morrow was "Classification of radical hysterectomy." Probably, Piver–Rutledge–Smith did not intend to classify radical hysterectomy itself but they intended to show the surgical margin of each extended hysterectomy depending on the cervical cancer lesion. However, the name of Class III radical hysterectomy started to be used independently in each institution as if the Class III radical hysterectomy was the standard for radical hysterectomy.

Querler & Morrow's classification was on radical hysterectomy using alphabets such as Type A, B, C, and D. Type A is a simple extrafascial total hysterectomy with minimum resection of the paracervix. In their classification, the terminology of paracervix is defined to include the cardinal ligament (Mackenrodt's ligament), parametrium, or paracolpium. This seems to again introduce ambiguity in the surgical margin by using a word with a wide range of meanings. In addition, they are also included a simple extrafascial total hysterectomy with less than 10 mm vaginal resection in the classification of radical hysterectomy with the name of Type A.

Type B is the surgery where the ureter is unroofed and rolled laterally, permitting transection of the paracervix at the level of the ureteric tunnel. This surgery does neither resect the cardinal ligament nor the deep uterine vein. Type B is almost the same as that of the original Wertheim's surgery. This surgery is rather a semi-radical hysterectomy. Querler & Morrow's classified Type B into two subtypes such as Type B1 or Type B2 depend on whether or not lymphadenectomy is performed. Type B2 surgery is the most common type of radical hysterectomy in Western countries.

Type C involves a transection of the paracervix at the junction with internal iliac vascular system. This entails the transection of the cardinal ligament with the deep uterine vein at the junction of the internal iliac vein; both Latzko–Meigs' and Okabayashi's radical hysterectomy described this step. Type C involves the transection of the uterosacral ligament at the rectum and vesicouterine ligament at the bladder and described the complete mobilization of the ureter, and the paracolpos with the corresponding length of vagina (15–20 mm from the tumor or the cervix) resected routinely. However, a detailed description on the anatomy of the vesicouterine ligament is lacking in the classification. Radical hysterectomy with nerve-sparing or without nerve sparing correspond to Type C1 and C2, respectively. The Type C radical hysterectomy corresponds to Latzko–Meigs' (Piver–Rutledge–Smith's Class III) radical hysterectomy, but in order to perform nerve-sparing radical hysterectomy (Type C1), the anatomy of Okabayashi's radical hysterectomy, particularly the anatomy of the posterior (dorsal) leaf of the vesicouterine ligament is essential. Type C1, nerve-sparing radical hysterectomy, describes the transection of uterine branch alone from the inferior hypogastric plexus and preserves bladder branch, hypogastric nerve, and pelvic splanchnic nerve with the plexus. It is not easy to accomplish this using the steps described in Latzko-Meigs' or Piver–Rutledge–Smith's Class III radical hysterectomy because they do not separate the posterior (dorsal) leaf of the vesicouterine ligament. Without careful separation of the posterior (dorsal) leaf of the vesicouterine ligament, identification of the complete structure of the inferior hypogastric plexus and transecting the uterine branch in isolation is difficult. Therefore, Type C1 surgery should be based on the Okabayashi's nerve-sparing radical hysterectomy. In 2011, Cibula-D, Querler, Morrow et al. in 2011 [8], published a paper entitled *"New classification system of radical hysterectomy: Emphasis on a three-dimensional anatomic template for parametrial resection."* This described the dissection in Type C1 where the ureter is unroofed, dissected from the cervix and from the parametria, but only partially from the ventral parametria. This anatomical description similarly does not allow easy identification of the inferior hypogastric plexus and transection of uterine branch in isolation. We recommend the use of consistent anatomical description on nerve-sparing radical hysterectomy for the better understanding of surgeons.

Type D is laterally extended resection. This category includes a super radical hysterectomy by Mibayashi in 1941 [9] or laterally extended parametrectomy (LEP) (Palifavi, Ungar [10]) or laterally extended endopelvic resection (LEER) (Hockel [11]).

## 2.3 Classification of Radical Hysterectomy and Corresponding Surgical Treatment Modalities

As shown in the Figure 2.1, each alphabetical category of Querler & Morrow's Classification corresponds to the existing surgical modalities for the different stage of cervical cancer (Figure 2.1). If we can reach a consensus on radical hysterectomy, the various classifications using classes or letters will become redundant.

A recent trend in surgical treatment of cervical cancer has been to reduce the surgical margins (less invasive) in order to achieve better quality of life following surgery. However, in order to accomplish a less invasive approach with reduced surgical margins, it is very important for us to have the skill and anatomical knowledge to accomplish the surgery of extended surgical margins.

Recently, some institutions have reported that the surgical outcomes following high quality radical hysterectomy or more extensive radical hysterectomy can achieve greater than 90% 5 year survival rate in patients with FIGO IB2 disease (Nam et al. [12, 13]) or invasive cervical cancer lesion having positive lymph node metastasis without giving any adjuvant radiotherapy, respectively (Ungar et al. [14]). In order for this to become a wider trend, it is imperative to have knowledge of precise pelvic anatomy to accomplish the most appropriate surgery for each patient.

**Classification of radical hysterectomy and corresponding surgical treatment modalities**

| Classification Piver et al 1974 | Classification Querler/Morrow (2008) | Surgical treatment modalities for cervical cancer |
|---|---|---|
| | | Conization |
| Type 1 | Type A | Extra-fascial simple total hysterectomy |
| Type II-III | Type B | Extended simple total hysterectomy or Semi-Radical hysterectomy |
| | | Radical Trachelectomy |
| | Type C1 | Radical hysterectomy with Nerve-sparing |
| Type III? | Type C2 | Radical hysterectomy (Latzko's or Meigs' surgery) Okabayashi's radical hysterectomy (not equal) |
| | Type D1 | Laterally extended parametrectomy(LEP) (Mibayashi: su per-rasical hysterectomy (TEIIBS)) |
| | D2 | D1 + adjacent fascial or muscular structure: laterally extended endopelvic resection(LEEP) |
| | | Pelvic Exenteration |

**Figure 2.1** Relationship between the classification and surgical treatment modalities for cervical cancer. *TEIIBS* Total extirpation of the internal iliac blood vessel system with the cardinal ligament

## References


1. Meigs JV. Surgical treatment of cancer of the cervix. New York: Grune & Stration; 1954.
2. Yabuki Y, Sasaki H, Hatakeyama N, Murakami G. Discrepancies between classic anatomy and gynecologic surgery on pelvic connective tissue structure: harmonization of those concepts by collaborative cadaver dissection. Am J Obstet Gynecol. 2005;193:7–15.
3. Yabuki Y, Asamoto A, Hoshiba T, Nishimoto H, Kitamura S. Dissection of the cardinal ligament in radical hysterectomy for cervical cancer with emphasis on the lateral ligament. Am J Obstet Gynecol. 1991;164:7–14.
4. Yabuki Y, Asamoto A, Hoshiba T, Nishimoto H, Satou N. A new proposal for radical hysterectomy. Gynecol Oncol. 1996;62:370–8.
5. Yabuki Y, Asamoto A, Hoshiba T, Nishimoto H, Nishikawa Y, Nakajima T. Radical hysterectomy: an anatomic evaluation of parametrial dissection. Gynecol Oncol. 2000;77:155–63.
6. Piver MS, Rutledge F, Smith JP. Five classes of extended hysterectomy for women with cervical cancer. Obstet Gynecol. 1974;44:265–72.
7. Querleu D, Morrow CP. Classification of radical hysterectomy. Lancet Oncol. 2008;9:297–303.
8. Cibula D, Abu-Rustam NR, Benedetti-Panici P, Kohler C, Raspagliesi F, Querleu D, Morrow CP. New classification system of radical hysterectomy: emphasis on a three-dimensional anatomical template for parametrial resection. Gynecol Oncol. 2011;122:264–8.
9. Mibayashi R. A surgical film of super-radical hysterectomy presented at the 39th Scientific Meeting of Japan Society of Gynecology in Nagoya; 1941 (original film is owned by Kyoto University).
10. Palfalvi L, Ungar L. Laterally extended parametrectomy (LEP), the technique for radical pelvic side wall dissection: feasibility, technique and results. Int J Gynecol Cancer. 2003;13:914–7.
11. Hockel M, Horn LC, Einenkel J. (Laterally) extended endopelvic resection: surgical treatment of locally advanced and recurrent cancer of the uterine cervix and vagina based on ontogenetic anatomy. Gynecol Oncol. 2012;127:297–302.
12. Park JY, Kim DY, Kim JH, Kim YM, Kim YT, Nam JH. Laparoscopic versus open radical hysterectomy in patients with stage IB2 and IIA2 cervical cancer. J Surg Oncol. 2013;108(1):63–9.
13. Park JY, Kim DY, Kim JH, Kim YM, Kim YT, Kim YS, Kim HJ, Lee JW, Kim BG, Bae DS, Huh SJ, Nam JH. Comparison of outcomes between radical hysterectomy followed by tailored adjuvant therapy versus primary chemoradiation therapy in IB2 and IIA2 cervical cancer. J Gynecol Oncol. 2012;23:226–34.
14. Ungár L, Pálfalvi L, Tarnai L, Horányi D, Novák Z. Surgical treatment of lymph node metastases in stage IB cervical cancer. The laterally extended parametrectomy (LEP) procedure: experience with a 5 year follow-up. Gynecol Oncol. 2011;123:337–41.

# 3 Concept of the Original Okabayashi's Radical Hysterectomy

## 3.1 Principles of Okabayashi's Radical Hysterectomy

This surgery is designed for the treatment of invasive cervical cancer. The principle is the removal of the whole uterus with enough length of vaginal cuff dissecting the most distal portion of the uterine supportive tissues (Figures 3.1, 3.2, and 3.3). Surgically, Okabayashi developed three major supportive tissue bundles between the uterus and the pelvic wall. The concept of the three supportive tissues was introduced by Latzko in 1919. Okabayashi also developed anterior, middle, and posterior supportive tissues (Figure 3.4). The anterior (ventral) supportive tissue is composed of the anterior (ventral) and posterior (dorsal) leaves of the vesicouterine ligament. The middle supportive tissue includes the cardinal ligament and pelvic splanchnic nerve. The posterior (dorsal) supportive tissue contains the uterosacral ligament, hypogastric nerve, and rectovaginal ligament. The cardinal ligament is visualized by the development of the pararectal space and the paravesical space. For the removal of the uterus, Okabayashi independently divided the paracolpium (vaginal blood vessels).

After separation of the urinary bladder from the cervical/vaginal fascia, the vesicouterine ligament surrounding the ureter is revealed between the sidewall of the cervix/vagina and the paravesical space. We call the ventral side of the ureter as the anterior (ventral)-leaf of the vesicouterine ligament and the dorsal side as the posterior (dorsal)-leaf of the vesicouterine ligament. By the complete separation of each leaf of the vesicouterine ligament, the ureter and the urinary bladder can be separated from the cervix/upper vagina as much as one wishes. In addition, this procedure allows us to identify the paracolpium (vaginal blood vessels and the connective tissue). The dissection level of the paracolpium depends on the level of disease and the length of the lateral vaginal cuff. Moreover, dissection of the rectovaginal ligament enables the surgeon to decide the appropriate vaginal cuff length of the dorsal vagina (Figure 3.5). In addition to the division of the distal portion of the three major supportive tissues, pelvic lymph nodes are systematically removed.


S. Fujii, K. Sekiyama, *Precise Neurovascular Anatomy for Radical Hysterectomy*,
https://doi.org/10.1007/978-981-13-8098-3_3

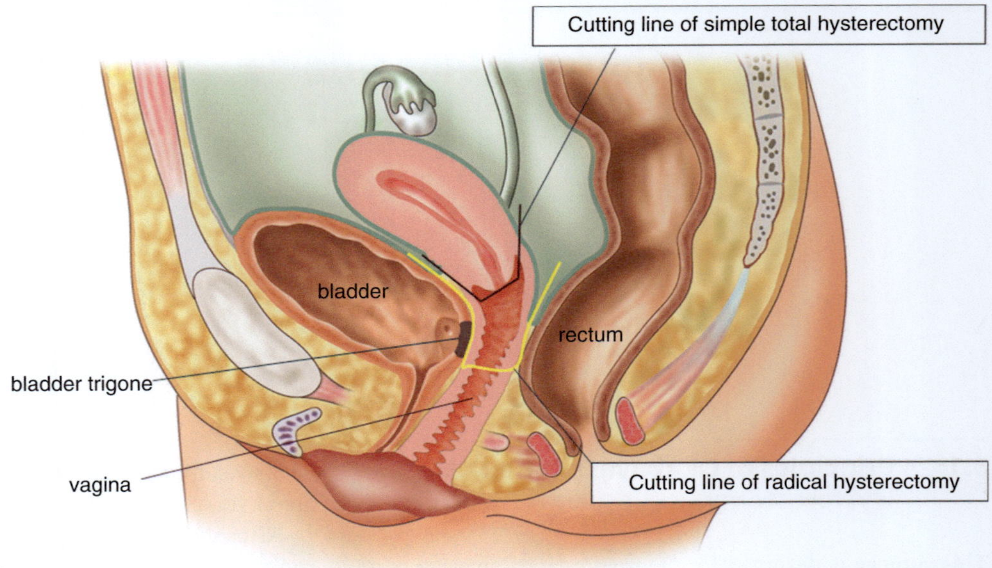


**Figure 3.1** Sagittal section view of the pelvic cavity is showing the different cutting line of the vagina of simple total hysterectomy and radical hysterectomy

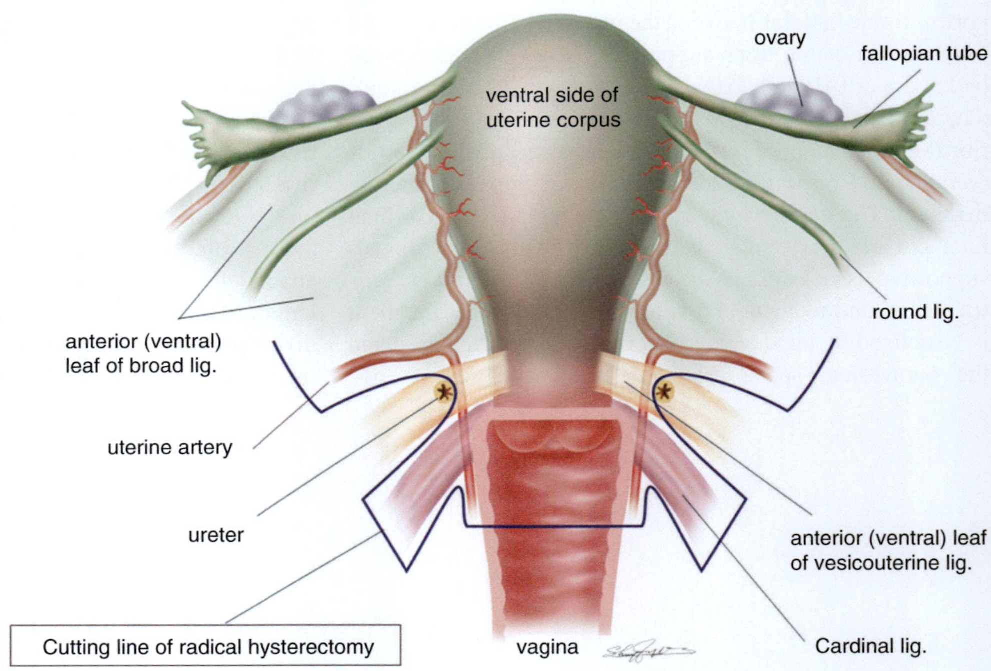


**Figure 3.2** Ventral side view of the uterus, vagina, and their associated supportive ligaments, showing the resection line of the uterine supportive tissues (the anterior (ventral) leaf of the vesicouterine ligament, the cardinal ligament) and the vagina at radical hysterectomy

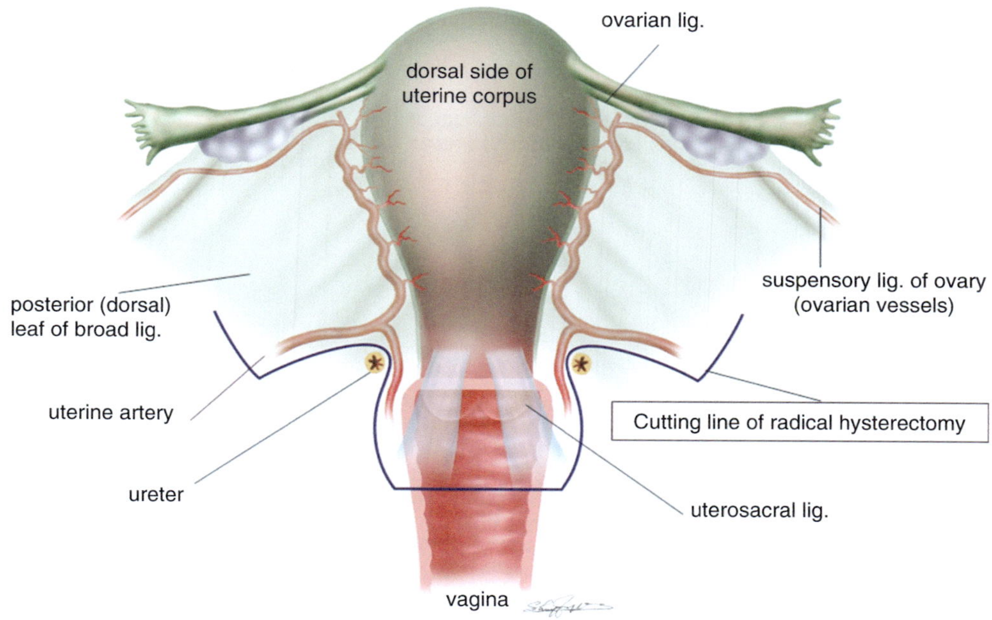


**Figure 3.3** Dorsal side view of the uterus, vagina, and the uterosacral ligament showing the resection line of the uterosacral ligament and the vagina at radical hysterectomy

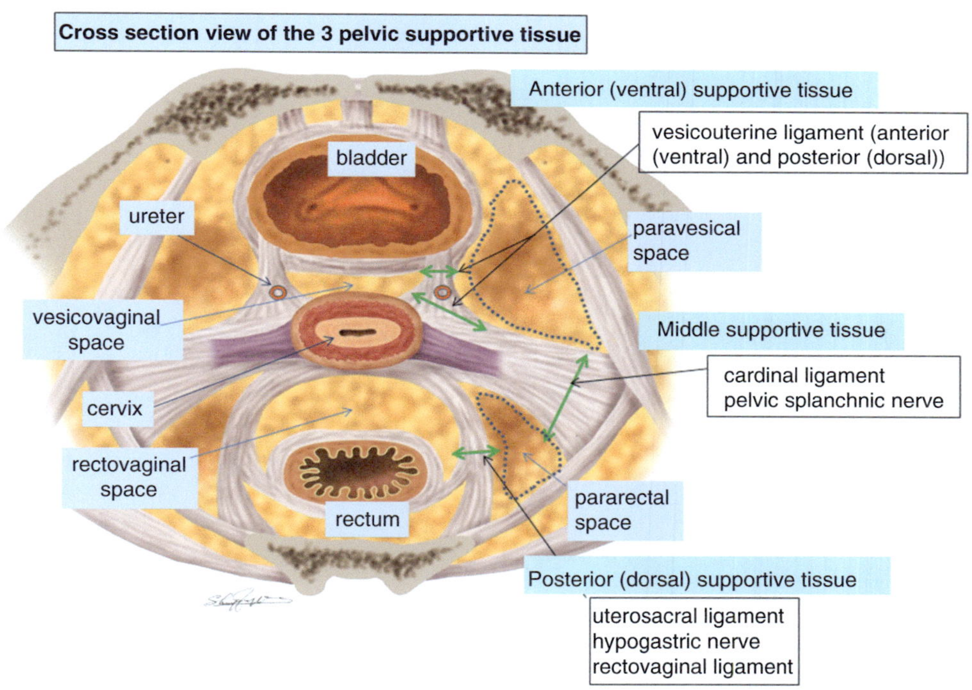


**Figure 3.4** A cross-sectional view of the pelvic cavity is showing three (anterior (ventral), middle, and posterior (dorsal)) pelvic supportive tissues and their cutting line at radical hysterectomy

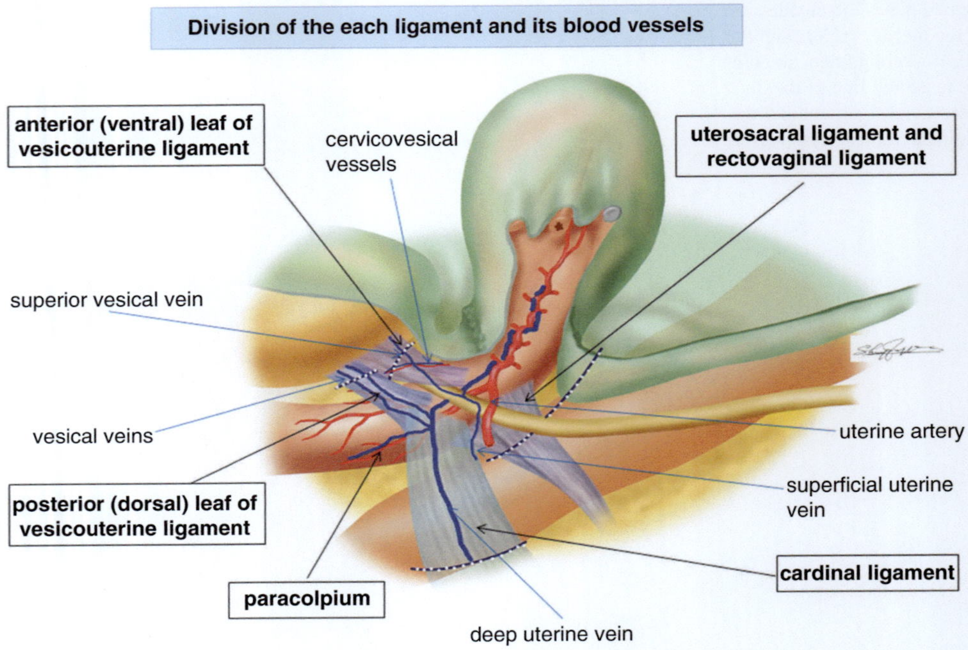


**Figure 3.5** A lateral side view of the resection line of the anterior (ventral) and posterior (dorsal) leaf of the vesicouterine, the cardinal, and the uterosacral ligaments. Major blood vessels are shown in each ligament and the paracolpium

# Atlas of the Original Okabayashi's Transabdominal Radical Hysterectomy

# 4

## 4.1 Surgical Steps of Original Okabayashi's Radical Hysterectomy

### 4.1.1 Opening of the Abdominal Cavity

The abdomen is opened by a midline incision which should be made a sufficient length to secure free exposure of the operative field. (This usually extends from the symphysis to above the umbilicus.)

### 4.1.2 Exposure of the Pelvic Cavity

After examination of the upper abdominal cavity, the intestine is packed out of the pelvis with large abdominal towels moistened with saline water and the uterus and both ovaries/fallopian tubes are exposed in the pelvic cavity.

### 4.1.3 Visual and Manual Examination of the Spread of the Disease and Judgment of Operability

The peritoneal surface of the pelvic cavity is inspected. The uterus and surrounding organs are examined to determine the extent of disease and the operability of the case. Bimanually, examination of the cervical lesion and surrounding tissues determines whether there is invasion outside of the cervix. Mobility of the uterus from the surrounding organs and pelvic wall is the most important determinant of operability.

### 4.1.4 Traction of the Uterus

The uterus is held on traction by a stout tenaculum on the fundus (Figure 4.1).


S. Fujii, K. Sekiyama, *Precise Neurovascular Anatomy for Radical Hysterectomy*,
https://doi.org/10.1007/978-981-13-8098-3_4

## 4.2 Illustrated Surgical Steps of Original Okabayashi's Radical Hysterectomy

### 4.2.1 Ligation and Division of the Round Ligament to Reveal the Connective Tissue of the Broad Ligament (Figure 4.1)

The uterus is drawn cranial (upward) left, then the right round ligament becomes tense. The ligament is picked up and the uterine side is clamped by Kocher forceps. The pelvic side is ligated. The round ligament is divided between the Kocher forceps and ligature. Then, picking up the peritoneum on the cut edge of the foot side of the broad ligament, the peritoneum is separated and incised toward the urinary bladder. Then, the peritoneum of the cranial side is separated and incised to open the retroperitoneal space of the broad ligament. This will expose the loose connective tissue within the retroperitoneal space.

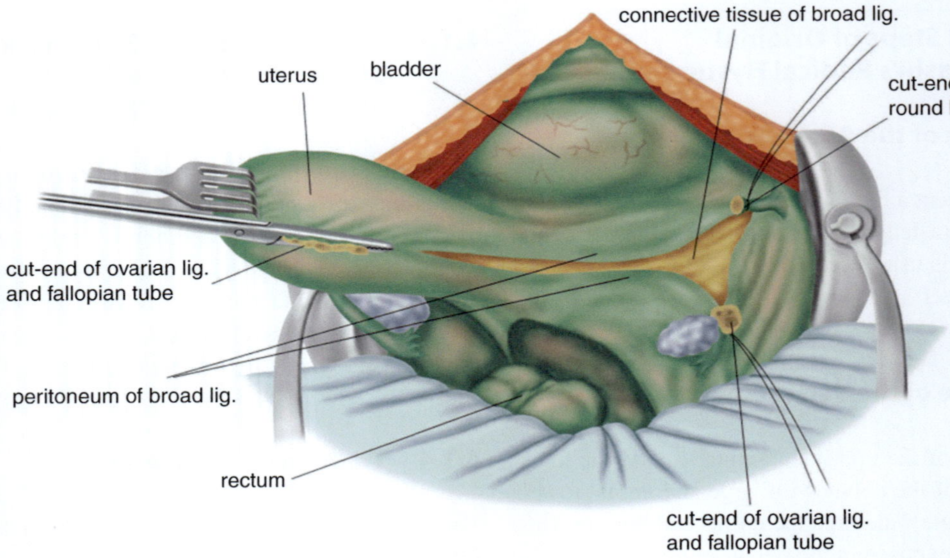


**Figure 4.1** Ligation and division of the round ligament to reveal the connective tissue of the broad ligament

### 4.2.2 Ligation and Division of the Ovarian Ligament (Propria Ovarii) and the Fallopian Tube for the Preservation of the Ovary (Figure 4.2)

With the uterus held over to the pelvic sidewall, long Kocher forceps are placed to clamp the uterine side of the ovarian ligament and the fallopian tube. The ovarian side of the ovarian ligament and the fallopian tube is ligated, and then between the long Kocher forceps and the ligature, a dissection is made. (*In case there is need to remove the ovary and the fallopian tube*, the suspensory ligament of ovary (ovarian vessels) is isolated, doubly ligated, and divided.)

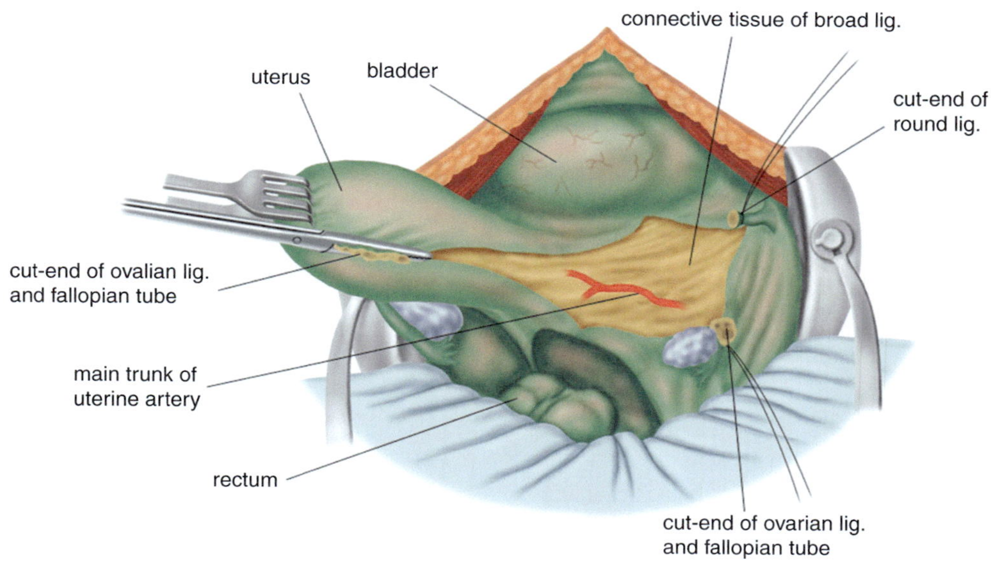


**Figure 4.2** Ligation and division of the ovarian ligament (propria ovarii) and the fallopian tube for the preservation of the ovary

### 4.2.3 Isolation, Ligation, and Division of the Uterine Artery (Figure 4.3)

Gradual separation of the loose connective tissue in the retroperitoneal space reveals the main trunk of the uterine artery and its junction with the internal iliac artery. The main trunk of the uterine artery is tied first, close to the origin from the internal iliac artery and second, near the uterus, and divided between the two ligatures.

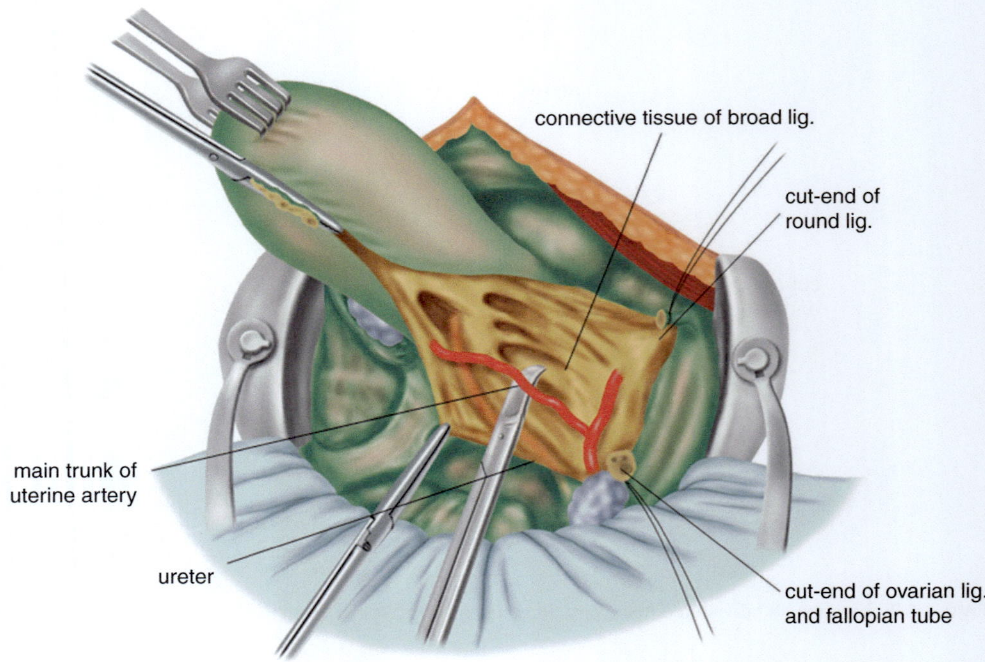


**Figure 4.3** Isolation, ligation, and division of the uterine artery

### 4.2.4 Separation of the Ureter from the Dorsal Peritoneal Layer of the Broad Ligament (Figure 4.4)

The ureter running along the dorsal peritoneal layer of the broad ligament is isolated. Kocher forceps are placed on the leading edge of the dorsal peritoneal layer and held cranially on traction, and the loose connective tissue of the retroperitoneal side of the broad ligament is separated. Then, the peristaltic ureter sheath becomes visible. The connective tissues surrounding the ureter including the feeding blood vessels are separated and isolated from the retroperitoneal side of the broad ligament using scissors. It is better to separate and trace the ureter as close as possible to the uterine side of the cut-end of the uterine artery.

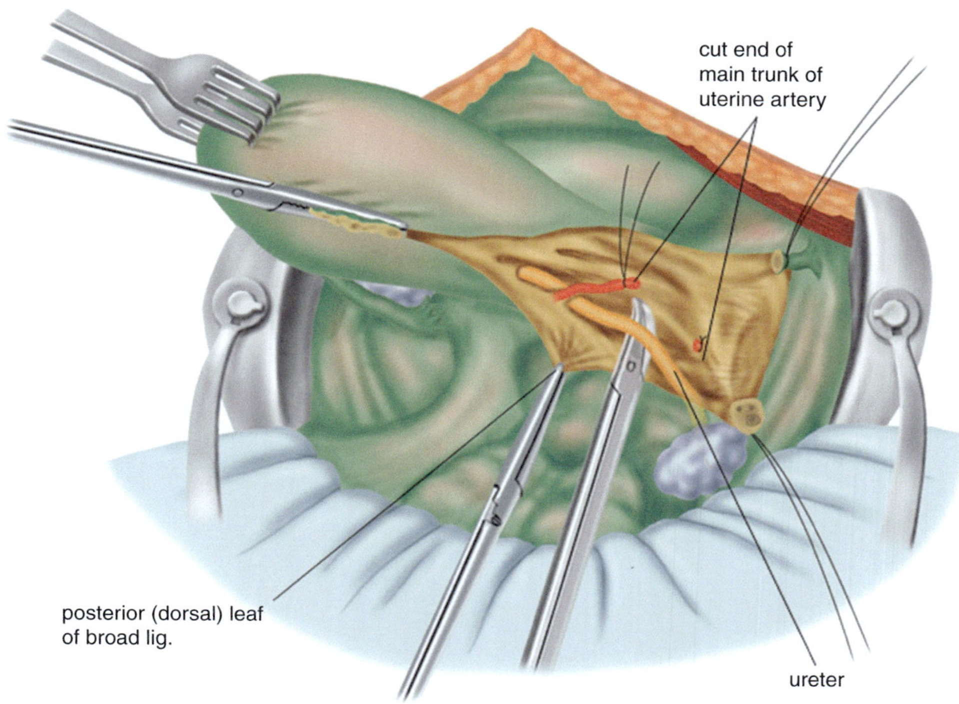


**Figure 4.4** Separation of the ureter from the dorsal peritoneal layer of the broad ligament

### 4.2.5 The Same Procedures on the Opposite Side

The same procedures Sects. 4.2.1–4.2.4 are performed on the opposite side.

### 4.2.6 Separation of the Peritoneal Layer of the Pouch of Douglas (Figure 4.5)

The uterus is tilted toward the pubic arch and the rectum with its peritoneal surface is stretched with the hand toward the cranial side. Then, the peritoneum between the uterus and the rectum is lifted from the bottom of the pouch of Douglas. The incision is made on the lifted-up peritoneum and carried with scissors across the dorsal side (back) of the cervix. The step connects the exposed retroperitoneal spaces on both sides of the broad ligament. With the uterus held over to the pubic arch and the rectum stretched toward the cranial portion with hand, a loose connective tissue layer appears between the rectum and the cervix/vagina. This is the landmark of the rectovaginal space. After the connective tissue of the rectovaginal space is separated, the rectum is gently freed from the cervical/vaginal wall.

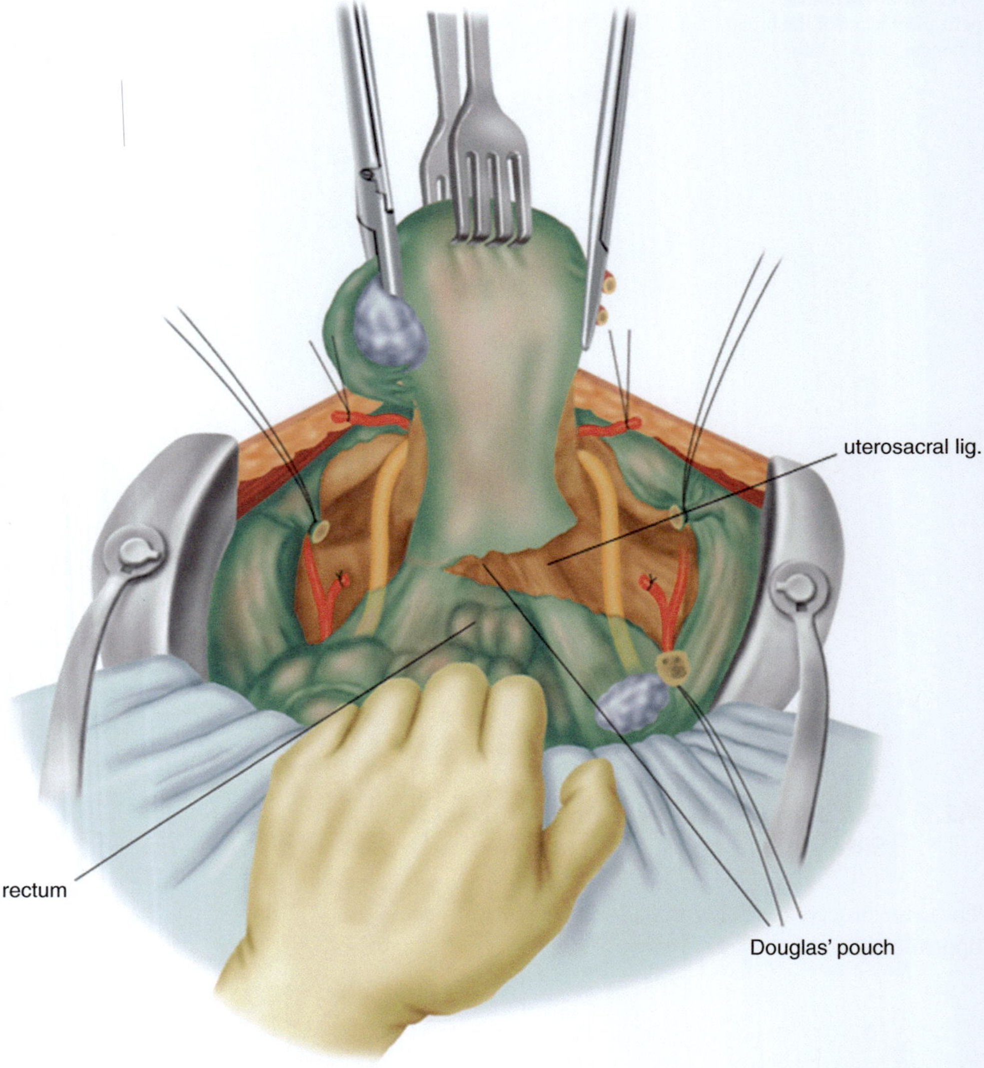


**Figure 4.5** Separation of the peritoneal layer of the Pouch of Douglas

### 4.2.7 Development of the Retrovaginal Space and Dissection of the Uterosacral Ligament (Figure 4.6)

If there is no infection-related adhesion or tumor invasion, the loose connective tissue layer between the rectum and cervical fascia is easily separated and can develop the rectovaginal space. Pressing the tips of scissors against the cervical fascia, the rectum is bluntly detached from the cervix/upper part of the vagina. This separation should be carried in the correct plane, to avoid the risk of injury to the rectum, which can occur if the dissection is close to the rectal wall. By this procedure, the bilateral thick connective tissue bundles (uterosacral ligament) become clear between the rectovaginal space and the retroperitoneal space of the broad ligament. The uterosacral ligament on either side is stretched forward and dissected at the base of the rectal sidewall.

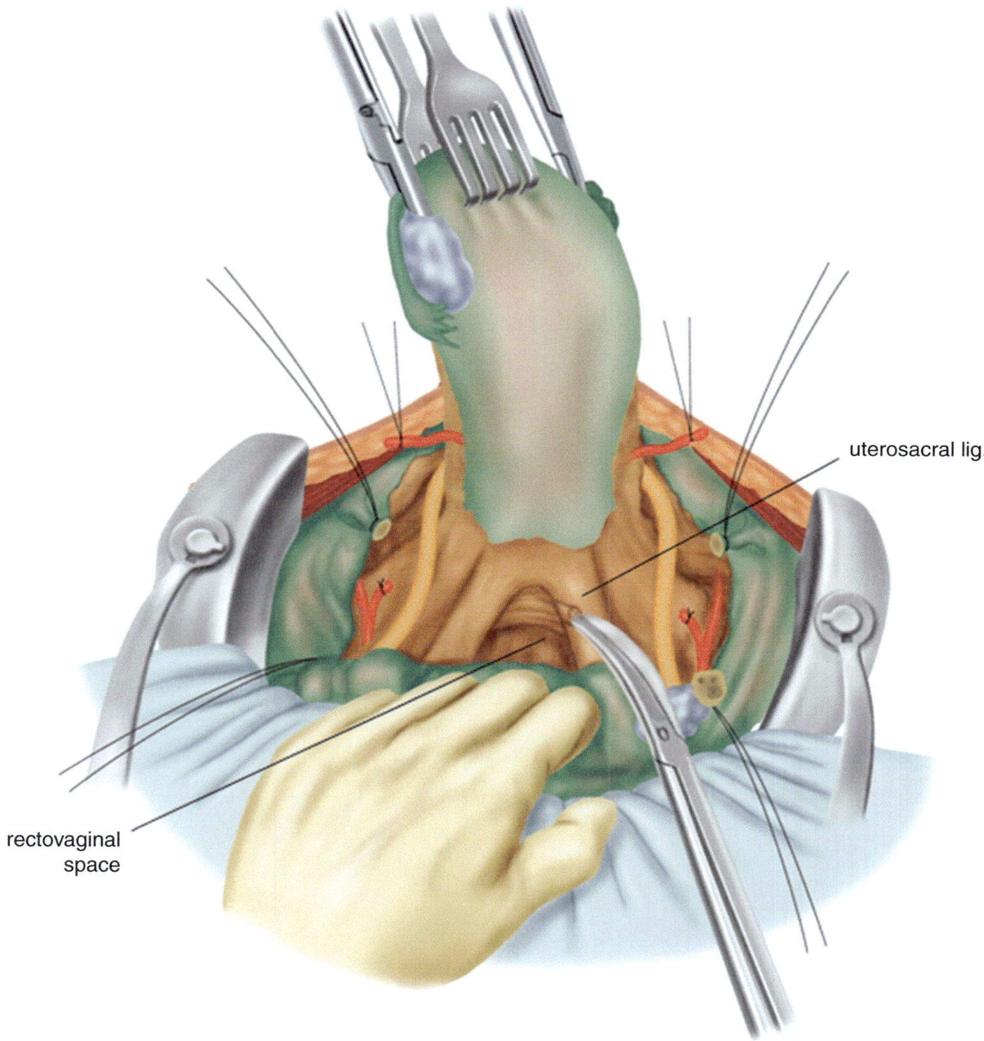


**Figure 4.6** Development of the retrovaginal space and dissection of the uterosacral ligament

### 4.2.8 Further Division of the Uterosacral Ligament and the Development of Okabayashi's Pararectal Space (Figure 4.7)

Further division of the uterosacral ligament with connective tissue of the rectal sidewall toward the base of the pelvis usually reveals a space filled with cobweb-like connective tissues between the rectal wall and the connective tissue layer in which the ureter is included. This is an entrance of the *Okabayashi's pararectal space*.

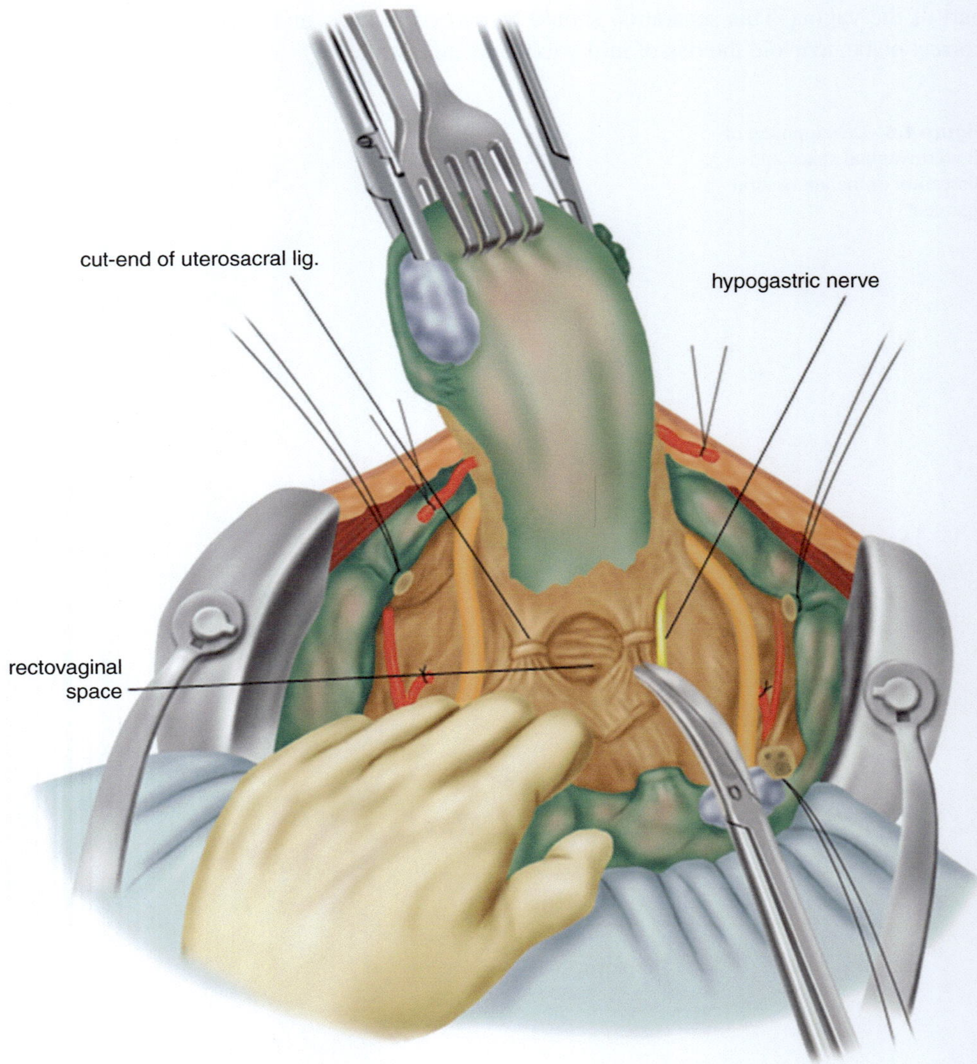


**Figure 4.7** Further division of the uterosacral ligament and the development of Okabayashi's pararectal space

**(Notes) Definition of the Spaces Developed During Radical Hysterectomy**

1. **Rectovaginal space** (Loose connective tissue between the rectum and cervical/vaginal fascia)
   After the separation of the peritoneum in the pouch of Douglas, the loose connective tissue along the dorsal center of the cervical fascia is easily separated from the rectum. This is the entrance of the rectovaginal space.
2. **Latzko's pararectal space and Okabayashi's pararectal space**
   The pararectal space can be defined as a loose connective tissue space surrounded by the rectal sidewall (uterine side), the internal iliac blood vessels (pelvic sidewall), the sacral bone (cranial side), and blood vessels and connective tissue of the cardinal ligament (inguinal side).
   There are two types of surgical approaches for the development of the pararectal space. One approach is the separation of the connective tissue between the rectum/ureter and the internal iliac artery/vein by retracting medially the rectal sidewall with the ureter. Then a space filled with cobweb-like connective tissues is revealed. This is a space called as **Latzko's pararectal space** (Figures 4.8 and 4.9). Another approach is from the division of the uterosacral ligament and separating the connective tissue of the rectal sidewall toward the base of the pelvis (Figure 4.10a, b). Then another space filled with cobweb-like connective tissues is revealed (Figure 4.10a, b). This is a space called as **Okabayashi's pararectal space** (Figures 4.8 and 4.10a, b). Okabayashi's pararectal space is a space between the rectal sidewall and the pelvic-side connective tissue layer in which the ureter and hypogastric nerve reside (Figure 4.10a, b). The ureter and the hypogastric nerve are in the same connective tissue plane, and the hypogastric nerve runs 2–3 cm dorsal to the ureter. Because Okabayashi's pararectal space is developed very close to the rectum, the pelvic side connective tissue plane becomes an obstacle for the expansion of Okabayashi's pararectal space. After isolation and retraction of the ureter toward the pelvic sidewall, it becomes necessary to sacrifice the hypogastric nerve. In order to increase the mobility of the uterus, Okabayashi preferred to open the space from the uterosacral ligament. In Particular, the mobility of the uterus is increased by the division of the hypogastric nerve, and the Okabayashi's pararectal space is extended laterally toward the space called Latzko's pararectal space (Figure 4.8). Therefore, the pararectal space developed by the Okabayashi's approach is usually wider and deeper than that of the Latzko's approach. Consequently, the extended Okabayashi's pararectal space (original Okabayashi's pararectal space + Latzko's pararectal space) (Figure 4.8) is surrounded by the rectal sidewall (uterine side), the internal iliac blood vessels (pelvic sidewall), the sacral bone (cranial side), and blood vessels and connective tissue of the cardinal ligament (inguinal side). The pararectal space is filled with the loose connective tissues to the base of the pelvis. In order to perform nerve-sparing radical hysterectomy, it is not necessary to develop the Okabayashi's pararectal space, and the Latzko's pararectal space is enough (Chapter 8).
3. **Paravesical space**
   Separation of the connective tissue between the obliterated umbilical artery and the external iliac vein at 2–3 cm cranial to the pubic bone reveals a cobweb-like loose connective tissue structure. The loose connective tissue that is deep into the base of the pelvis is separated. This is the paravesical space surrounded by the obliterated umbilical artery (urinary bladder side), rectal/vaginal wall (rectal side), external iliac vein (inguinal side), public bone (foot side), and the connective tissue of the cardinal ligament (cranial side) (Figures 4.8 and 4.9). The most dorsal part of the cardinal ligament is composed of loose connective tissue. By penetrating the dorsal side of the cardinal ligament with scissors, the paravesical space and the pararectal space are connected.
4. **Vesicocervical/vaginal space**
   At the center of the dorsal wall of the urinary bladder and the ventral cervical fascia/vaginal wall is composed with a loose connective tissue, and easily separated by the cranial level of the trigone of the urinary bladder. This is the vesicocervical/vaginal space (Figure 4.8). By picking up the urinary bladder with the covering peritoneum, the hollow loose connective tissue is appreciated between the dorsal side of the urinary bladder and ventral side of the cervical fascia at the center of both organs. Press the tip of scissors on the cervical fascia and push down toward the hollow, then the bladder is easily separated from central wall of the cervical/upper vaginal fascia by the cranial level of the trigone of the urinary bladder, and the connective tissue bundle (the vesicouterine ligament) is formed on each lateral side of the cervix.

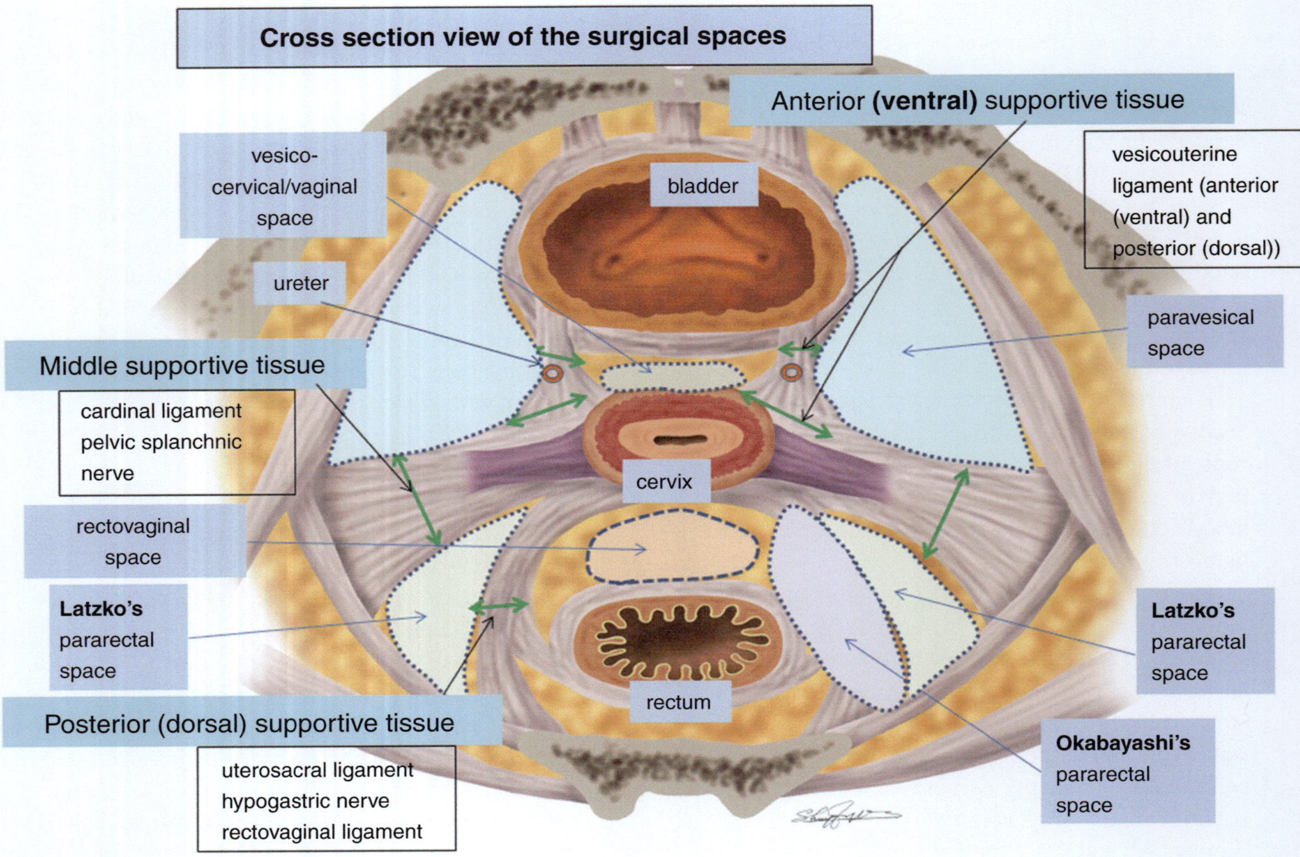


**Figure 4.8** Cross-sectional view of the pelvis at the level of cervix showing major three supportive tissues and their corresponding ligaments

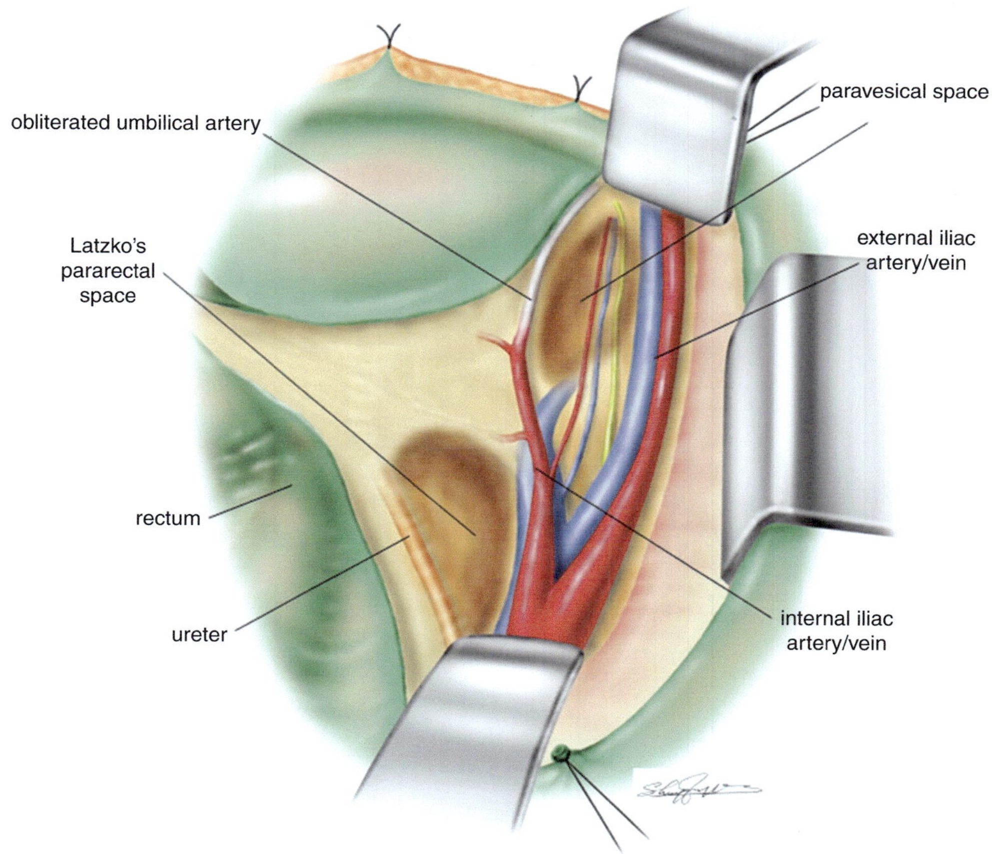


**Figure 4.9** Location of Latzko's pararectal space and paravesical space during surgery

The surgical spaces created between these supportive tissues and between the pelvic organs are also illustrated. The difference of the Latzko's pararectal space and Okabayashi's pararectal space is also illustrated.

Figure 4.10a is showing the entrance of Okabayashi's paravesical space between the rectum and the hypogastric nerve, Figure 4.10b is showing the location of Okabayashi's pararectal space as a photo during surgery.

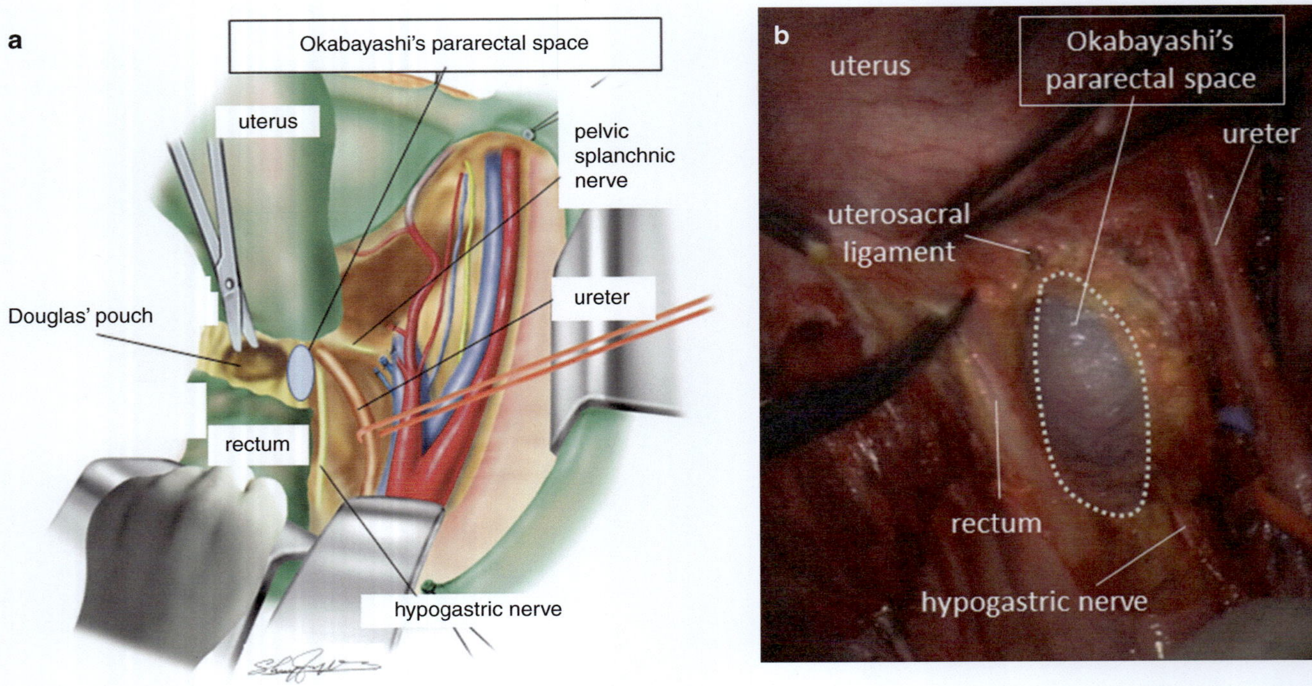


**Figure 4.10** Okabayashi's pararectal space

### 4.2.9 Further Development of the Pararectal Space (Figure 4.11)

Okabayashi's pararectal space is very close to the rectum, and hence, during the opening processes of the space the hypogastric nerve is usually divided and the space is extended toward Latzko's pararectal space. The boundaries of the pararectal space include the rectal sidewall (uterine side), the internal iliac blood vessels (pelvic sidewall), the sacral bone (cranial side) and, blood vessels and connective tissue of the cardinal ligament (inguinal side). The pararectal space is filled with the loose connective tissues to the base of the pelvis. The development of the pararectal space can be achieved using fingers inserted between the rectum and the internal iliac artery/vein. The direction of insertion is toward the pelvic axis.

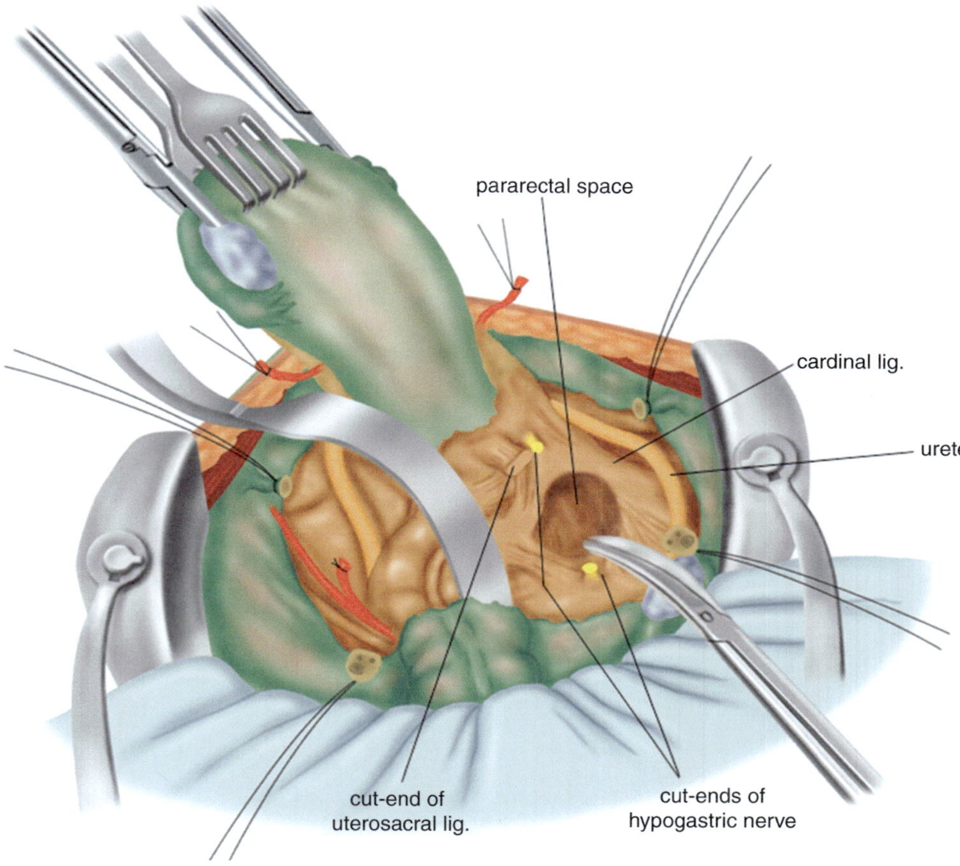


**Figure 4.11** Further development of the pararectal space

### 4.2.10 Development of the Paravesical Space and Separation of the Connective Tissue of the Base of the Cardinal Ligament (Figures 4.8, 4.9, and 4.12)

Separation of the connective tissue between the obliterated umbilical artery and the external iliac vein at a point 2–3 cm cranial to the pubic bone reveals a cobweb-like loose connective tissue structure. Separate the loose connective tissue deep into the base of the pelvis. This is the paravesical space, the boundaries of which include the obliterated umbilical artery (urinary bladder side), rectal/vaginal wall (rectal side), external iliac vein (inguinal side), public bone (foot side), and the connective tissue of the cardinal ligament (cranial side). The most dorsal part of the cardinal ligament is composed of loose connective tissue. By penetrating the dorsal side of the cardinal ligament with scissors, the paravesical space and the pararectal space are connected.

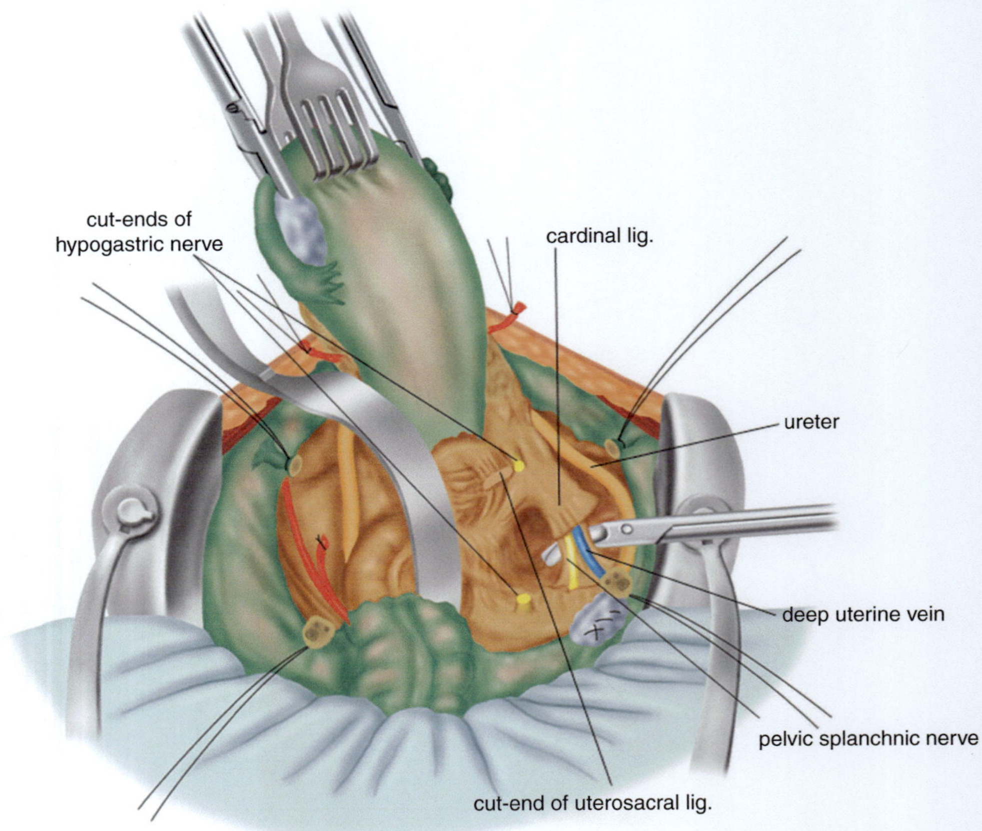


**Figure 4.12** Development of the paravesical space and separation of the connective tissue of the base of the cardinal ligament

### 4.2.11 Clamp the Cardinal Ligament (Figure 4.13)

The connective tissue of the cardinal ligament is separated to make it as narrow as possible. The deep uterine vein and the pelvic splanchnic nerve usually lie within the cardinal ligament. A long Pean forceps is placed close to ***the pelvic sidewall*** (see the following **Notes**) and another forceps is placed to the uterine side of the cardinal ligament.

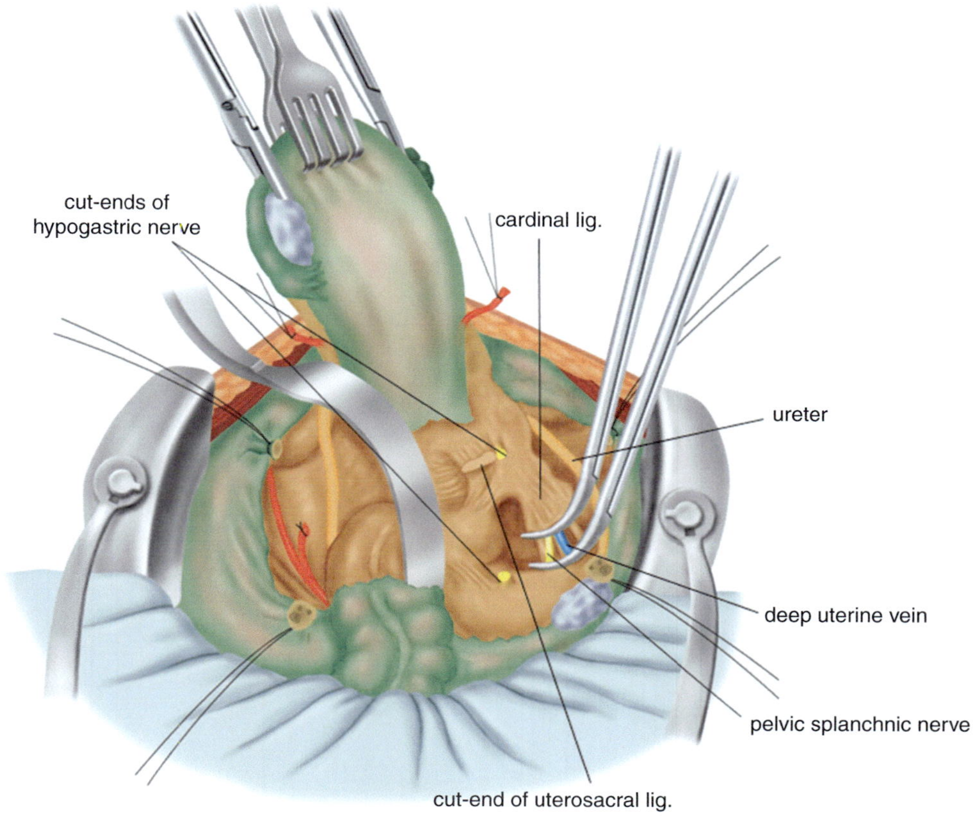


**Figure 4.13** Clamp the cardinal ligament

**Notes:** The term *pelvic sidewall* is very confusing. Surgical anatomy of the *pelvic sidewall* means the draining site of the deep uterine vein into the internal iliac vein. The procedure of Okabayashi's original approach to the cardinal ligament usually clamps both the deep uterine vein and the pelvic splanchnic nerve. However, it is not recommended to clamp the cardinal ligament too close to the *pelvic sidewall*. If the clamp is placed too close to the pelvic sidewall, there is a possibility of clamping the internal iliac vein itself including the inflow of the deep uterine vein. Dividing the cardinal ligament close to the pelvic sidewall can lead to terrible bleeding from the internal iliac vein itself, which is often very difficult to control. In order to avoid this mistake, it is better to perform pelvic lymphadenectomy first. Then the base of the cardinal ligament becomes well defined and the inflow of the deep uterine vein into the internal iliac vein is better exposed (Figure 4.14).

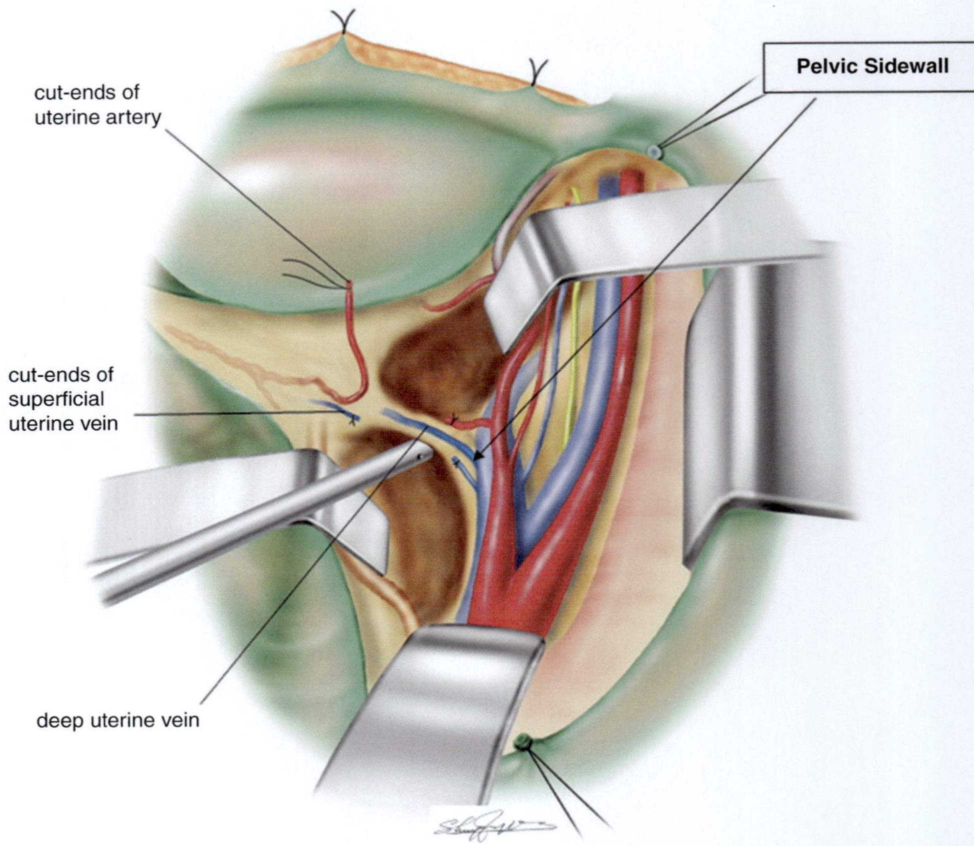


**Figure 4.14** Surgical anatomy of the pelvic sidewall means the draining sites of the deep uterine vein into the internal iliac vein

### 4.2.12 **Dissection of the Cardinal Ligament** (Figure 4.15)

The base of the cardinal ligament is divided between the two clamps, near the forceps on the pelvic side. The pelvic side forceps is replaced with a suture ligation and the uterine side forceps is left for a marker of the cut-end of the cardinal ligament. Okabayashi described that now the muscles of the pelvic floor are seen and the rectum is laid bare. (**Notes**: The divided cardinal ligament usually contains the superficial uterine vein, the deep uterine vein, and the pelvic splanchnic nerve.)

**Figure 4.15** Dissection of the cardinal ligament

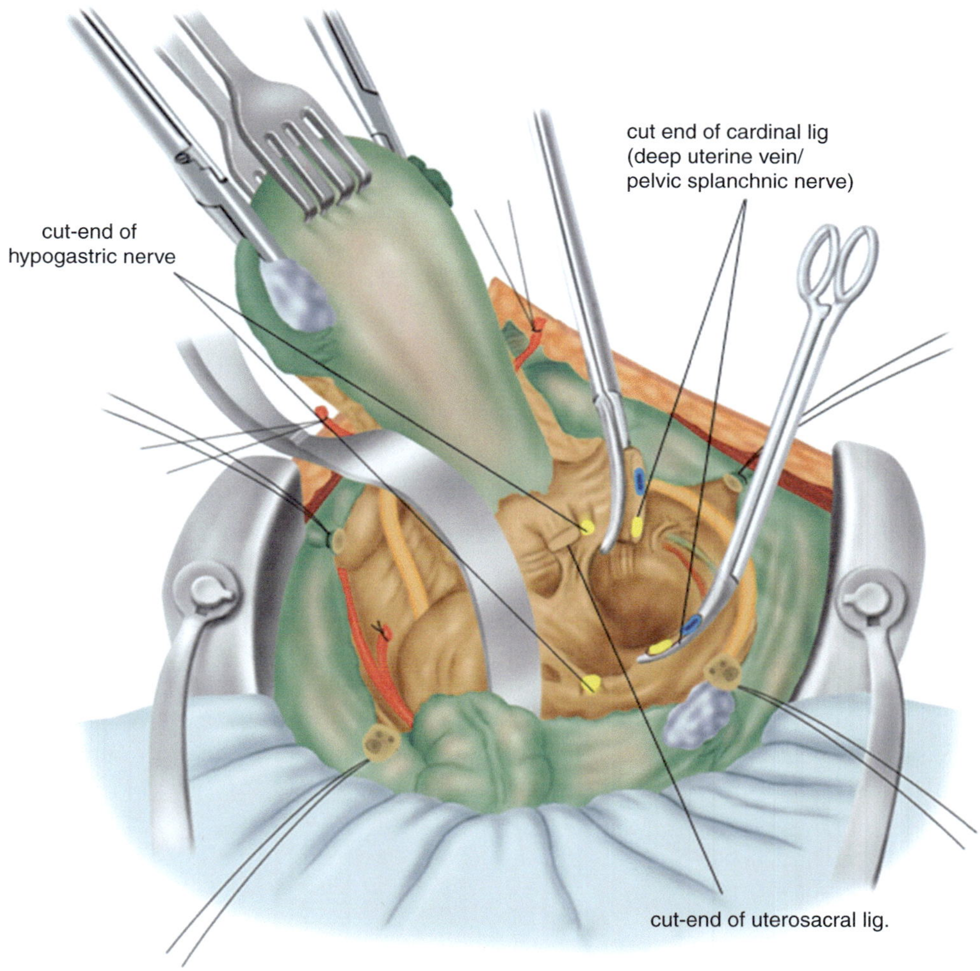


### 4.2.13 **The Procedures on the Opposite Side**

The same procedures Sects. 4.2.6–4.2.12 are performed on the opposite side.

### 4.2.14 Separation of the Peritoneum Between the Urinary Bladder and the Uterus (Figure 4.16)

In order to stretch the vesicouterine fold of peritoneum, the uterus is drawn toward the cranial side. The peritoneum of the bladder side is lifted with forceps. The peritoneum, just 1–2 cm inferior to the vesicouterine fold where scissors can separate the peritoneum easily without any damage to the urinary bladder, is divided across the ventral side of the cervix. Separation of the peritoneum too close to either the urinary bladder or vesicouterine fold can lead to bleeding.

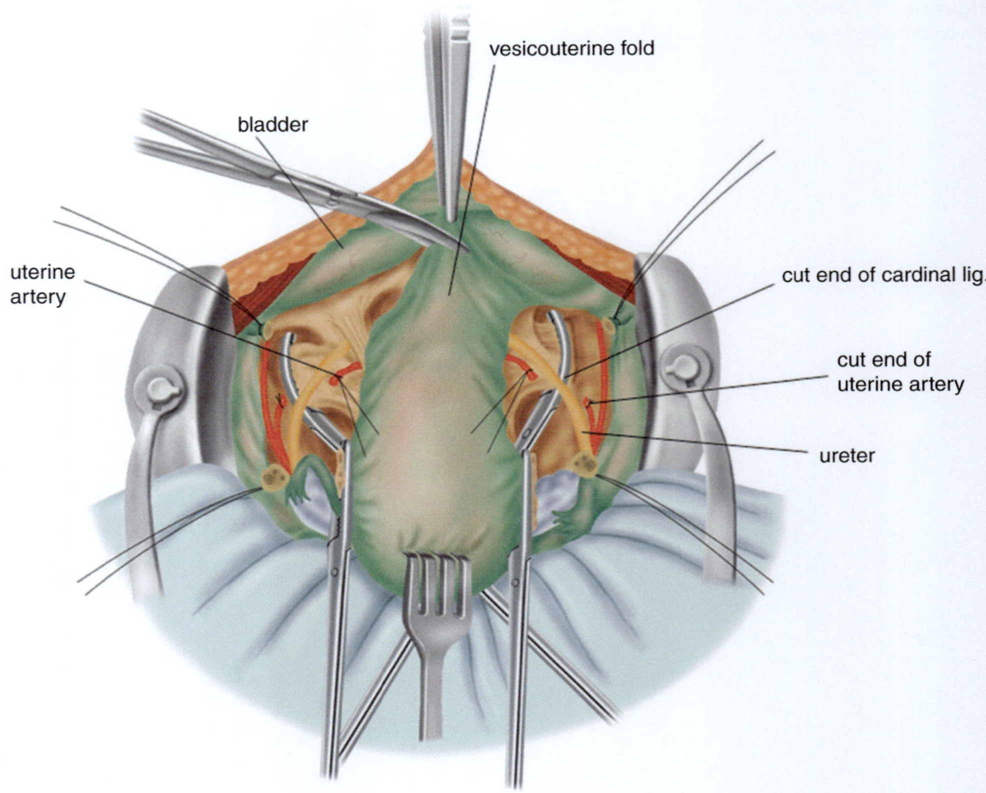


**Figure 4.16** Separation of the peritoneum between the urinary bladder and the uterus

### 4.2.15 Separation of the Connective Tissue Between the Urinary Bladder and the Ventral-Side of the Cervical Fascia (the Vesicocervical Space) (Figure 4.17)

By picking up the urinary bladder along with its peritoneum in an up-and-down motion, the hollow of the loose connective tissue is formed between the dorsal side of the urinary bladder and ventral side of the cervical fascia at the midline of both organs. Press the tip of scissors on the cervical fascia and push down toward the hollow in order to separate the bladder easily from the central wall of the cervical/upper vaginal fascia. Inferiorly, the trigone of the urinary bladder (vesicocervical space) and the connective tissue bundle (vesicouterine ligament) are formed on each lateral side of the cervix.

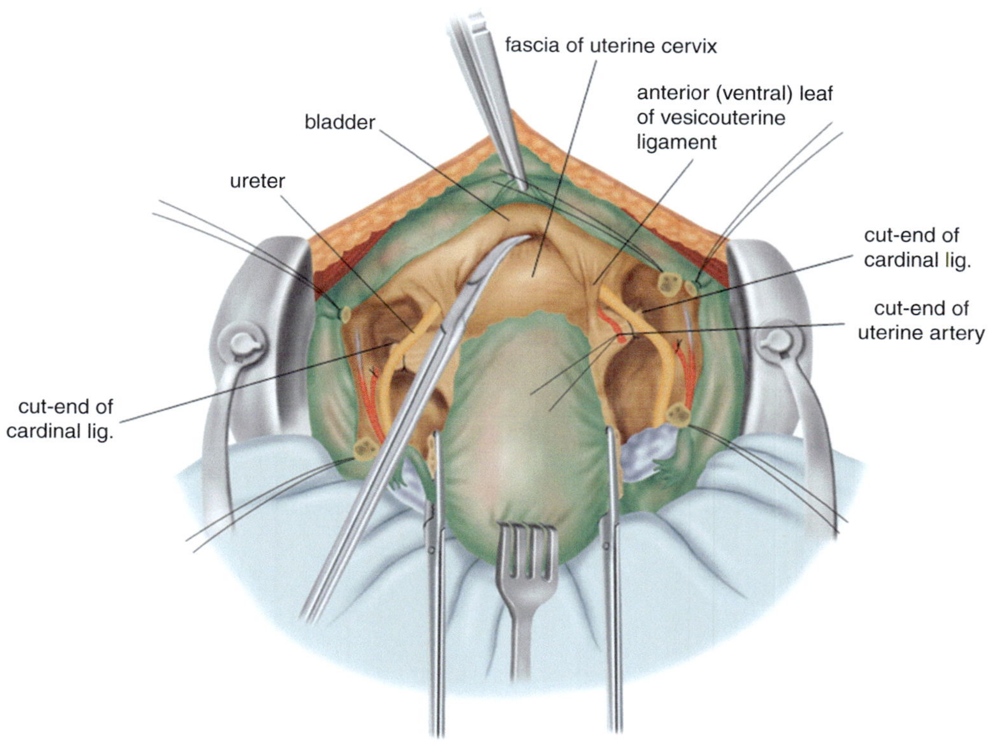


**Figure 4.17** Separation of the connective tissue between the urinary bladder and the ventral side of the cervical fascia (the vesicocervical space)

### 4.2.16 Separation of the Anterior (Ventral) Leaf of the Vesicouterine Ligament (Left Side) (Figure 4.18)

The uterus is drawn cranially right. The cut-end of the uterine artery on the uterine side is lifted with forceps and the connective tissue between the ureter and the uterine artery is carefully separated. The entrance of the ureter tunnel now comes into view. The curved scissors with the concave side pointing dorsally are insinuated into the tunnel and the ureter is pressed dorsal side with it. This movement allows the tunnel to be enlarged and the ventral side of the connective tissues covering the ureter is separated through the tunnel. (**Notes**: If this step does not produce the desired result, the trigone side connective tissue of the anterior (ventral) leaf of the vesicouterine ligament should be opened. From the trigone side of the anterior (ventral) leaf of the vesicouterine ligament, the ureter can be shelled out.)

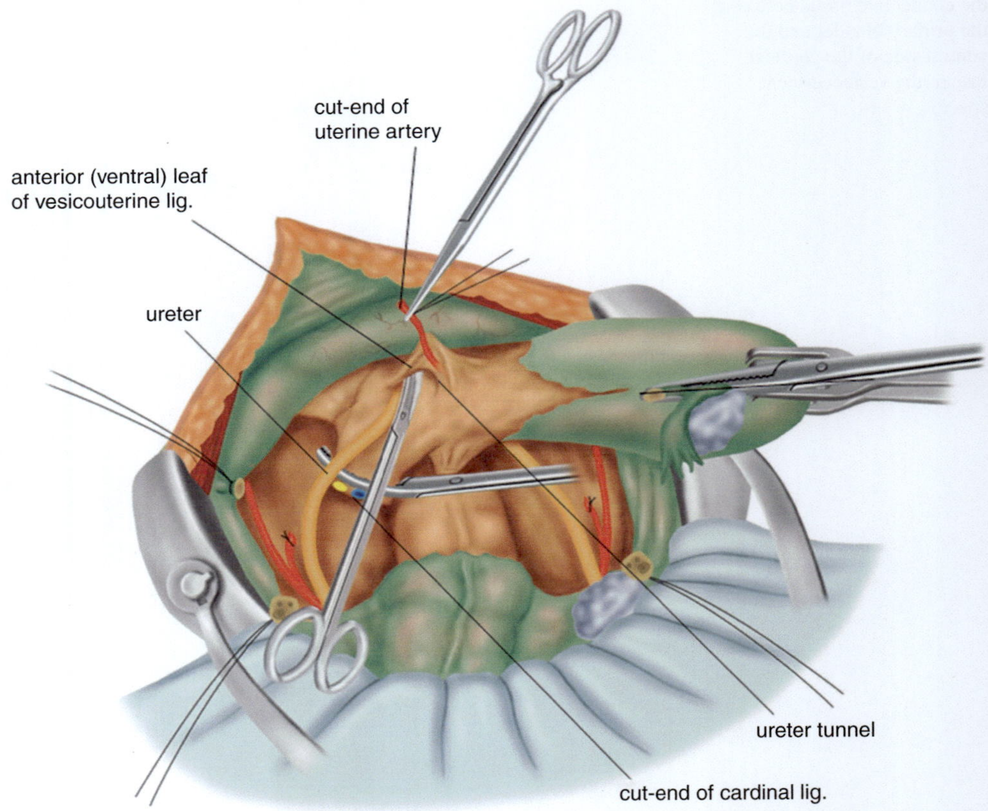


**Figure 4.18** Separation of the anterior (ventral) leaf of the vesicouterine ligament (left side)

### 4.2.17 Clamp and Dissect the Anterior (Ventral) Leaf of the Vesicouterine Ligament (Figure 4.19)

Protecting the ureter with the scissors, place two forceps on the anterior (ventral) leaf of the vesicouterine ligament along the course of the insinuated scissors. Incision is made with scissors between the two forceps. The forceps are replaced by ligatures.

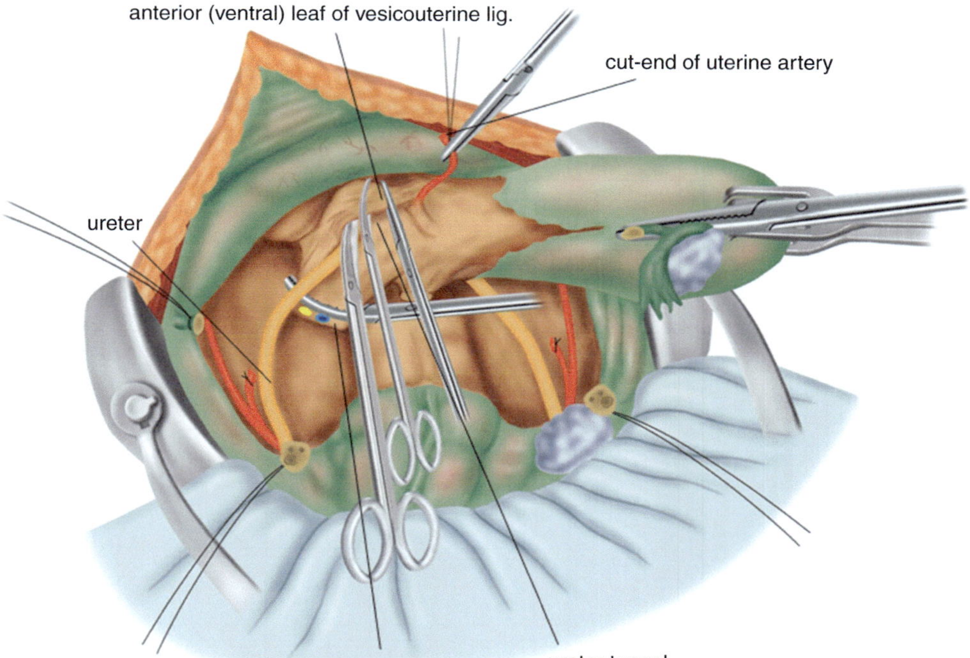


**Figure 4.19** Clamping and dissection of the anterior (ventral) leaf of the vesicouterine ligament

### 4.2.18 Separation of the Posterior (Dorsal) Leaf of the Vesicouterine Ligament and the Paravaginal Space (Figure 4.20)

By the separation of the connective tissues in the anterior (ventral) leaf of the vesicouterine ligament, the ureter is completely freed of its attachment to the posterior (dorsal) leaf of the vesicouterine ligament. Consequently, the ureter is separated from the surface of the posterior (dorsal) leaf of the vesicouterine ligament and shifted inferiorly. Following this, the urinary bladder with the ureter is separated from the cervix/upper vagina. The extent to which dissection is desirable varies in different cases, but it should certainly be no less than 1.5–2 cm below the lowest level/extent of tumor visualized. The insertion of a broad L-shaped retractor to reflect the bladder above the line of the separation is very useful. Then, try to find a space in the posterior (dorsal) leaf of the vesicouterine ligament named as "a paravaginal space" by Okabayashi. The entrance to the paravaginal space is marked using a circle line.

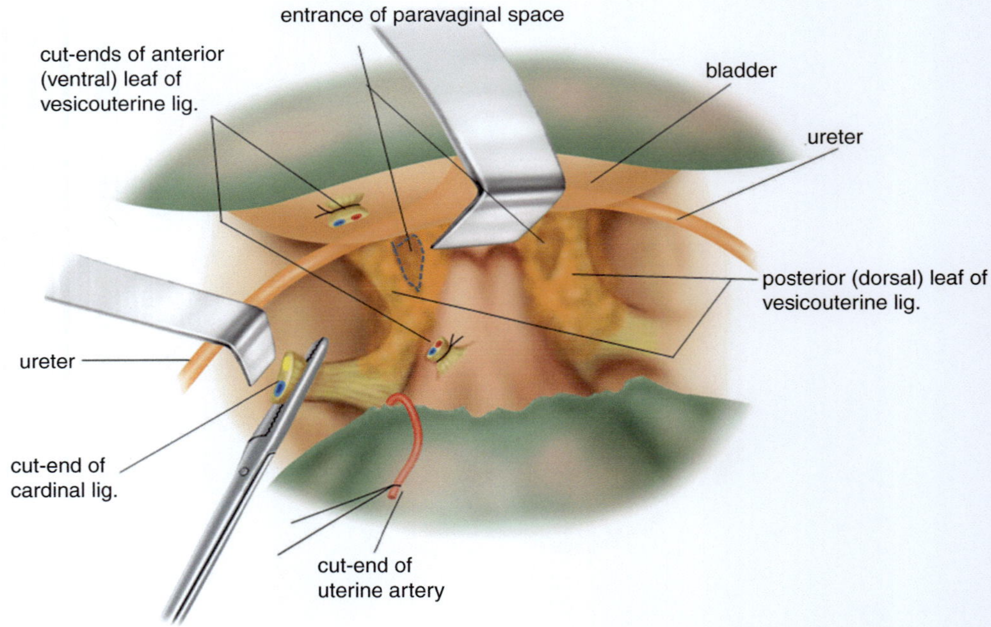


**Figure 4.20** Separation of the posterior (dorsal) leaf of the vesicouterine ligament and the paravaginal space

### 4.2.19 Separation of the Posterior (Dorsal) Leaf of the Vesicouterine Ligament Through the Paravaginal Space (Figure 4.21)

Draw the uterus cranially, and give tension to the cut-end of the cardinal ligament laterally and to the L-shaped retractor holding the bladder with ureter toward the foot side, then the connective tissue of the posterior (dorsal) leaf of the vesicouterine ligament becomes tense. At a level 2–3 cm cranial from the insertion of the ureter into the bladder, there exists a loose connective tissue area (paravaginal space) between the posterior (dorsal) leaf of the vesicouterine ligament and the paracolpium (vaginal vessels). The curved scissors insinuated into this area is rather easily penetrated into the paravesical space and recognized as a paravaginal space. (**Notes:** If the curved scissors are not insinuated appropriately into the paravesical space, a large amount of bleeding can occur at this stage.)

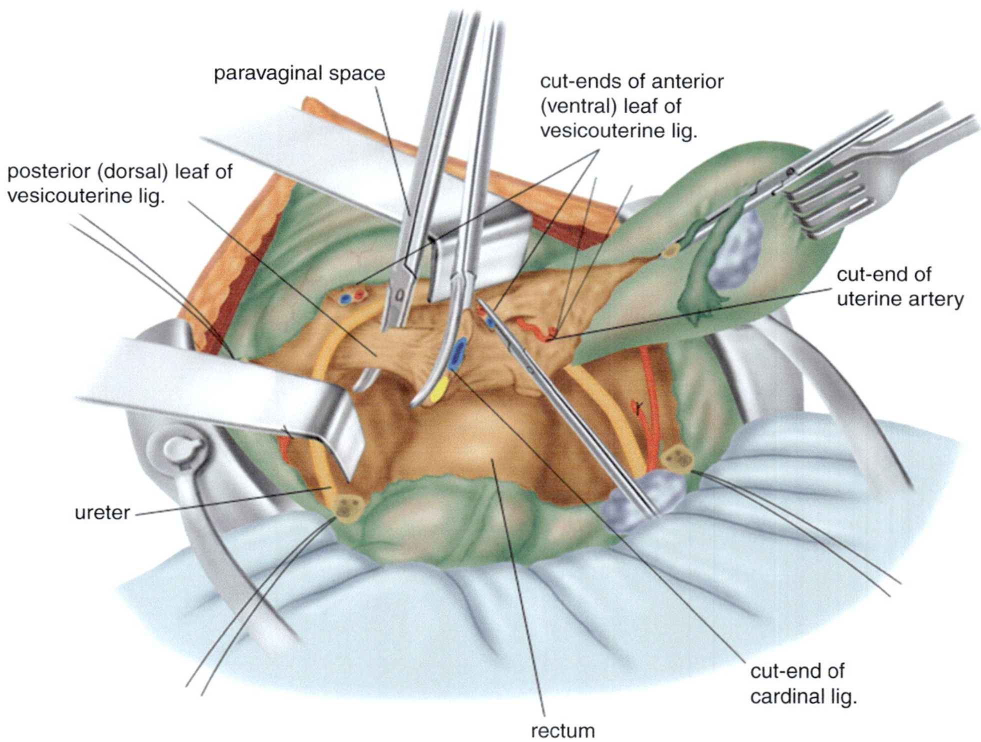


**Figure 4.21** Separation of the posterior (dorsal) leaf of the vesicouterine ligament through the paravaginal space

### 4.2.20 Division of the Posterior (Dorsal) Leaf of the Vesicouterine Ligament from the Paracolpium (Figure 4.22)

Giving tension to the cut-end of the cardinal ligament, two straight long pressure forceps are inserted along the line of the scissors. Place one toward the bladder side and the other toward the uterine side of the posterior (dorsal) leaf of the vesicouterine ligament. Then divide and ligate between the two forceps. This step separates the posterior (dorsal) leaf of the vesicouterine ligament from the vaginal vessels (paracolpium). Moreover, the urinary bladder with the ureter becomes free from the vaginal wall. Therefore, by separating the connective tissue between the vaginal wall and the bladder, the urinary bladder with ureter is separated from the vaginal wall for whatever length one wishes.

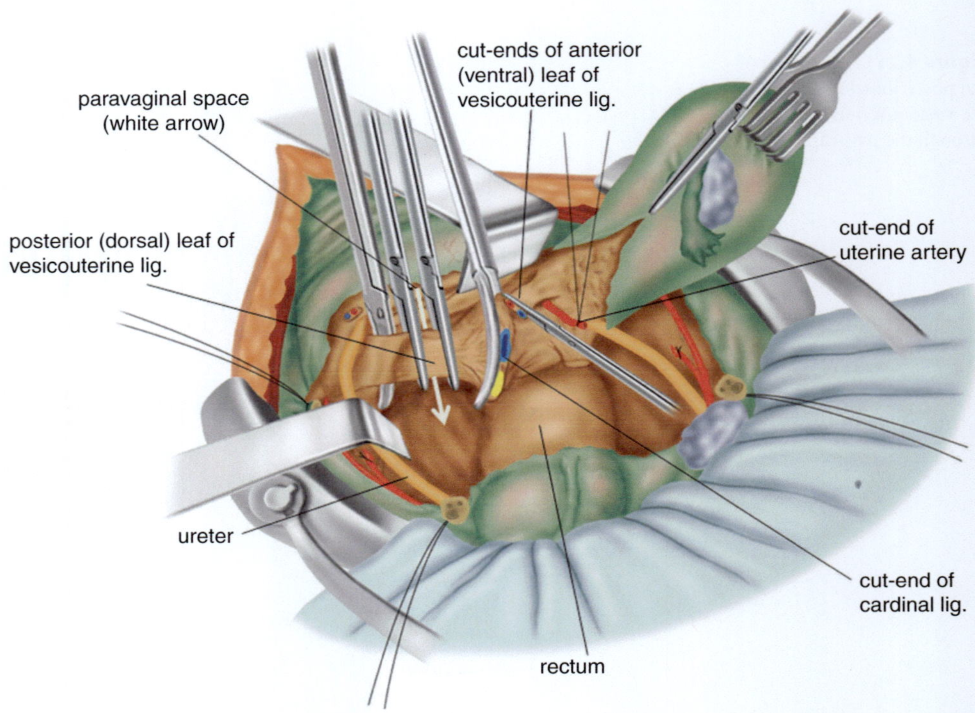


**Figure 4.22** Division of the posterior (dorsal) leaf of the vesicouterine ligament from the paracolpium

### 4.2.21 The Same Procedures on the Opposite Side

The same procedures Sects. 4.2.14–4.2.20 are performed on the opposite side.

### 4.2.22 Treatment of the Rectovaginal Ligament (Figure 4.23)

The uterosacral ligament is already divided bilaterally, and only the connective tissue bundles are recognized bilaterally between the vagina and the rectum. Draw the uterus to the ventral/pubic bone side and stretch the rectum toward cranial portion with hand, then the connective tissue bundles become clear between the rectum and vagina. These are the rectovaginal ligaments. Okabayashi tried to ligate and divide the rectovaginal ligaments. Therefore, in this illustration the stitch to the rectovaginal ligament is appreciated. However, it is not necessary to ligate the rectovaginal ligament because the use of electrocautery, such as monopolar or bipolar instruments, is usually enough for the division of the rectovaginal ligament. By the division of the rectovaginal ligament, the dorsal side of the vaginal wall becomes free. Therefore, the length of the vaginal cuff can now be selected and tailored to be as long as one wishes.

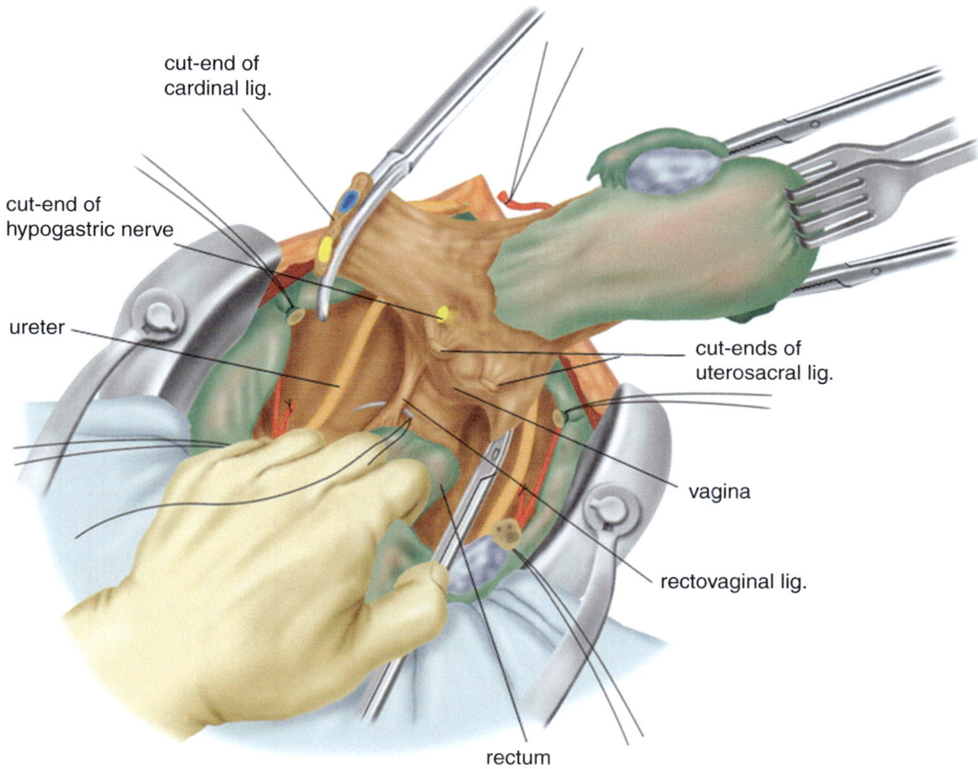


**Figure 4.23** Treatment of the rectovaginal ligament

### 4.2.23 A Figure of the Both Cut-Ends of the Cardinal Ligament, the Uterosacral Ligaments, and the Rectovaginal Ligaments (Figure 4.24)

The pelvic view from the cranial side of the pelvis is demonstrating both cut-ends of the cardinal ligament, the uterosacral ligament including the hypogastric nerve, and the rectovaginal ligament. Now, the uterus is connected only with the bilateral vaginal blood vessels (paracolpium) and the vaginal wall. Next step is ligation and division of the paracolpium.

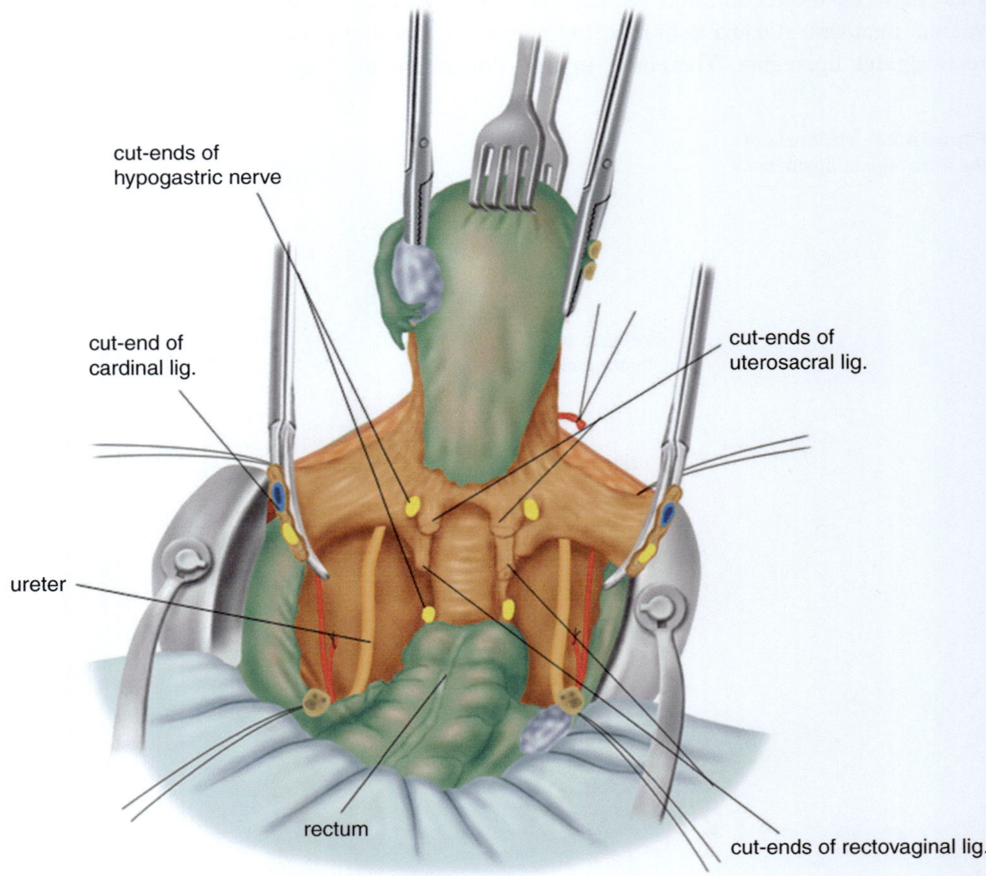


**Figure 4.24** A figure of the both cut-ends of the cardinal ligament, the uterosacral ligaments, and the rectovaginal ligaments

### 4.2.24 Ligation and Dissection of the Paracolpium (Figure 4.25)

The uterus with its surrounding tissues such as cut-ends of the cardinal ligament and the vesicouterine ligament are appreciated. Now only the lateral vaginal tissue (the paracolpium) is connected with the vagina and is ready to be ligated. The paracolpium is ligated where we wish to amputate the vaginal wall.

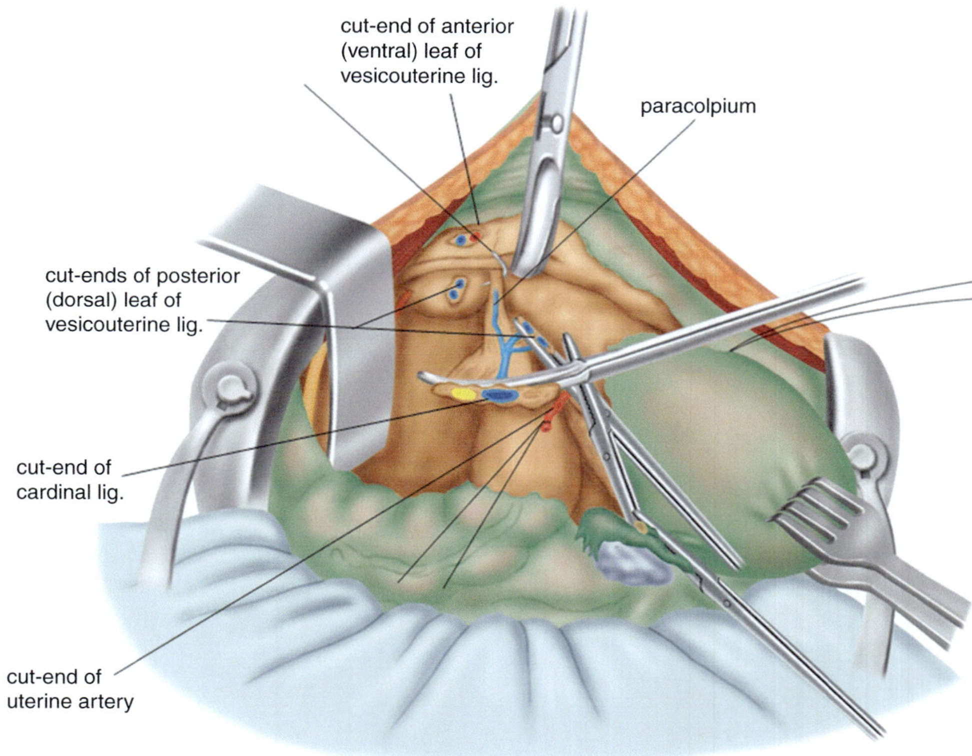


**Figure 4.25** Ligation and dissection of the paracolpium

#### 4.2.24.1 Division of the Vagina and Extirpation of the Uterus (Figure 4.26)

The vaginal wall is divided. Now the uterus is attached only with the vaginal wall. A hot Paquelin cautery (Okabayashi's original description) or a monopolar device is used to open the vaginal cavity. Then, a piece of gauze is pushed into the opened vaginal cavity in order to expel the discharge from the uterus. Tincture of iodine is painted over the inner surface of the vaginal wall. After this, the vaginal wall is divided completely around. The bleeding parts of the cut edge of the vaginal wall are grasped with forceps and the forceps are replaced by ligatures. Then, the ventral side and dorsal side of the vaginal stump are closed with suture material.

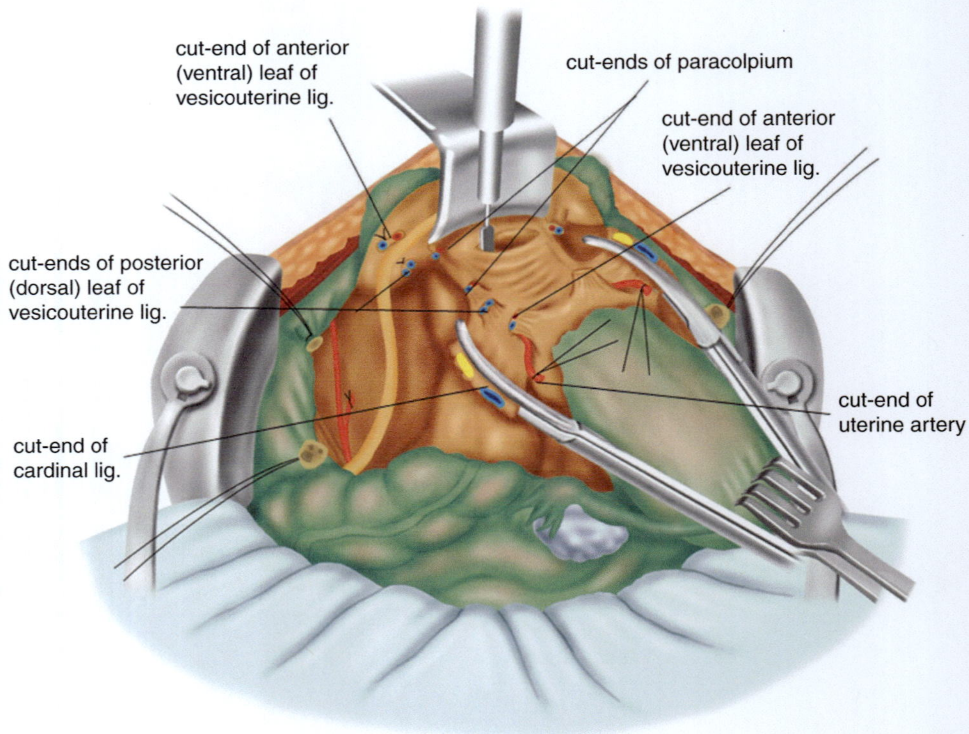


**Figure 4.26** Division of the vagina and extirpation of the uterus

### 4.2.25 A View of the Pelvic Cavity After the Removal of the Uterus and Lymphadenectomy and Closure of the Abdominal Cavity (Figure 4.27)

Okabayashi usually performed pelvic lymphadenectomy after the removal of the uterus. However, the procedure of lymphadenectomy is not clearly described in his atlas. In the atlas of original Okabayashi's radical hysterectomy, only a view of the pelvic cavity after the division of the vagina (Figure 4.27) is illustrated. On the detail of the pelvic lymphadenectomy, readers can refer to the procedure of pelvic lymphadenectomy described in Chap. 6.

Following closure of the ventral abdominal peritoneum and the fascia, interrupted skin suture is undertaken. Using a vaginal speculum, the packed gauze is removed from the vagina and the vaginal stump suture is checked. The surgery is now finished.

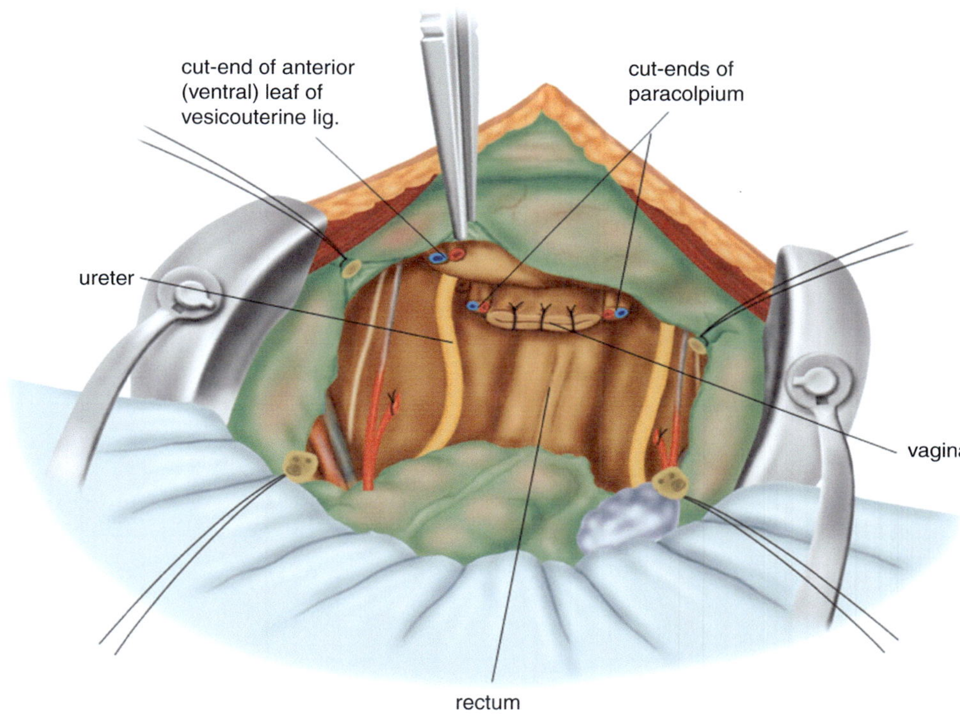


**Figure 4.27** A view of the pelvic cavity after the removal of the uterus and lymphadenectomy

# 5 Novel Points of Okabayashi's Radical Hysterectomy

## 5.1 Novel Points of the Okabayashi's Radical Hysterectomy

### 5.1.1 Clarification of the Anatomy of the Paravaginal Space Between the Posterior (Dorsal) Leaf of the Vesicouterine Ligament and the Paracolpium

In the tissue of the paracervix, Okabayashi found a loose connective tissue space. The space is named as Okabayashi's paravaginal space (Figure 5.1a, b). By insinuation of scissors into the space, the paracervix is separated into the posterior (dorsal) leaf of the vesicouterine ligament and the vaginal blood vessels (paracolpium).

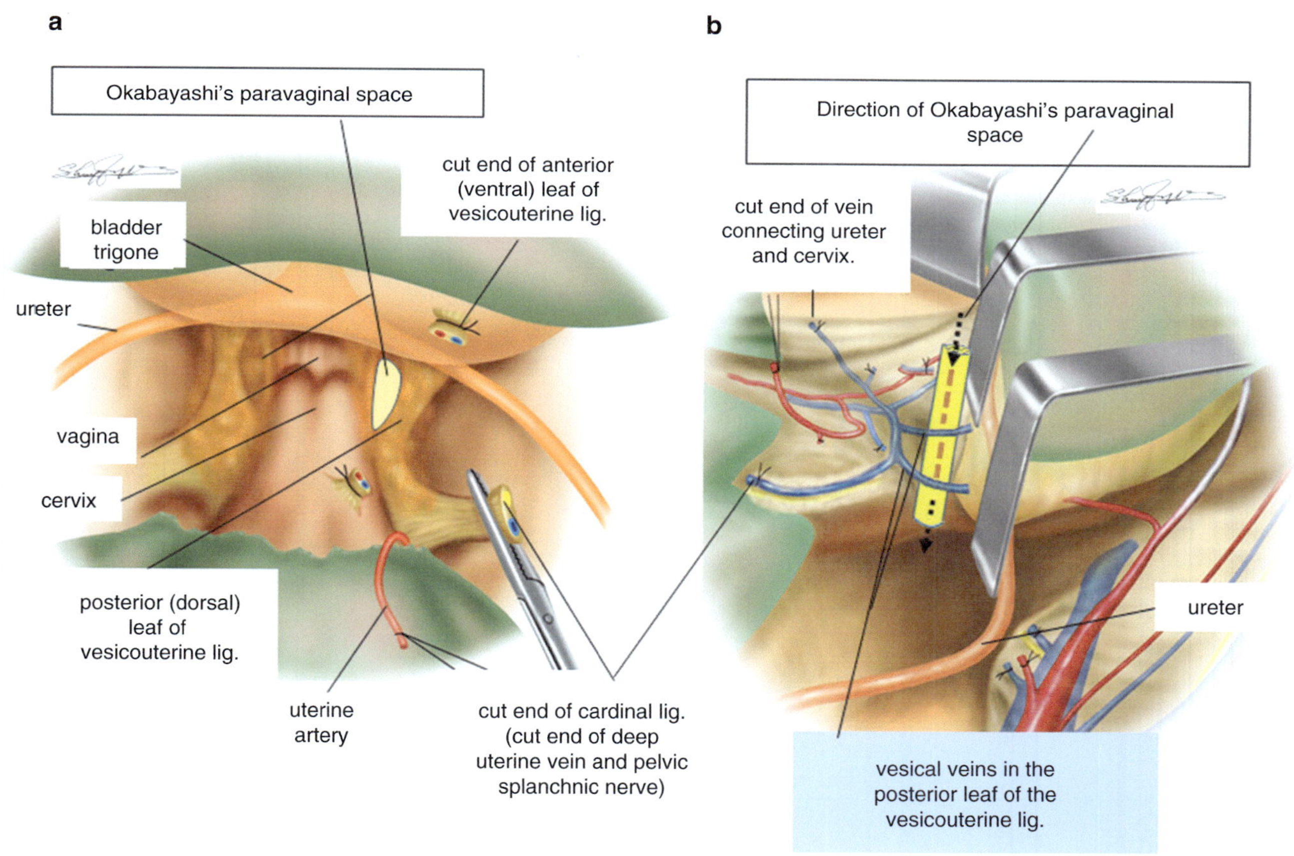


**Figure 5.1** Anatomical location of Okabayashi's paravaginal space. (**a**) Anatomical location of the entrance of Okabayashi's paravaginal space (a yellow color area surrounded by a blue line) in the posterior (dorsal) leaf of the vesicouterine ligament. (**b**) In the skeletonized view of the posterior (dorsal) leaf of the vesicouterine ligament from the lateral side of the cervix, the location of the paravaginal space is illustrated as a yellow band with two black arrow heads


S. Fujii, K. Sekiyama, *Precise Neurovascular Anatomy for Radical Hysterectomy*,
https://doi.org/10.1007/978-981-13-8098-3_5

Recently, our clarification of the posterior (dorsal) leaf of the vesicouterine ligament revealed that at least two to three venous blood vessels from the dorsal side of the urinary bladder run in the posterior leaf of the vesicouterine ligament and drain into the deep uterine vein in the cardinal ligament (Figures 5.1b and 5.2a, b).

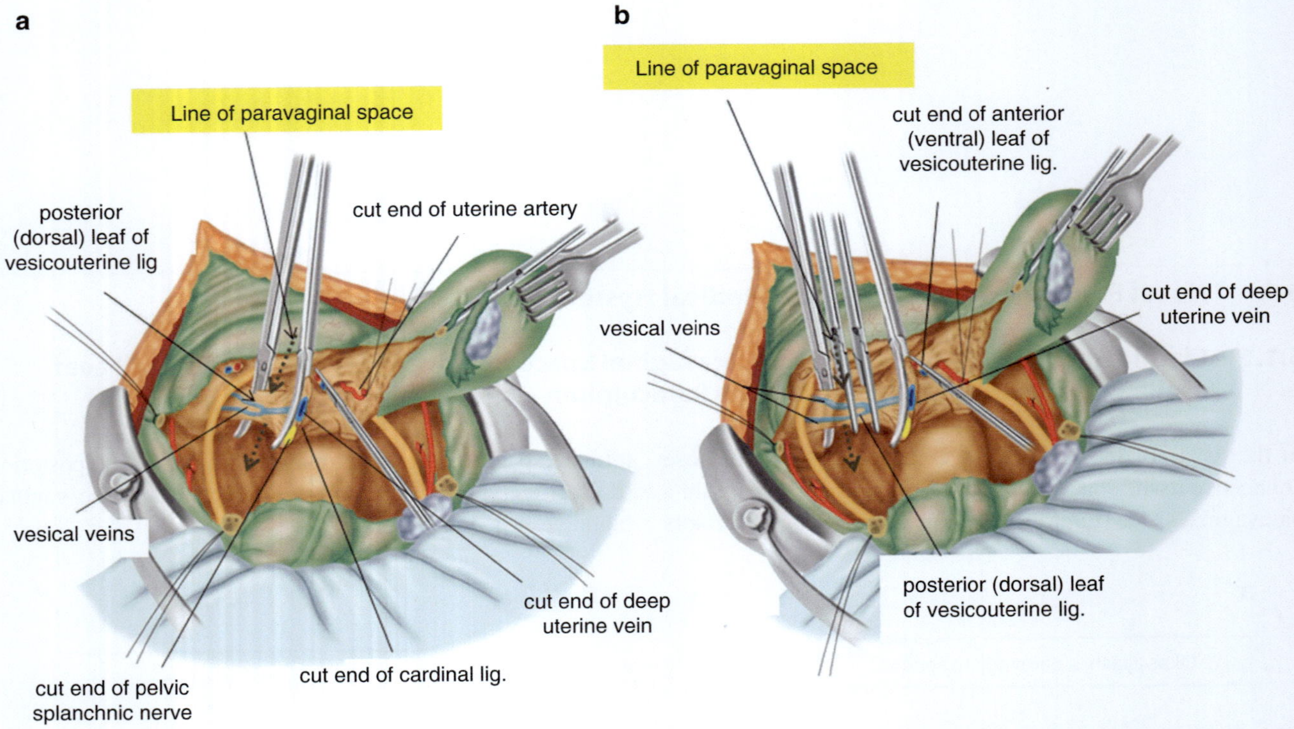


**Figure 5.2** Lateral view of the venous blood vessels in the posterior (dorsal) leaf of the vesicouterine ligament. (**a**) Insinuation of scissors into Okabayashi's paravaginal space. Two dotted arrow lines are indicating the direction of insinuation. (**b**) Using two Kocher forceps, the posterior (dorsal) leaf of the vesicouterine ligament is clamped through Okabayashi's paravaginal space

The separation and division of the posterior (dorsal) leaf of the vesicouterine ligament enables the urinary bladder with ureter to be completely free from the cervix and the vaginal wall (with the vaginal vein that also drains into the deep uterine vein). It resembles the picture of an open book (Figure 5.3a, b).

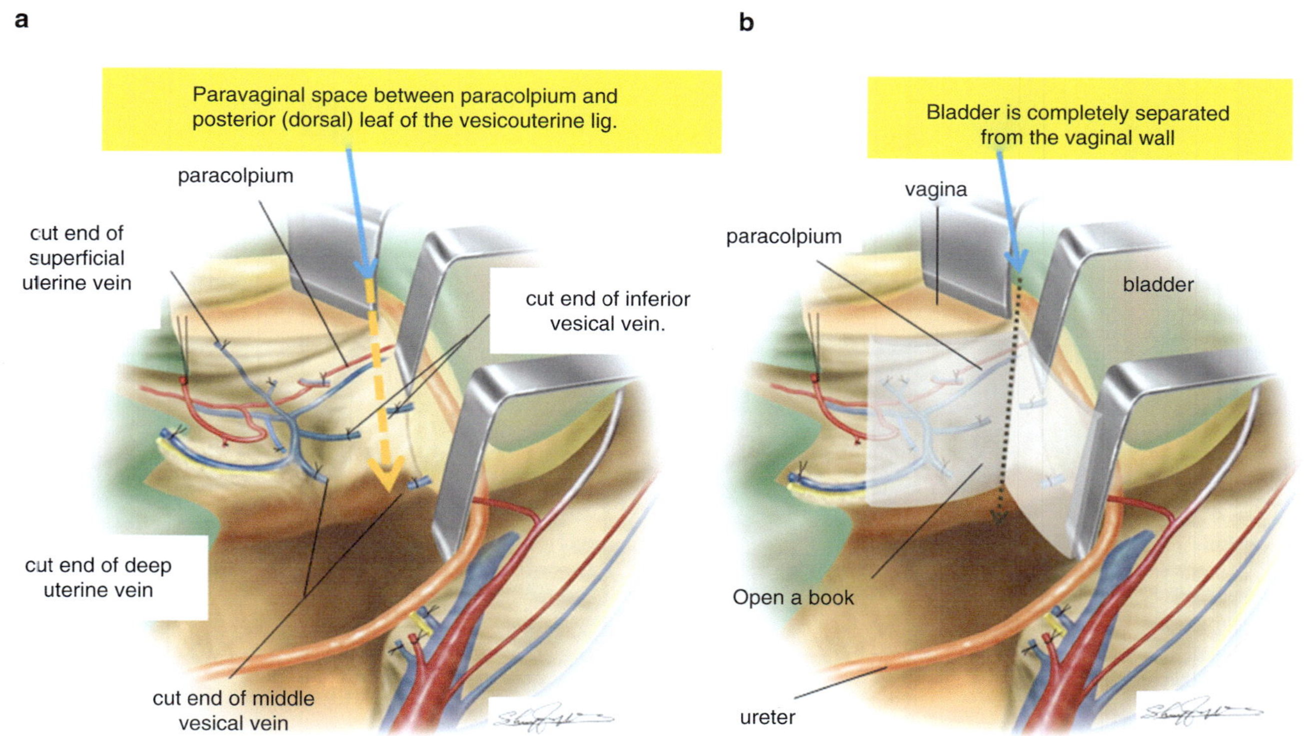


**Figure 5.3** The result of the division of the posterior (dorsal) leaf of the vesicouterine ligament. (**a**) The relationship between the divided blood vessels in the posterior (dorsal) leaf of the vesicouterine ligament and the vaginal blood vessels of the paracolpium (a yellow dotted arrow line is indicating the direction to the paravaginal space). (**b**) The relationship between the urinary bladder with the ureter and the vaginal tissues with the paracolpium. As if we open a book, the urinary bladder with the ureter is completely separated from the vaginal tissues with the paracolpium

Then, by the separation of the trigone portion of the urinary bladder from the vaginal wall, we can select the level at which the vagina is divided. Consequently, the vaginal blood vessels (paracolpium) are independently ligated and divided where the surgeon wishes to amputate (Figure 5.4a). The uterus is removed with any length of the vaginal cuff deemed appropriate for the extent of disease (Figure 5.4b).

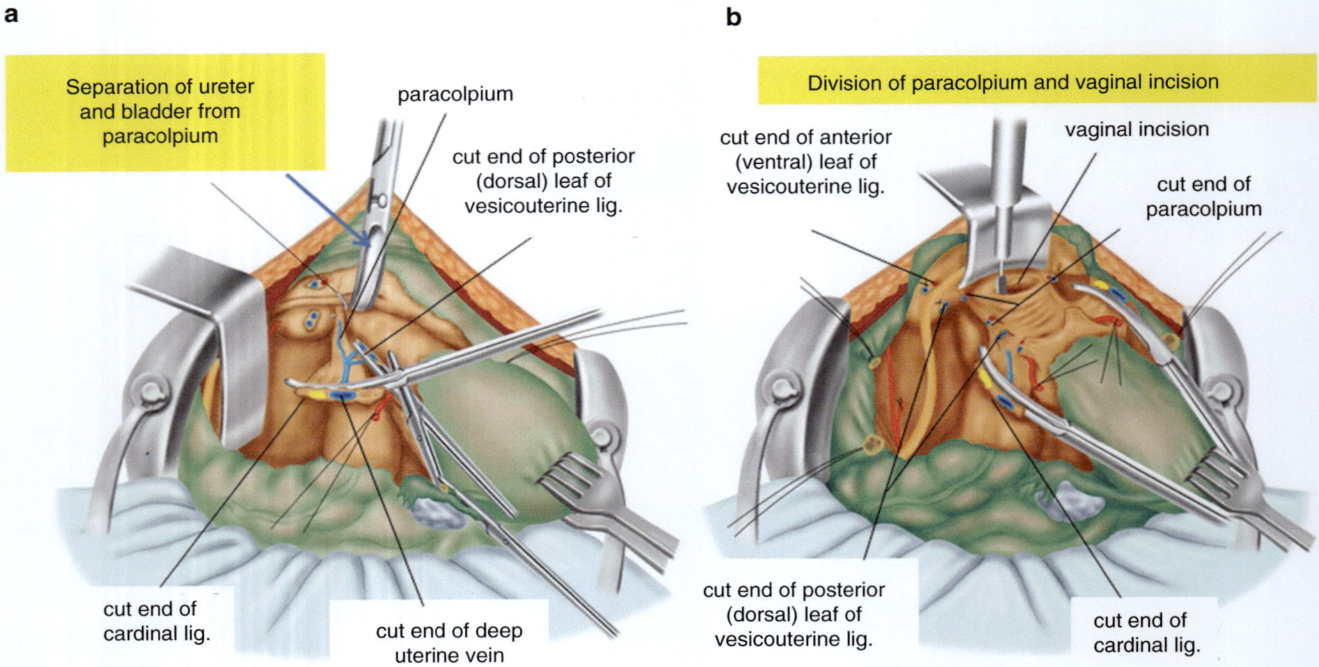


**Figure 5.4** The treatment of the paracolpium and the division of the vaginal wall. (**a**) The vaginal blood vessels (paracolpium) have a connection with the deep uterine vein (cardinal ligament). The paracolpium is ligated. (**b**) By the division of the blood vessels in the paracolpium, the uterus is connected only with the vagina. The incision to the vagina is made with enough vaginal cuff for the treatment of cervical cancer

### 5.1.2 Clarification of the Anatomy of the Posterior (Dorsal) Leaf of the Vesicouterine Ligament

A novel point of Okabayashi's radical hysterectomy is the independent separation and division of the posterior (dorsal) leaf of the vesicouterine ligament and the paracolpium. In Wertheim's or Meigs' operation (Piver et al. Class III), the posterior (dorsal) leaf of the vesicouterine ligament is treated as a mass of the parametrial tissues with the vaginal blood vessels (the paracolpium) under the name of the paracervix. During the process of the removal of the uterus with the vaginal cuff, all other types of radical hysterectomies have to divide tissues in conjunction with venous blood vessels from the urinary bladder and the vagina together as a mass (Figure 5.5a, b). However, only Okabayashi's radical hysterectomy divides the vesical veins separating from the vaginal blood vessels and can select the length of vaginal cuff deemed appropriate for each case (Figure 5.5c). This is the most sophisticated section of Okabayashi's radical hysterectomy.

Through Okabayashi's radical hysterectomy, we learnt the following anatomical truths:

1. *The venous blood vessels from the urinary bladder are running in the posterior (dorsal) leaf of the vesicouterine ligament and they drain into the deep uterine vein in the cardinal ligament.*
2. *The venous drainage from the vaginal wall is running parallel with the vaginal wall and drains into the deep uterine vein in the cardinal ligament.*

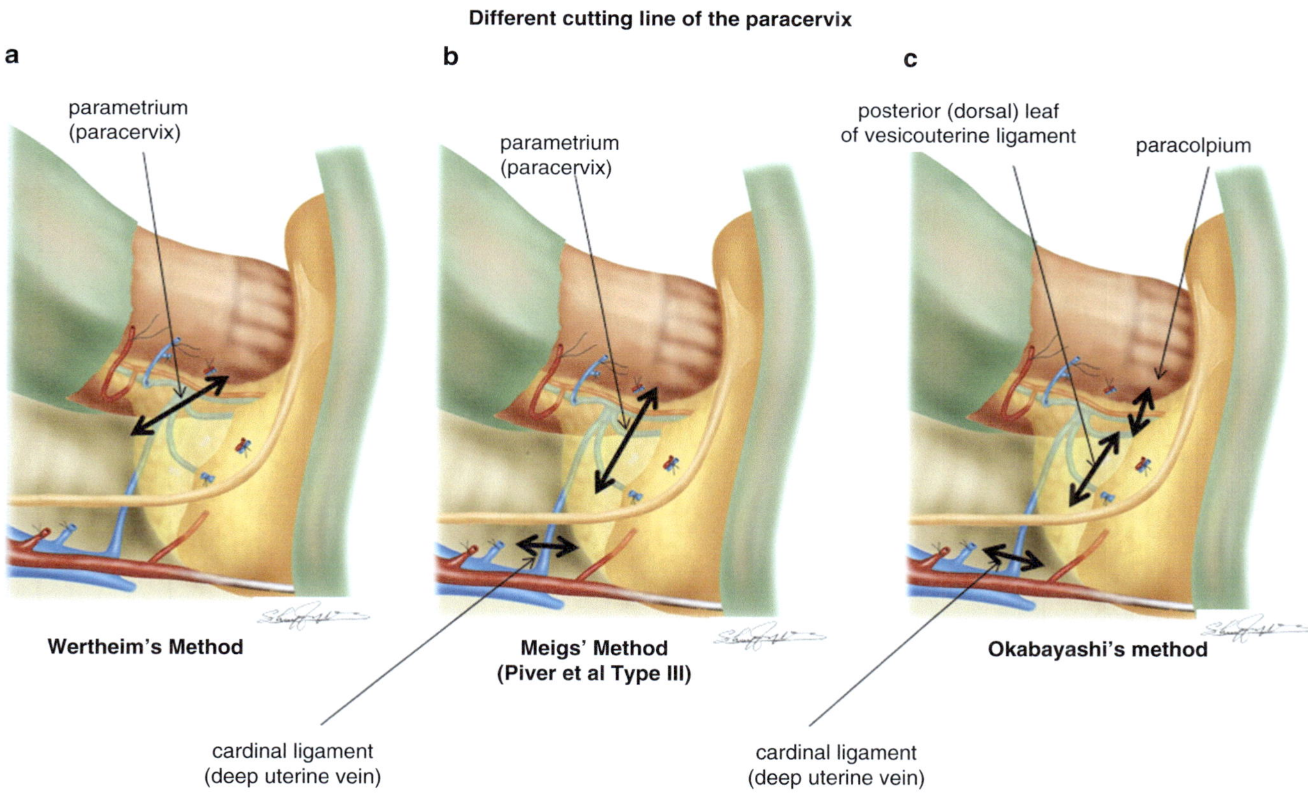


**Figure 5.5** Different cutting lines (two-directional arrow lines) of the paracervix among three different radical hysterectomies such as Wertheim's method (**a**), Meigs' method (Piver et al. Type III) (**b**) and Okabayashi's method (**c**)

# Step-by-Step Radical Hysterectomy with Pelvic Lymphadenectomy (Without Nerve-Sparing)

# 6

## 6.1 Surgical Process of the Step-by-Step Radical Hysterectomy

### 6.1.1 Open the Abdominal Cavity

### 6.1.2 Exposure of the Pelvic Cavity

### 6.1.3 Visual and Manual Examination of the Spread of the Disease and Operability

### 6.1.4 Traction of the Uterus (Figure 6.1)

Long Kocher forceps are placed close to the bilateral uterine body including the round ovarian ligaments as well as the fallopian tubes. The Kocher forceps are tied by a ribbon to use as a uterine retractor.

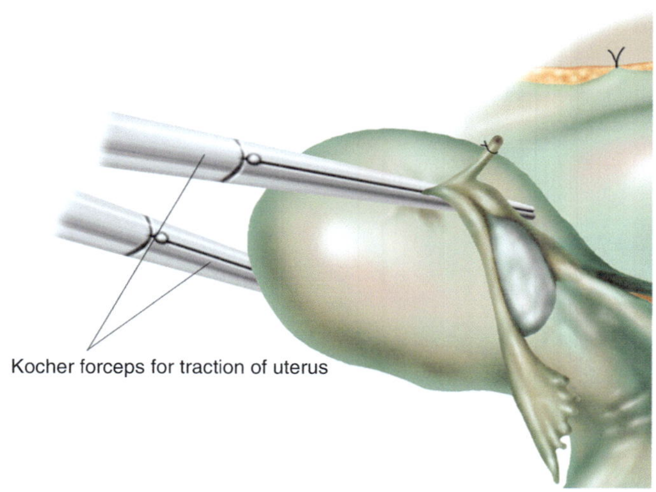


**Figure 6.1** Traction of the uterus using two long Kocher forceps


S. Fujii, K. Sekiyama, *Precise Neurovascular Anatomy for Radical Hysterectomy*,
https://doi.org/10.1007/978-981-13-8098-3_6

### 6.1.5 Ligation and Division of the Round Ligament (Figure 6.2)

The uterus is drawn cranially left, then the right round ligament becomes tense. The ligament is picked up and two ligatures, one to the uterine side and the other to the inguinal side, are placed on the round ligament through the broad ligament. The round ligament is divided between the two ligatures. Then an incision to the anterior peritoneal layer of the broad ligament is made toward the urinary bladder and cranially toward the common iliac artery to expose the loose connective tissue in the broad ligament (the retroperitoneal connective tissue).

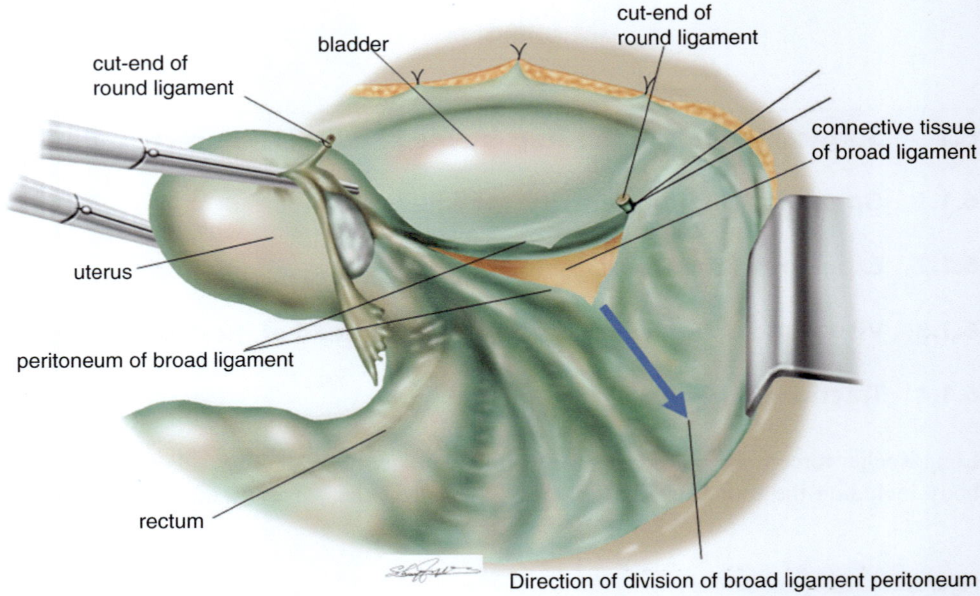


**Figure 6.2** Ligation and division of the round ligament and the direction of the separation of the peritoneum of the broad ligament (blue arrow line)

### 6.1.6 Ligation and Division of the Suspensory Ligament of the Ovary (Ovarian Vessels) (Figure 6.3)

With the uterus held over to the left side, long Kocher forceps are already placed to clamp the uterine side of the ovarian ligament and fallopian tube. The suspensory ligament of the ovary (ovarian vessels) is isolated, doubly ligated, and divided. (**For the preservation of the ovary and the fallopian tube**, ovarian side of the ovarian ligament and fallopian tube is ligated, then dissected between the long Kocher forceps and the ligature.)

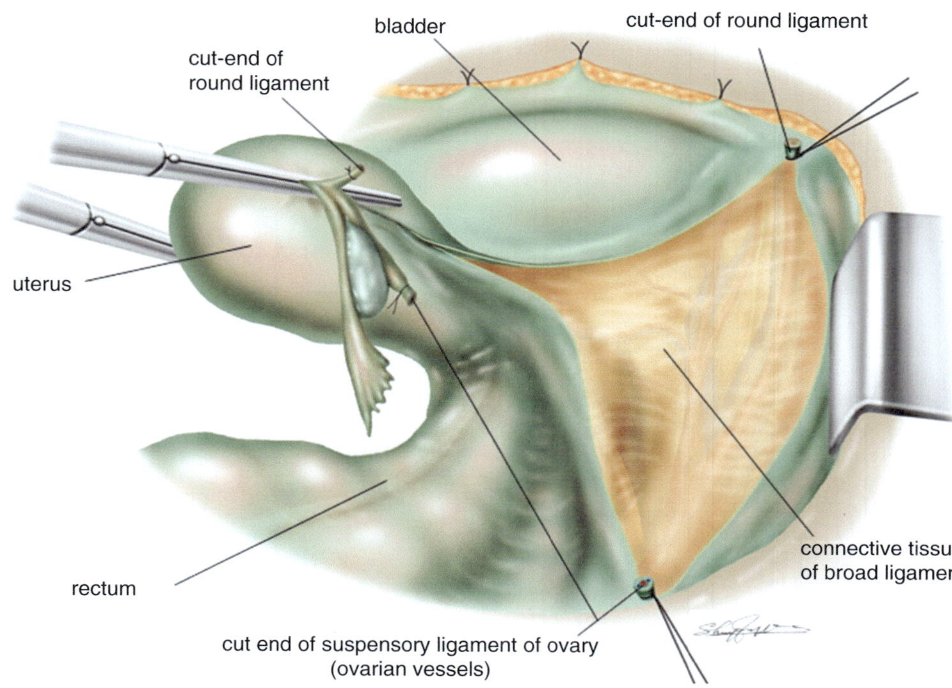


**Figure 6.3** Ligation and division of the suspensory ligament of the ovary (ovarian vessels). The retroperitoneal space beneath the broad ligament is widely separated

### 6.1.7 **Confirmation of the Ureter** (Figure 6.4)

Usually, in the connective tissue of the dorsal side of the cut-end of the suspensory ligament of the ovary, a long tubular structure can be appreciated running toward the urinary bladder. Tapping the tubular structure stimulates a vermiculation movement. This is a characteristic feature of the ureter. Manually, firmly press the tubular structure between the thumb and middle finger, which should lead to the tubular structure slipping from your fingers with a "snapping sensation." The snapping sensation is characteristics of the ureter.

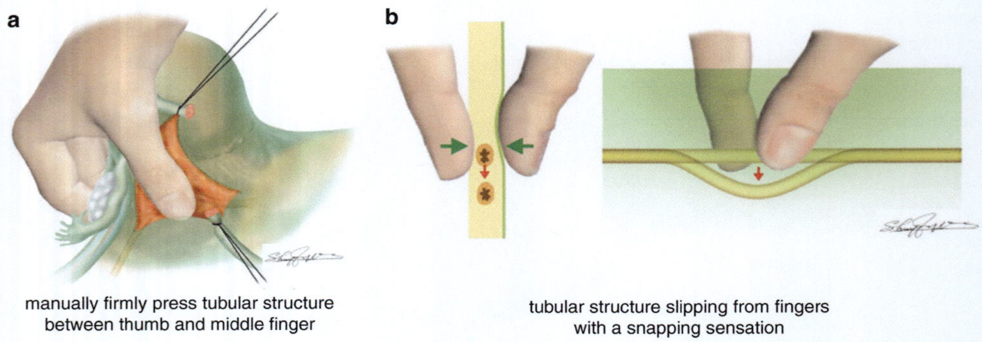


**Figure 6.4** Manual confirmation of the ureter with fingers using thumb and middle fingers. (**a**) Putting the connective tissues of the broad ligament between thumb and middle fingers, search the tubular structure. (**b**) Press firmly the tubular structure with two fingers, then the ureter usually slips between the fingers and creates a snap sound (snapping sensation)

### 6.1.8 Isolation of the Ureter (Figure 6.5)

The ureter running along the posterior peritoneal layer of the broad ligament is separated from the connective tissue of the retroperitoneal side of the peritoneum. The ureter is easier to isolate from the surrounding connective tissue, when approached as cranially at the level of the common iliac artery and caudally at the level where the ureter crosses the uterine artery.

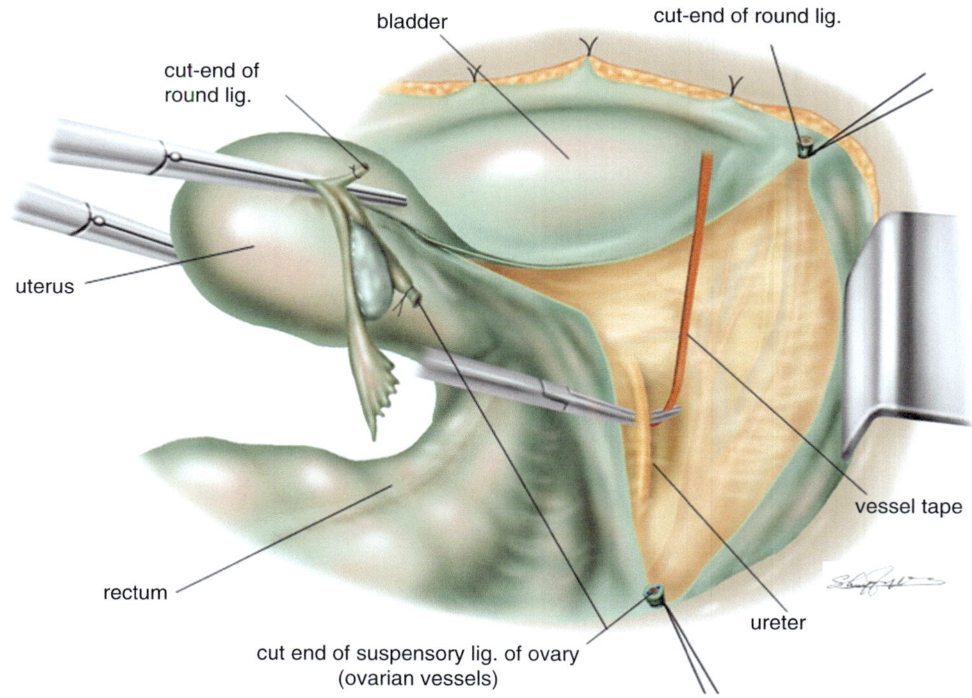


**Figure 6.5** Isolation of the ureter. The ureter is isolated from the loose connective tissues beneath the rectal side of the broad ligament peritoneum

### 6.1.9 Application of a Vessel Tape for a Marker of the Ureter (Figure 6.6)

A vessel tape is applied to act as a marker of the isolated ureter. It is very important to maintain the ureter with a marker during a radical hysterectomy. There are many opportunities to divide or damage the ureter as a result of a careless mistake during surgery. The marker of the vessel tape can help to avoid injuries to the ureter.

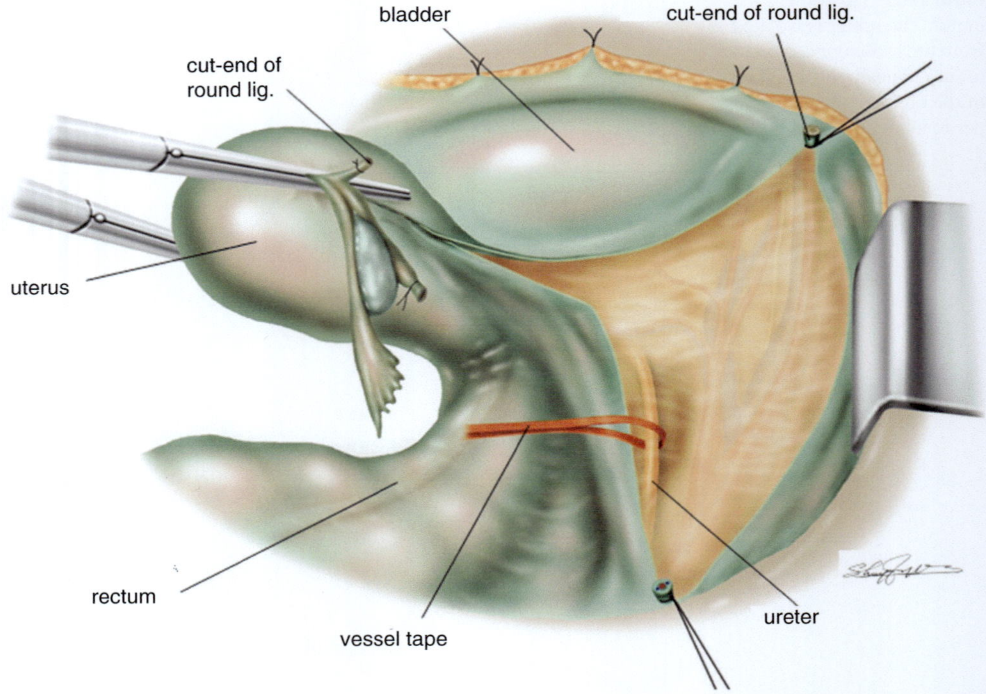


**Figure 6.6** Application of a vessel tape for a marker of the ureter

### 6.1.10 Tentative Development of the Pararectal Space (Figure 6.7)

Between the posterior peritoneal layer and internal iliac vein/artery, the retroperitoneal connective tissue is dissected. This allows the loose connective tissue to be easily separated toward the pelvic floor along the pelvis axis between the rectum and the internal iliac artery/vein. This is the loose connective tissue of the pararectal space (**Latzko's pararectal space**).

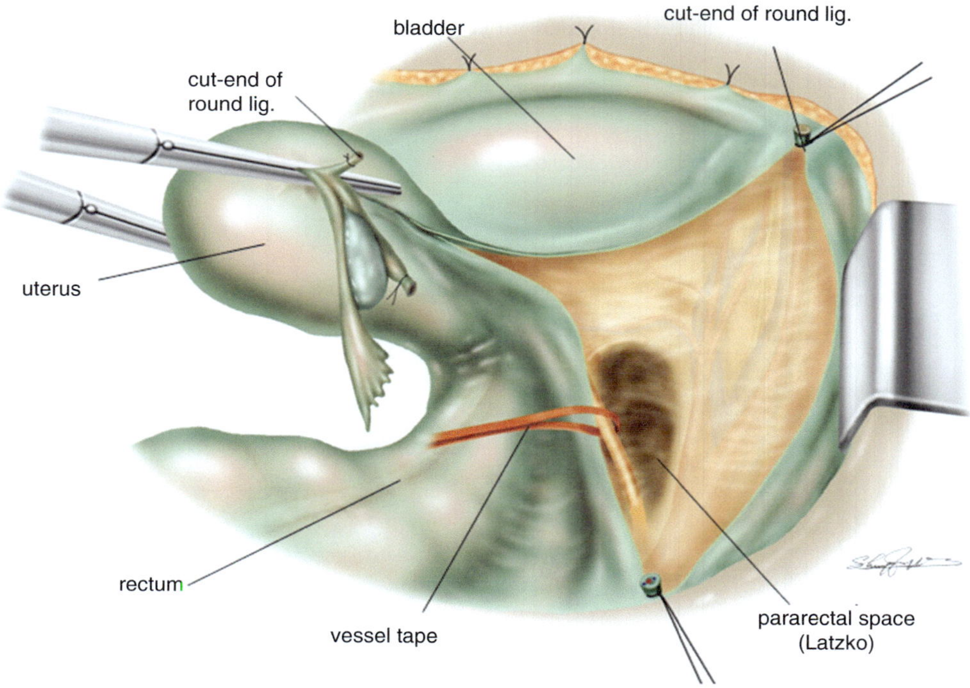


**Figure 6.7** Tentative development of the pararectal space (Latzko)

### 6.1.11 **Definition of the Pararectal Space** (Figures 6.8 and 6.9)

The pararectal space is a space surrounded by rectal sidewall (uterine side), internal iliac blood vessels (pelvic sidewall), sacral bone (cranial side), and blood vessels and connective tissue of cardinal ligament (inguinal side). The pararectal space is filled with the loose connective tissue to the base of the pelvis. The development of the pararectal space can be undertaken by inserting fingers into the loose connective tissue between the rectum and the internal iliac artery/vein. The direction of insertion is toward the pelvic axis. Separation of the connective tissue between the internal iliac artery and the ureter reveals a space called as *Latzko's pararectal space*.

a

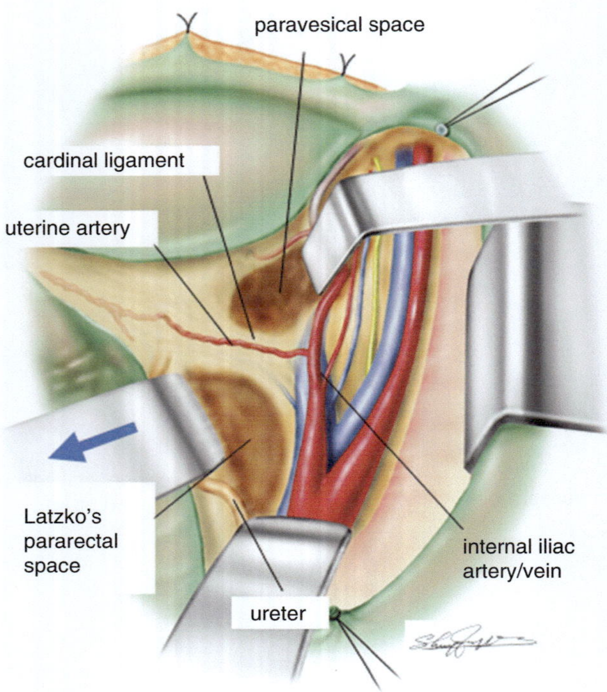


b

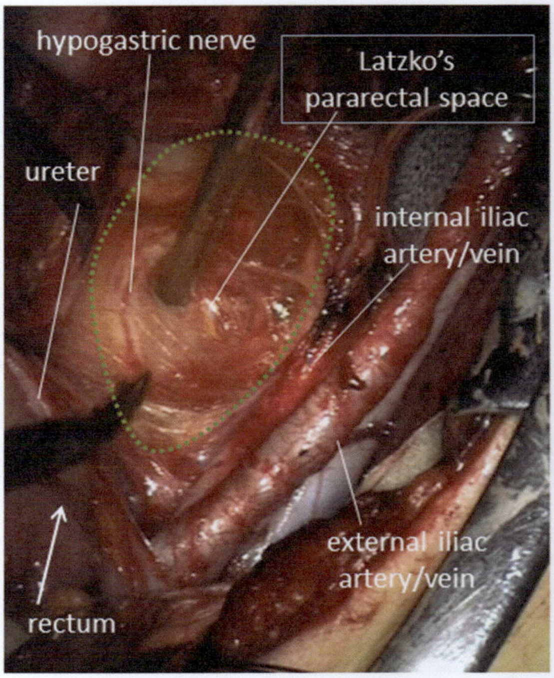


**Figure 6.8** Definition of the pararectal space. (**a**) The relationship among the paravesical space, the cardinal ligament and the pararectal space (Latzko). (**b**) A surgical photo of the developed pararectal space between the rectal sidewall with the ureter and the internal iliac artery/vein. On the rectal sidewall of the pararectal space the hypogastric nerve accompanied by a small blood vessel is appreciated

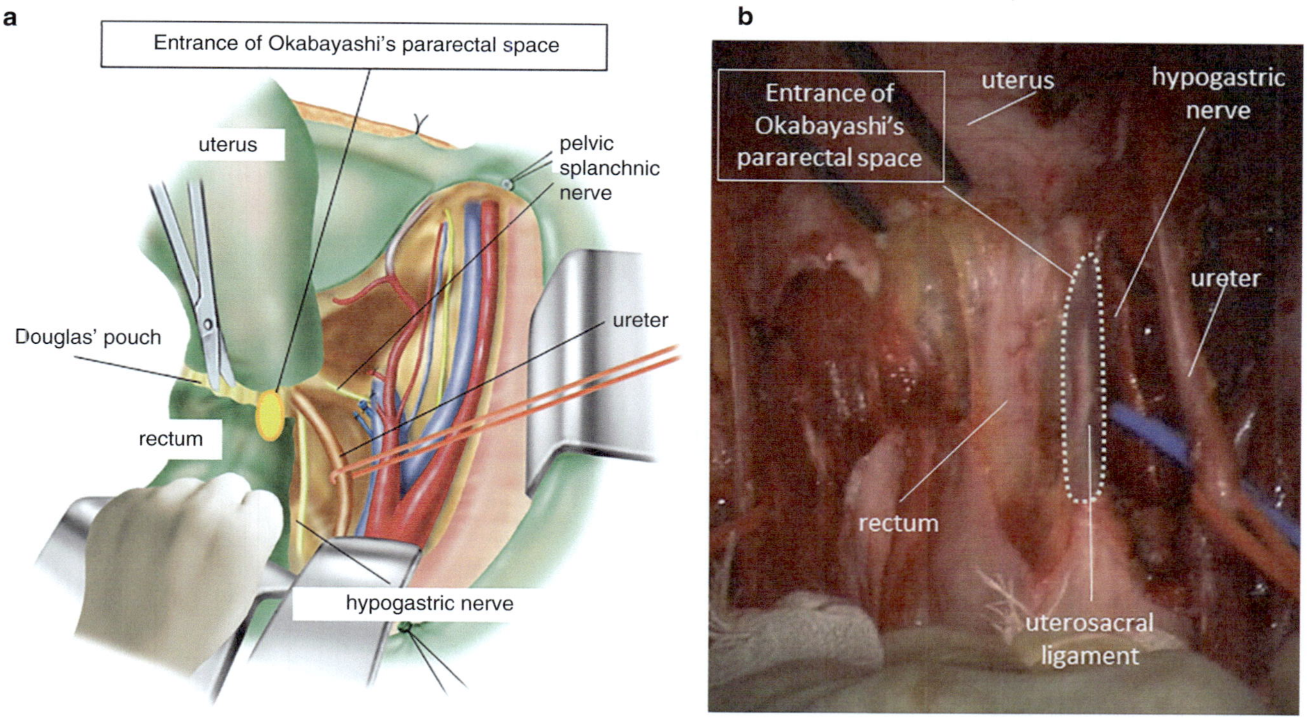


**Figure 6.9** Anatomical location of Okabayashi's pararectal space. (**a**) An oval-shaped orange circle filled with yellow color on the uterosacral ligament is the landmark of the entrance of Okabayashi's pararectal space. (**b**) A surgical photo of Okabayashi's pararectal space developed just between the rectal sidewall and the connective tissue plane that includes the ureter and the hypogastric nerve. This connective tissue plane resides between Okabayashi's pararectal and Latzko's pararectal space

In contrast, Okabayashi opened the pararectal space by the division of the uterosacral ligament and usually divided the hypogastric nerve. Therefore, **Okabayashi's pararectal space** is developed just close to the rectal sidewall retracting the isolated ureter to the pelvic sidewall (Figure 6.9a, b). In order to increase the mobility of the uterus, Okabayashi preferred to open the space from the uterosacral ligament. Between Latzko's and Okabayashi's pararectal space, the hypogastric nerve is appreciated parallel to the ureter as shown in Figure 6.8b. In order to extend Okabayashi's pararectal space toward Latzko's pararectal space, it is necessary to divide the hypogastric nerve, which in turn increases the mobility of the uterus.

### 6.1.12 The Ureter and the Hypogastric Nerve Are on the Same Connective Tissue Plane (Figure 6.10)

As shown in the photos during surgery (Figure 6.10a, b), if the two spaces are developed separately, the connective tissue plane containing the ureter is created between Okabayashi's pararectal space and Latzko's pararectal space. The hypogastric nerve runs at a level 2–4 cm dorsal to the ureter in the same connective tissue plane. Usually, the ureter is already isolated from the connective tissue plane. The division of the connective tissue plane with the hypogastric nerve can expand Okabayashi's pararectal space to reach Latzko's pararectal space. The expanded pararectal space is very wide and deep. ***When performing nerve-sparing radical hysterectomy, the development of Latzko's pararectal space is enough and development of the Okabayashi's pararectal space is not required.***

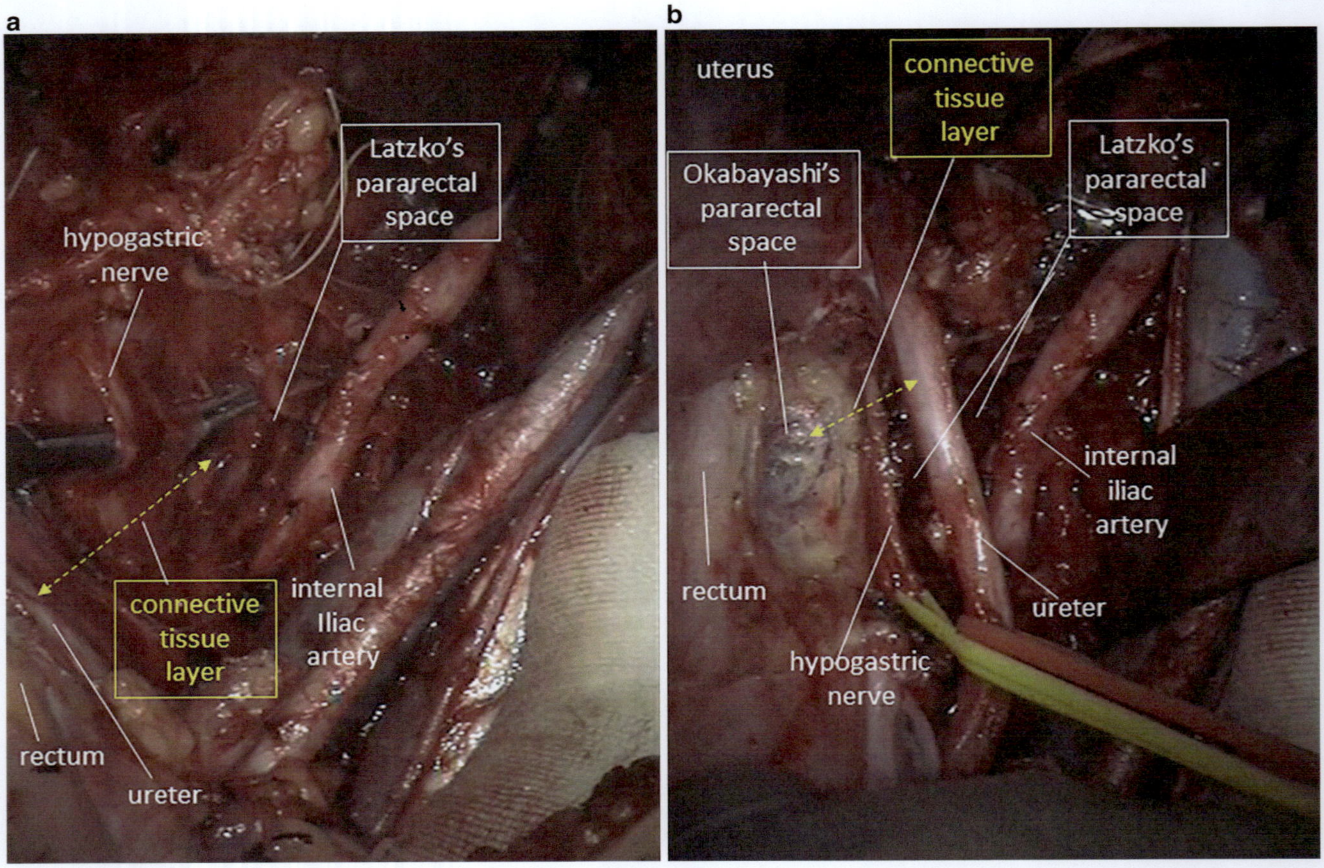


**Figure 6.10** Anatomical relationship between Okabayashi's pararectal space and Latzko's pararectal space. (**a**) On the rectal sidewall of Latzko's pararectal space, the ureter and the hypogastric nerve are appreciated on the same connective tissue plane (a dotted line with bidirectional arrow). (**b**) Okabayashi's pararectal space is medially developed between the rectum and the connective tissue plane of the ureter and hypogastric nerve that was the rectal sidewall of Latzko's pararectal space

### 6.1.13 Division of the Peritoneum at Pouch of Douglas (Figure 6.11)

The uterus is drawn toward the pubic arch and the rectum with its peritoneal surface is stretched with the hand toward the cranial side. The peritoneum between the uterus and the rectum is lifted from the base of the Pouch of Douglas. The incision is made on the elevated peritoneum and extended with scissors across the dorsal side (back) of the cervix. This step connects the retroperitoneal spaces of the broad ligament on both sides.

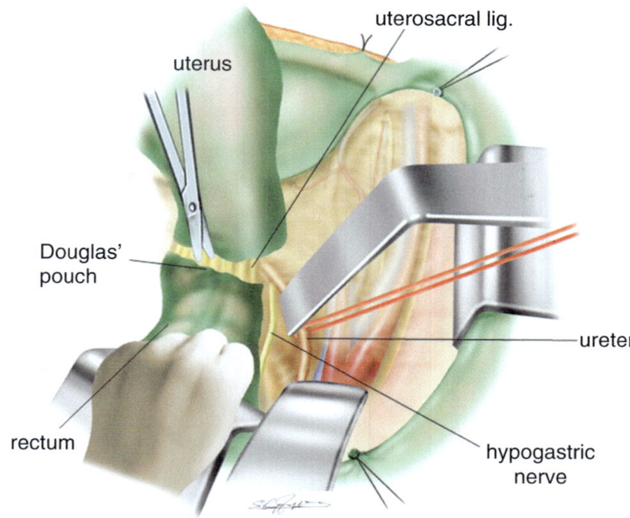


**Figure 6.11** Division of the peritoneum of the Douglas' pouch

### 6.1.14 Separation of the Peritoneum of the Vesicouterine Pouch (Figure 6.12)

The peritoneum is divided across the ventral side of the cervix, just 1–2 cm below the vesicouterine fold where scissors can insinuate and divide the peritoneum easily without any damage to the urinary bladder.

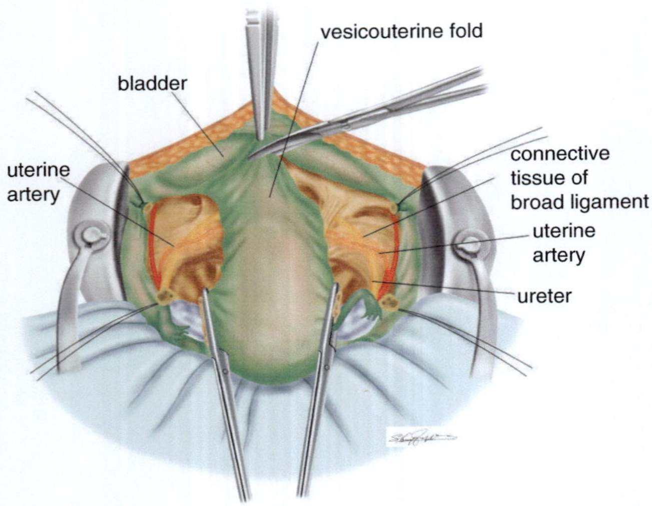


**Figure 6.12** Separation of the peritoneum of the vesicouterine pouch

## 6.2 Pelvic Lymphadenectomy

### 6.2.1 Lymph Nodes in the Pelvis (Figure 6.13)

Major lymph nodes in the pelvic cavity are illustrated in the Figure 6.13. We usually start the dissection of lymph nodes from the supra-inguinal area and finish cranially by the common iliac area. If we find positive nodes in the pelvic lymph nodes, we undertake paraaortic lymphadenectomy above the bifurcation of the aorta either till the level of the inferior mesenteric artery or till the level of the renal vein.

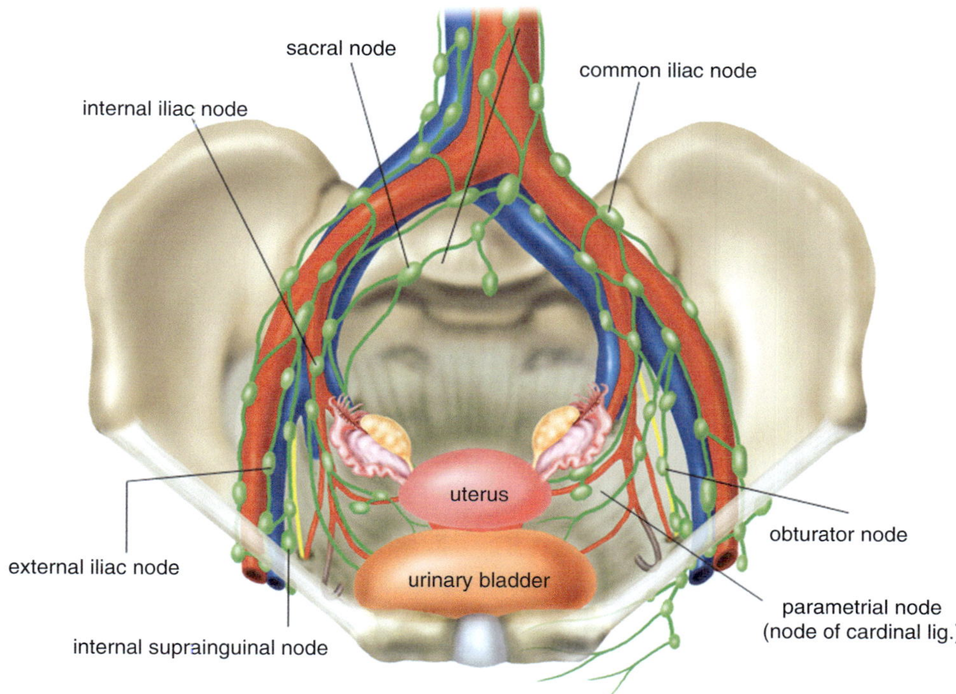


**Figure 6.13** Lymph nodes in the pelvis

## 6.2.2 Exposure of the Adipose Tissue in the Supra-Inguinal Area (Figure 6.14)

The adipose tissues are distributed in the retroperitoneal space of the pelvis on the external iliac/internal iliac/common iliac vessels as shown in Figure 6.14a. Including the incised abdominal wall and the cut-end of the round ligament, a retractor is applied to the abdominal wall on the inguinal side. Then, the retractor is pulled caudally, to expose the adipose tissue of the supra-inguinal area. Figure 6.14b shows a cross-sectional view of the retroperitoneal structures in the pelvis at the level of a two-directional arrow drawn in the Figure 6.14b. A dotted arrow line in Figure 6.14b shows the separation point of connective tissue from the iliopsoas muscle. In the following illustrations of cross-sectional view of lymphadenectomy, the dotted arrow line indicates the separation line of the connective tissue from muscle, blood vessels, or nerve.

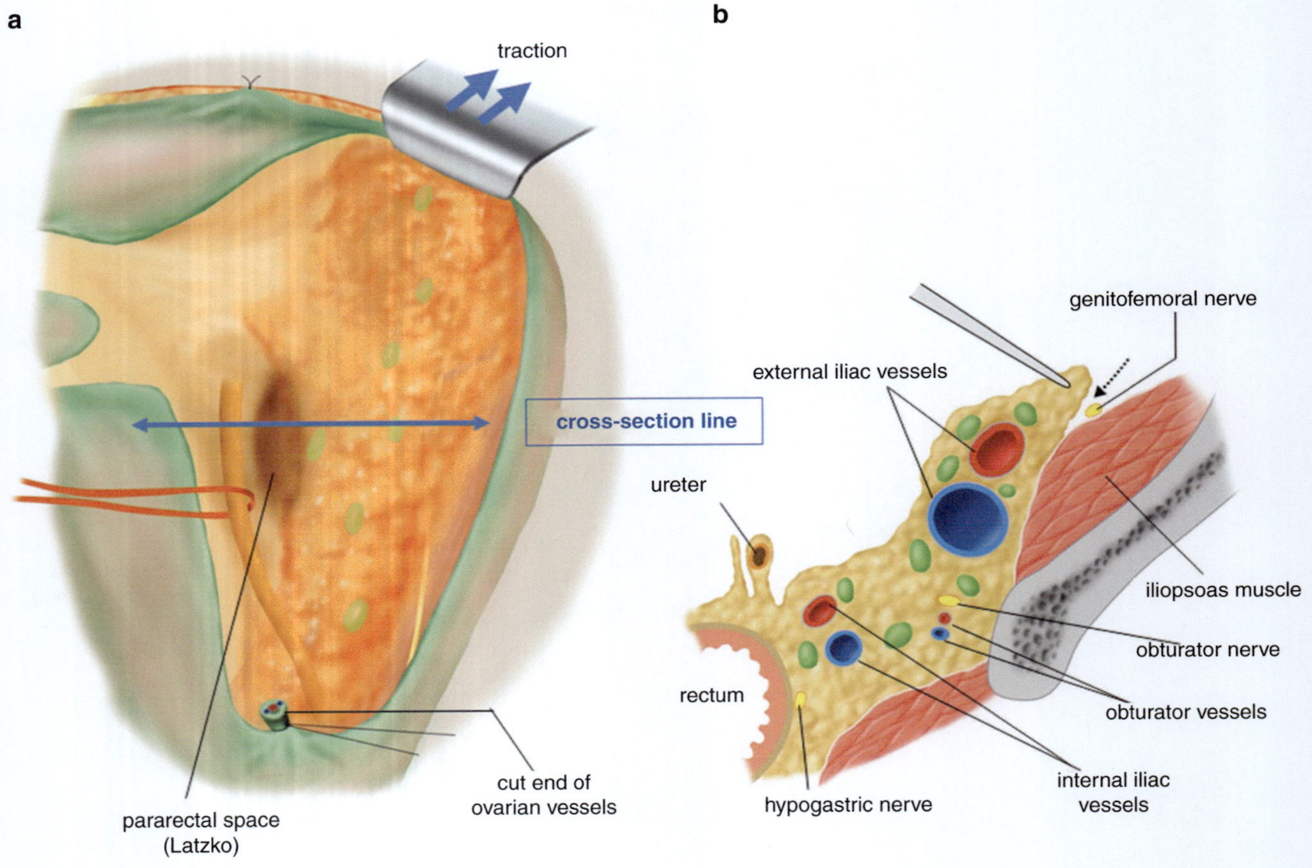


**Figure 6.14** Exposure of the adipose tissues in the supra-inguinal area. (**a**) Exposed retroperitoneal adipose tissues of the broad ligament. (**b**) A cross-sectional view of the retroperitoneal structures in the pelvis at the level of a two-directional arrow (cross-sectional line) drawn in Figure 6.14a. A dotted arrow line indicates the separation point of the connective tissue from the iliopsoas muscle

### 6.2.3 Exposure of the Iliopsoas Muscle (Figure 6.15)

By retracting the incised abdominal wall laterally from the supra-inguinal region to the region of the common iliac artery, the ventral side of the iliopsoas muscle is revealed. The connective tissue with adipose tissue is dissected from the surface of the iliopsoas muscle toward the ventral surface of the external iliac artery (Figure 6.15a). The genitofemoral nerve runs parallel to the external iliac artery. Usually, the genitofemoral nerve is preserved. A dotted arrow line in Figure 6.15b indicates the direction of separation of the adipose tissue on the external iliac artery.

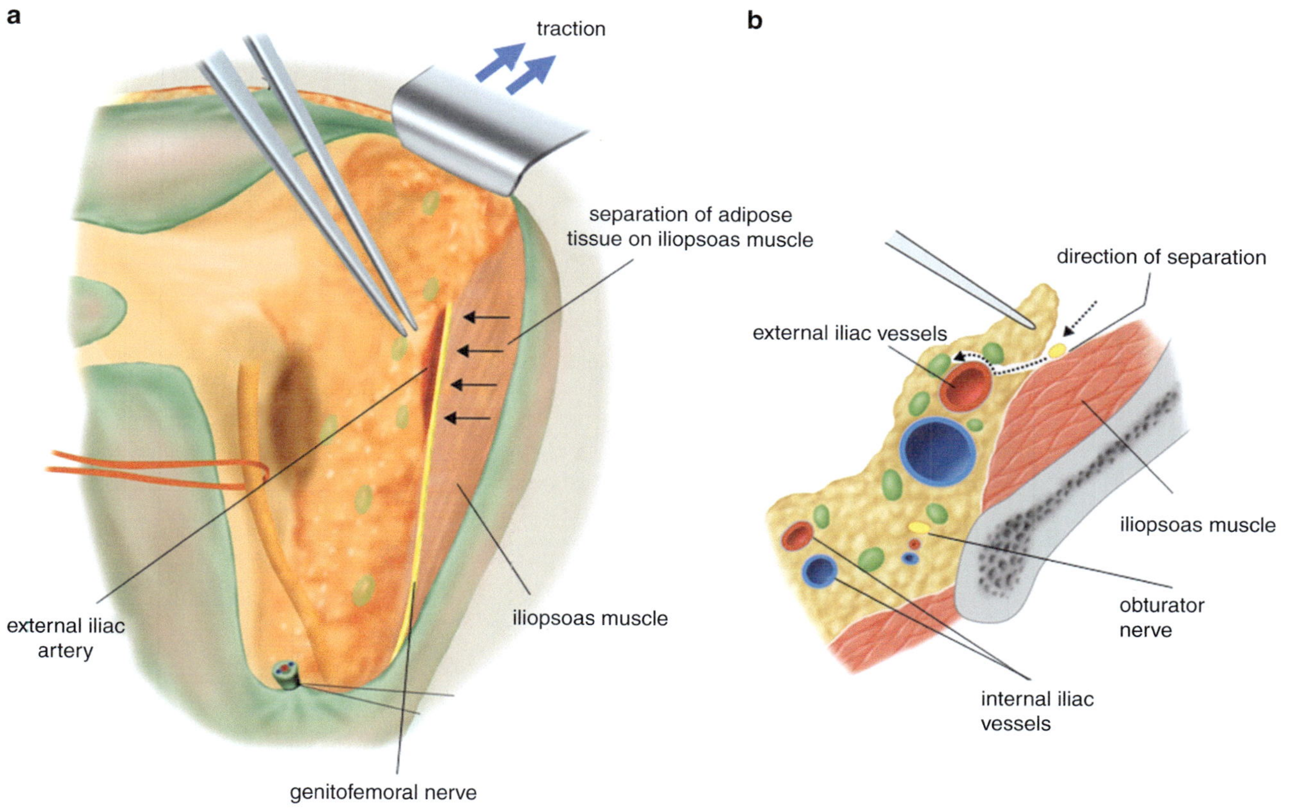


**Figure 6.15** Exposure of the iliopsoas muscle. (**a**) Four small arrows on the iliopsoas muscle are indicating the direction of the separation of the adipose tissues toward the external iliac artery. (**b**) Two dotted arrow lines are showing direction of the separation of the adipose tissues toward the external iliac artery

### 6.2.4 Separation of the External Supra-Inguinal Nodes from the Ventral Surface of the External Iliac Artery (Figure 6.16)

Retraction of the abdominal wall of the supra-inguinal area distally (arrow in Figure 6.16a) exposes the adipose tissue of the supra-inguinal region. Picking up the adipose tissue on the external iliac artery, the adipose tissue including supra-inguinal node is separated from the ventral surface of the external iliac artery. In the supra-inguinal region, usually the deep circumflex iliac vein runs across the external iliac artery. Avoiding a deep circumflex iliac vein, the adipose tissue with lymph nodes is dissected up from the ventral surface of the external iliac artery. A dotted arrow line in Figure 6.16b indicates the direction of separation that reaches to the ventral surface of the external iliac vein. Paying attention to the deep circumflex iliac vein, the adipose tissues with the external supra-inguinal nodes are removed.

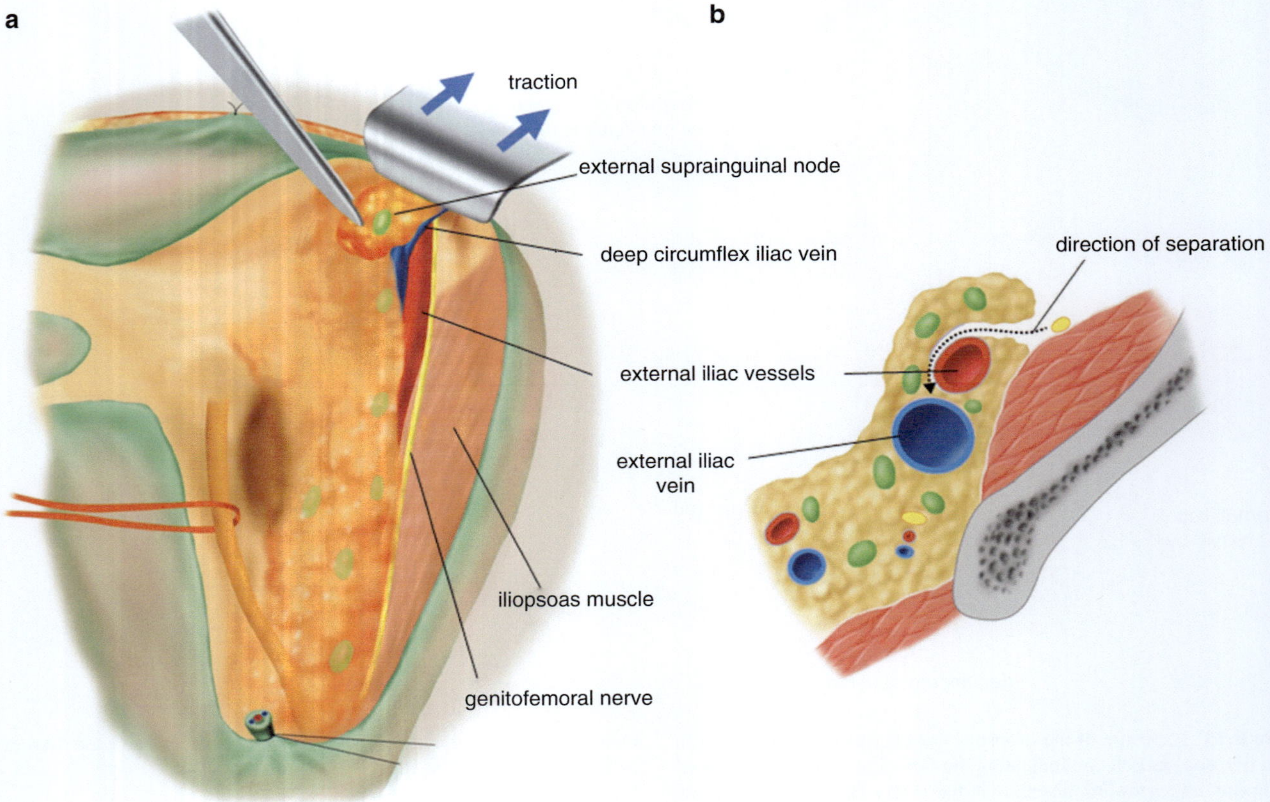


**Figure 6.16** Separation of the external supra-inguinal nodes from the ventral surface of the external iliac artery. (**a**) By the traction of the abdominal wall of the supra-inguinal area distally (arrow), the adipose tissue including supra-inguinal nodes is separated from the ventral surface of the external iliac artery. (**b**) A dotted arrow line indicates the direction of separation of the adipose tissues that reaches to the ventral surface of the external iliac vein

### 6.2.5 Tentative Development of the Paravesical Space (Figure 6.17)

By the separation of the connective tissue between the obliterated umbilical artery and the external iliac vein at a point 2–3 cm cranial to the pubic bone, the cobweb-like loose connective tissue becomes visible. This is the entrance of the paravesical space. The paravesical space is surrounded by the obliterated umbilical artery (urinary bladder side), rectal/vaginal wall (rectal side), external iliac vein (inguinal side), public bone (caudal side), the connective tissue of the cardinal ligament (cranial side), and pelvic floor (dorsal side). In the base of the pelvis, a yellow-white string running from the foramen obturatum is appreciated. This is the obturator nerve. The obturator nerve can be traced along the dorsal side of external iliac vein by the lateral side of the common iliac vein.

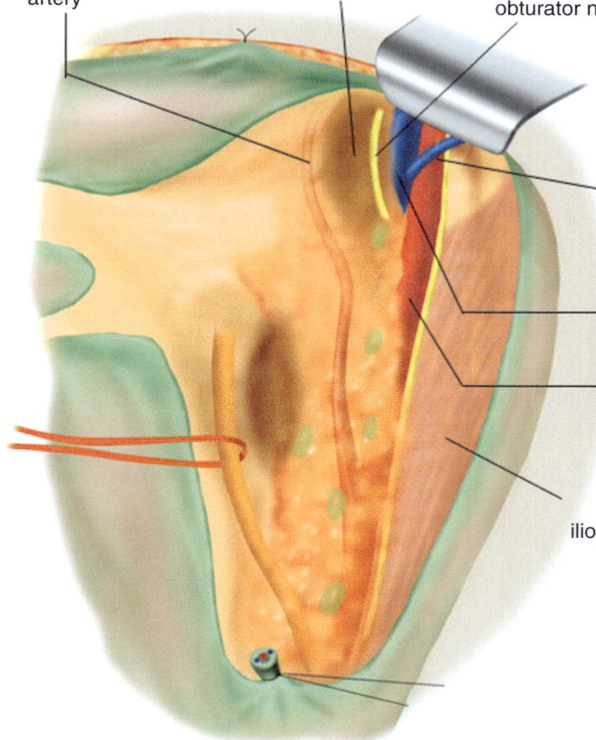


**Figure 6.17** Tentative development of the paravesical space

### 6.2.6 Separation of the Connective Tissue Between the External Iliac Artery and Iliopsoas Muscle (Figure 6.18)

The connective tissue surrounding the external iliac artery is separated by insertion of a small retractor and medial traction of the external iliac artery as shown in Figure 6.18. Giving tension to the connective tissue between the external iliac artery and iliopsoas muscle, the loose connective tissue sheath on the surface of the external iliac artery is dissected. This procedure opens the space between the iliopsoas muscle and external iliac vessels. It is possible to continue the dissection along the medial surface of the iliopsoas muscle deep into the obturator fossa.

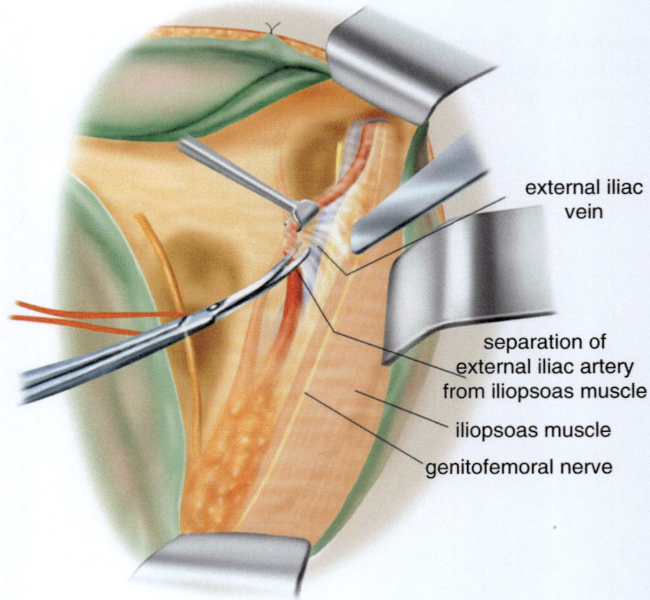


**Figure 6.18** Separation of the connective tissue between the external iliac artery and iliopsoas muscle

### 6.2.7 Separation of the Uterine Side Connective Tissue of the External Iliac Artery and Vein (Figure 6.19)

The dissection proceeds toward the medial side of the external iliac artery and continues to the sheath of the medial side of the external iliac vein.

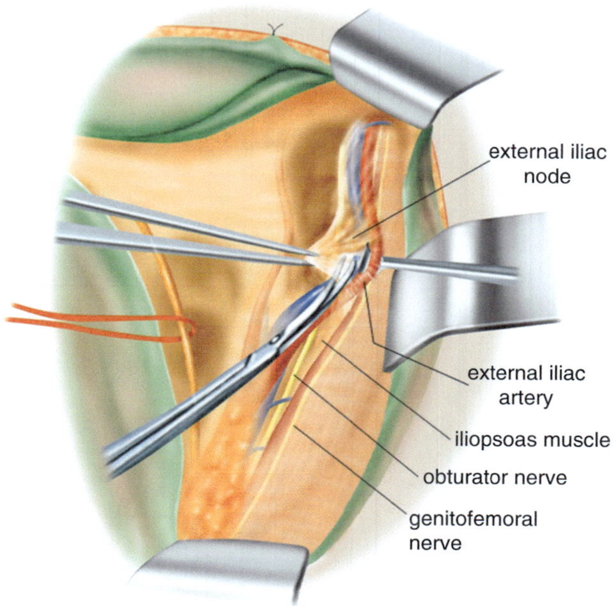


**Figure 6.19** Separation of the uterine side connective tissue of the external iliac artery and vein

### 6.2.8 Lymphadenectomy of the External Iliac Nodes of the Uterine Side (Figure 6.20)

Picking up the adipose tissue on the medial side, the external iliac lymph nodes are dissected from the external iliac artery and vein. The direction of the separation is illustrated using a dotted arrow line in Figure 6.20b.

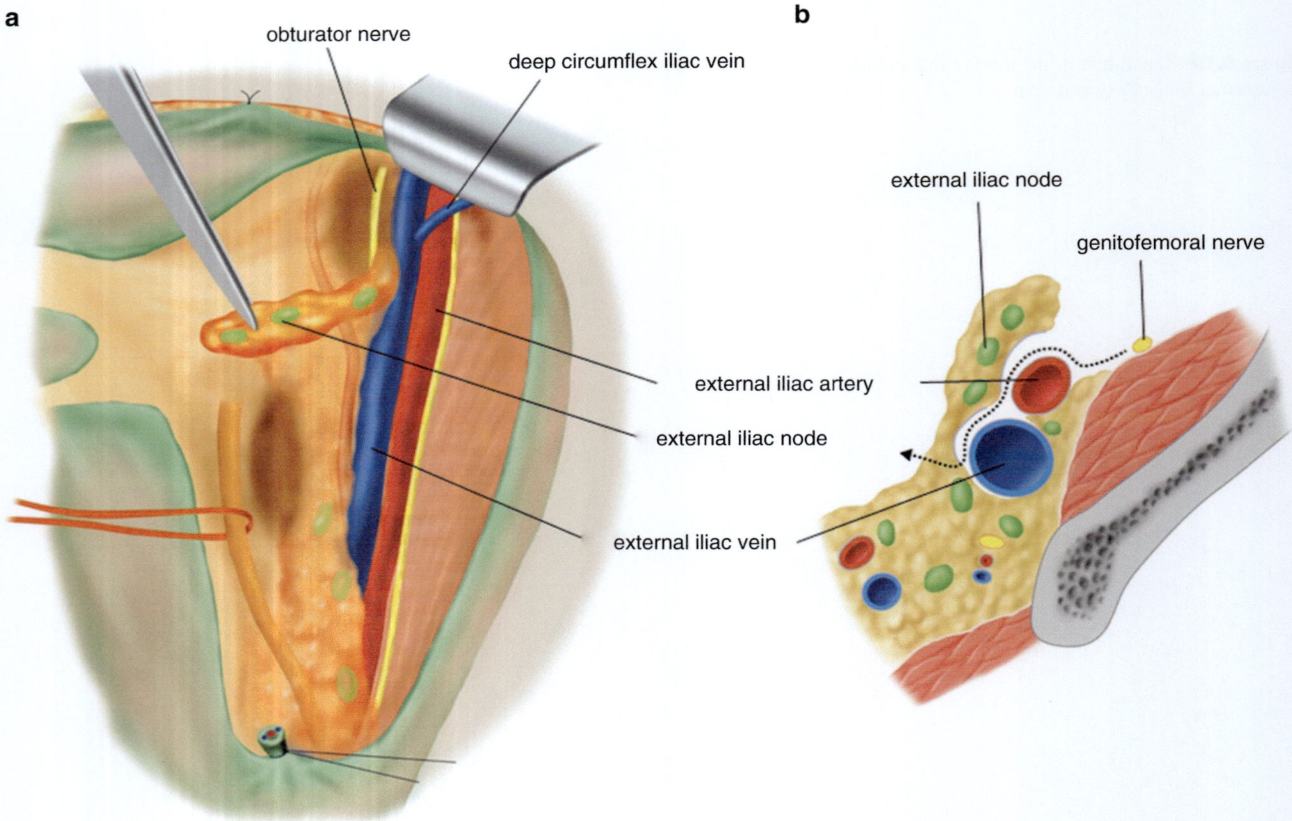


**Figure 6.20** Lymphadenectomy of the external iliac nodes of the uterine side. (**a**) Picking up the adipose tissue on the medial side, the external iliac lymph nodes are dissected from the external iliac artery and vein. (**b**) A dotted arrow line is the direction of the separation

### 6.2.9 Separation of the Connective Tissue Between the Iliopsoas Muscle and the External Iliac Vessels Toward the Pelvic Floor (Figure 6.21)

The ventral side of the adipose tissue on the iliopsoas muscle is already removed. The connective tissue of the external iliac artery side is picked up and scissors are advanced into the connective tissue along the medial side of the iliopsoas muscle (Figure 6.21a). The scissors are advanced dorsally into the obturator fossa. Moreover, the dissection should be extended deep enough to reach the base of the pelvic wall as shown in Figure 6.21b using a dotted arrow line.

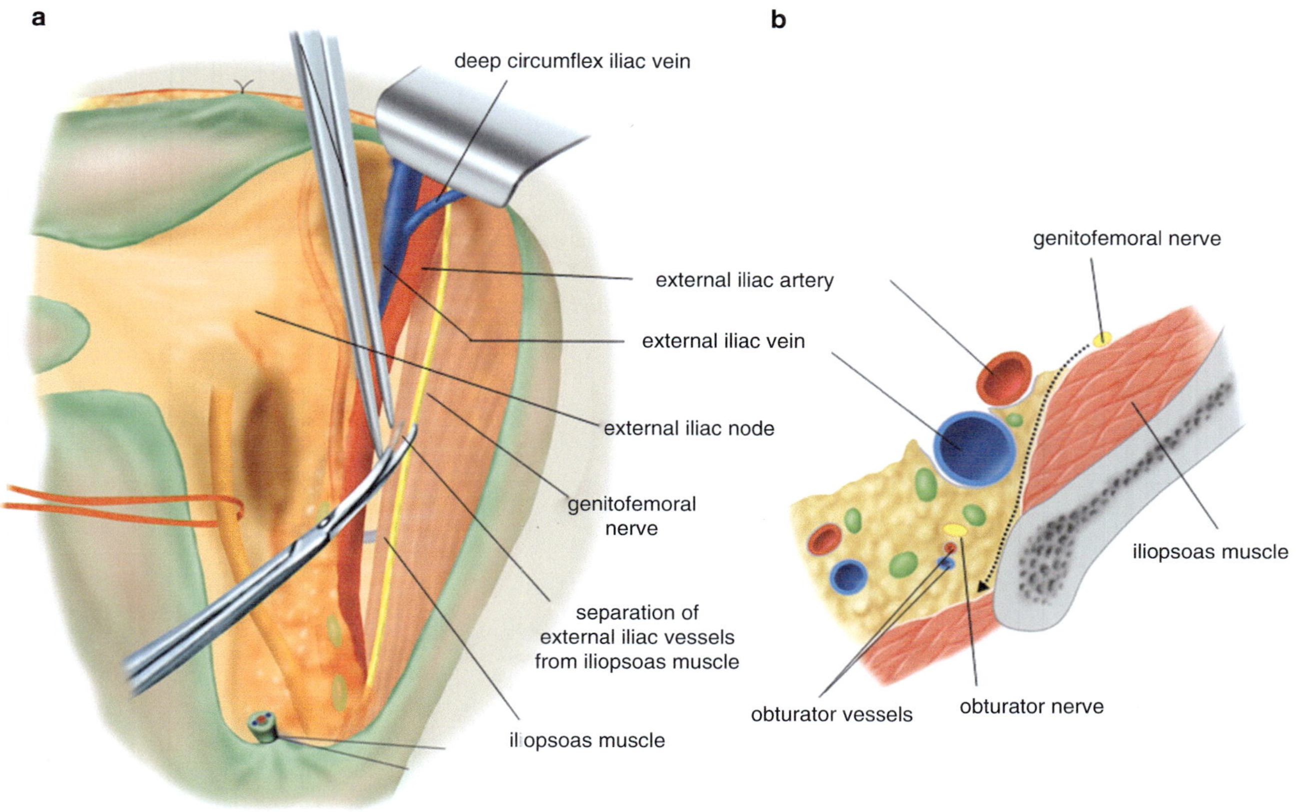


**Figure 6.21** Separation of the connective tissue between the iliopsoas muscle and the external iliac vessels. (**a**) The connective tissue of the external iliac artery side is picked up and scissors are advanced into the connective tissue along the medial side of the iliopsoas muscle. (**b**) A dotted arrow line is the direction of the scissors dorsally into the obturator fossa deep enough to reach the base of the pelvic sidewall

### 6.2.10 Dissection of the External Iliac Nodes (Figure 6.22)

Drawing the external iliac artery medially by a small retractor, the loose connective tissue sheath on the external iliac vein is separated toward the dorsal surface of the external iliac vein (Figure 6.22a). During this step, the connective tissue sheath with adipose tissue including the external iliac lymph nodes is separated from the external iliac vein (Figure 6.22b). The separated adipose tissues with lymph nodes are reflected medially to the obturator fossa or can be dissected at this point.

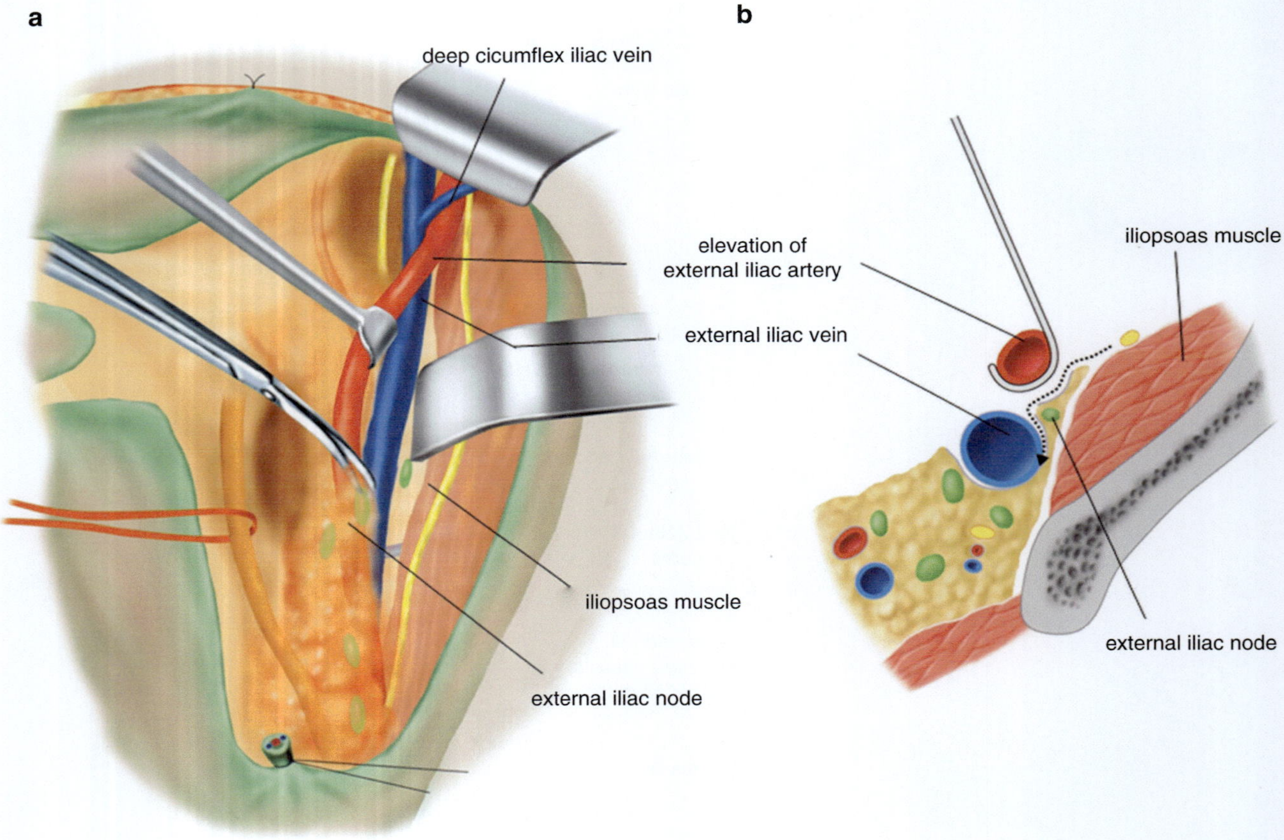


**Figure 6.22** Dissection of the external iliac nodes. (**a**) Drawing the external iliac artery medially by a small retractor, the loose connective tissue sheath on the external iliac vein is separated toward the dorsal surface of the external iliac vein. (**b**) The connective tissue sheath with adipose tissue including the external iliac lymph nodes is separated from the external iliac vein as illustrated using a dotted arrow line

### 6.2.11 Separation of the Connective Tissue on the Internal Iliac Artery (Figure 6.23)

The same kind of dissection is extended to both cranial side and caudal side of the external iliac vein. The adipose tissues with external iliac lymph nodes are separated from the external iliac vein and are collected in the obturator fossa (Figure 6.23a). Once the common iliac artery is identified, the internal iliac artery is found medially and the adipose and connective tissues are separated from the ventral side of the internal iliac artery (Figure 6.23b). The uterine artery and the obturator arteries often branch from the internal iliac artery. In order to avoid injuries to these arteries, it is better to start dissection from the ventral surface of the internal iliac artery.

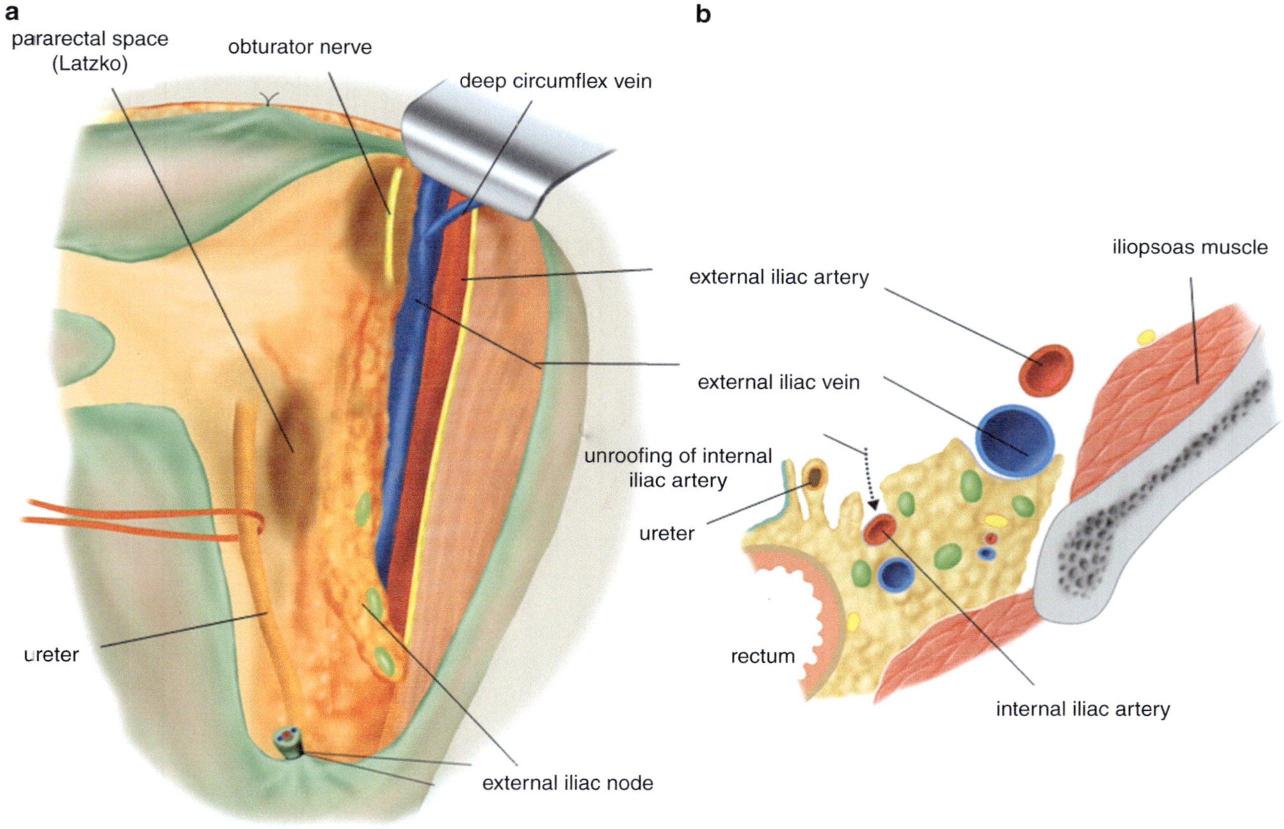


**Figure 6.23** Separation of the connective tissue on the internal iliac artery. (**a**) The dissection is extended to both cranial side and caudal side of the external iliac vein. The adipose tissues with external iliac nodes are separated from the external iliac vein and are collected in the obturator fossa. (**b**) Once the internal iliac artery is found medially, the adipose and connective tissues are separated from the ventral side of the internal iliac artery as illustrated using a dotted arrow line

### 6.2.12 **Confirmation of the Obturator Nerve in the Obturator Fossa** (Figure 6.24)

In the dorsal level of the external iliac vein, we usually appreciate a yellow-white solid string running in the obturator fossa. This is the obturator nerve. The obturator nerve becomes a landmark of the obturator fossa (Figure 6.24a). As shown in Figure 6.24b, the connective tissue with lymph nodes is separated toward the obturator nerve.

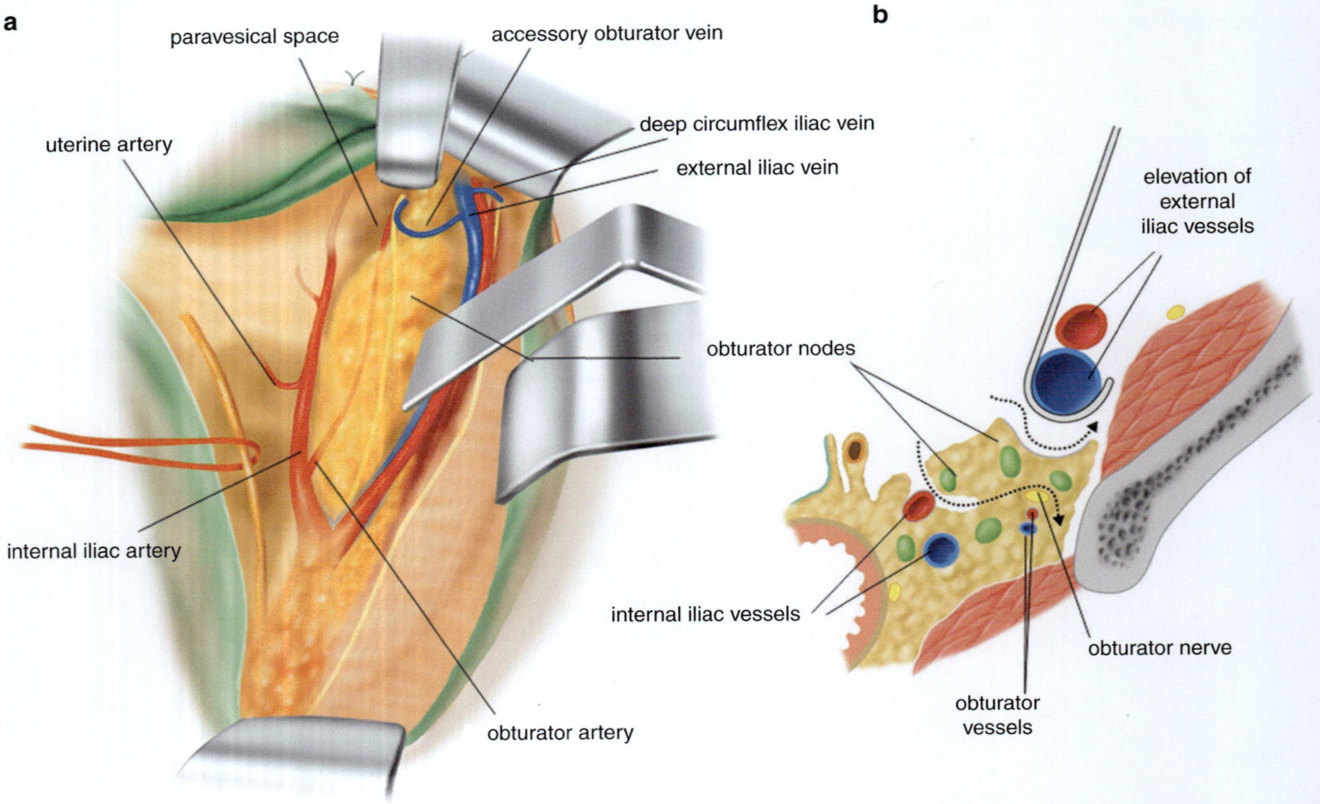


**Figure 6.24** Confirmation of the obturator nerve in the obturator fossa. (**a**) In the dorsal level of the external iliac vein, we usually appreciate a yellow-white solid string running in the obturator fossa. This is the obturator nerve. The obturator nerve becomes a landmark of the obturator fossa. (**b**) As illustrated using a dotted arrow line, the connective tissue with lymph nodes is separated toward the obturator nerve

### 6.2.13 Lymphadenectomy of the Obturator Fossa [1] (Figure 6.25)

Using a small retractor to lift up both the external iliac artery and vein at the pelvic wall side opens the space of the obturator fossa as widely as possible. Picking up the adipose tissues of the dorsal side of external iliac vein, the connective/adipose tissues surrounding the obturator nerve are separated. The obturator nerve is easily stripped from the adipose tissues (Figure 6.25a). It is better to trace the obturator nerve from the foot/caudal side (obturator canal) to the cranial side (between the common iliac vein and iliopsoas muscle). In the dorsal side of the obturator nerve, the obturator artery and vein are usually running parallel to the obturator nerve (Figure 6.25b). In order to avoid unnecessary hemorrhage, attention should be paid to these vessels.

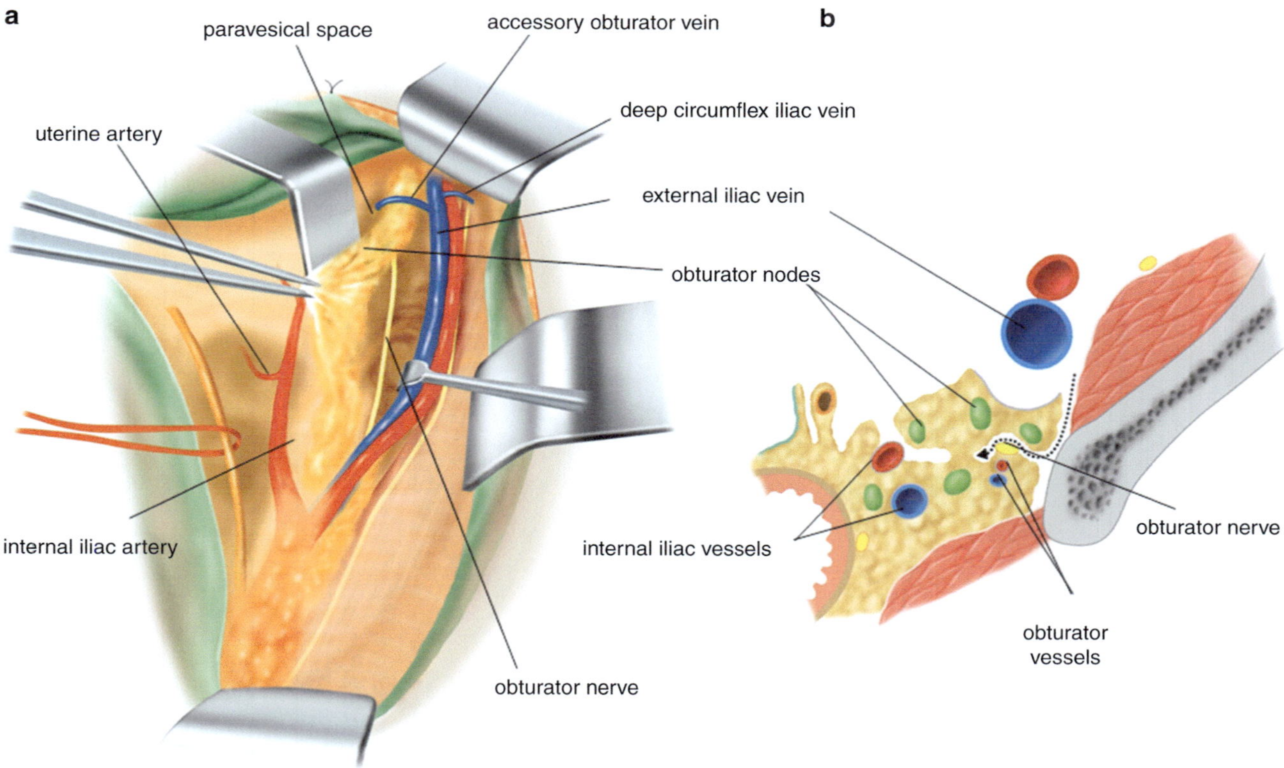


**Figure 6.25** Lymphadenectomy of the obturator fossa. (**a**) Stripping of the adipose tissues surrounding the obturator nerve. (**b**) A dotted arrow is showing the separation line from the iliopsoas muscle side. The relationship between the obturator nerve and obturator vessels are also illustrated

### 6.2.14 Lymphadenectomy of the Obturator Fossa [2] (Figure 6.26)

In the inguinal side of the external iliac vein, the internal supra-inguinal node is residing between the accessory obturator vein and iliopsoas muscle/pubic bone. From the foot side, the lymph node is separated and passed to the dorsal side of the accessory obturator vein. If this step is difficult, the accessory obturator vein can be divided and ligated. At this stage, the adipose tissues with lymph nodes on the side of the iliopsoas muscle can be separated from both the external iliac artery and vein.

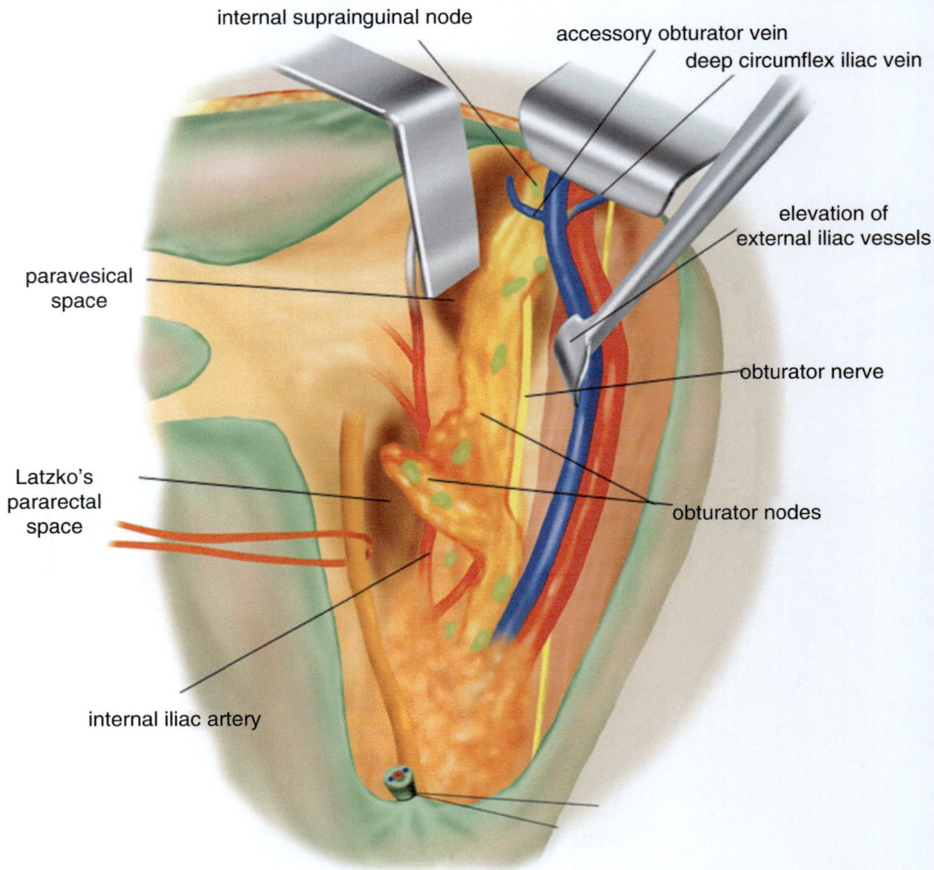


**Figure 6.26** The internal supra-inguinal node is separated and passed to the dorsal side of the accessory obturator vein

### 6.2.15 Lymphadenectomy of the Obturator Fossa [3] (Figure 6.27)

After the separation of the internal supra-inguinal node, the lymph nodes of the external iliac artery/vein are passed into the obturator fossa. Lifting up the passed internal supra-inguinal node, the adipose tissues with lymph nodes are separated from the obturator nerve. The denuded obturator nerve can be traced cranially along the external iliac vessels to the dorsal space between the iliopsoas muscle and the common iliac vessels.

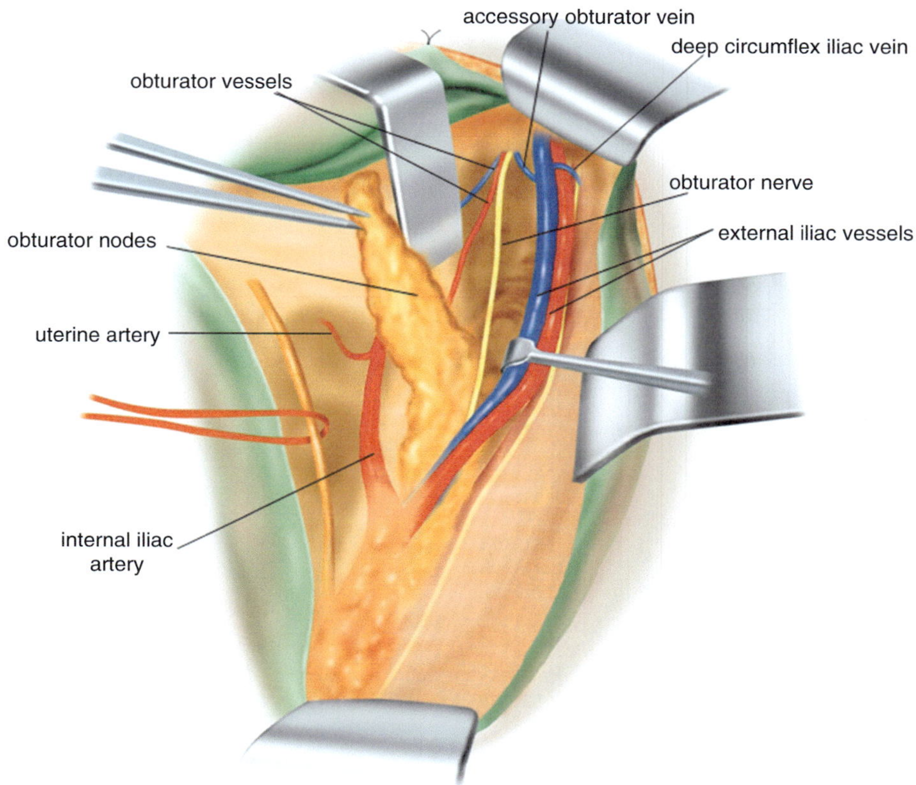


**Figure 6.27** Separation of the obturator lymph node from the obturator fossa

### 6.2.16 En Bloc Removal of the Lymph Nodes in the Obturator Fossa (Figure 6.28)

By separating the adipose tissue with lymph nodes surrounding the obturator nerve, lymph node dissection on the ventral side of the obturator nerve is completed. Using the metal tube suction, try to aspirate the adipose tissues surrounding the obturator nerve, which makes it easier to separate the connective tissues with lymph nodes from the obturator nerve and from the base of the pelvis. Usually the adipose tissue in the retroperitoneal space is easily aspirated and the network of the small blood/lymph vessels becomes visible. Confirming the anatomy of the network, en bloc removal of the lymph nodes in the obturator fossa is possible.

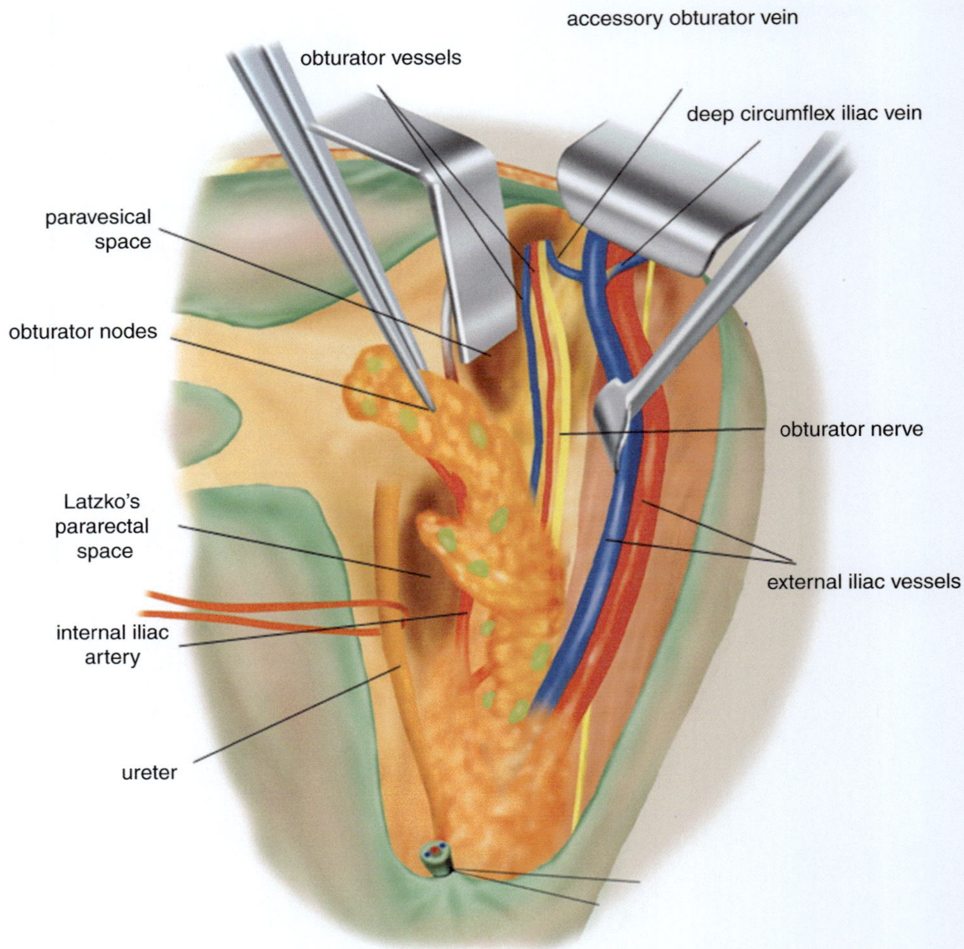


**Figure 6.28** En bloc removal of the lymph nodes in the obturator fossa

### 6.2.17 Lymphadenectomy for the Dorsal Side of the Obturator Nerve (Figure 6.29)

In the dorsal portion of the obturator nerve, the obturator artery and vein are usually running parallel to the obturator nerve. Therefore, in order to preserve these vessels, careful separation is necessary (Figure 6.29a). However, division of these vessels is necessary if lymph nodes are adherent to these blood vessels. Ligation and division of these vessels usually has no adverse side effects to the patient.

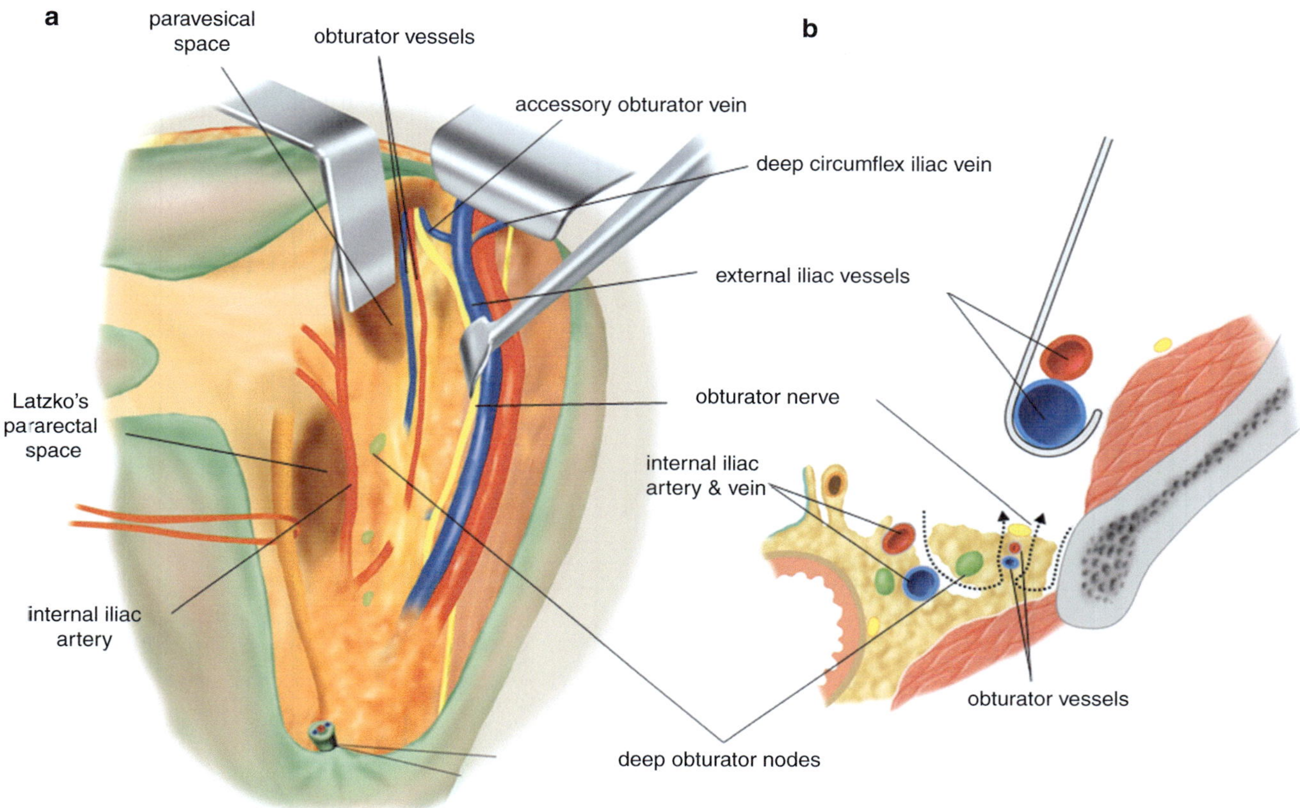


**Figure 6.29** Lymphadenectomy for the dorsal side of the obturator nerve. (**a**) Removal of the lymph nodes in the dorsal side of the obturator nerve can skeletonize the obturator artery and vein. (**b**) Two dotted arrow lines are indicating the separation point of the dorsal side of the obturator nerve

Cranially, separate the connective tissues with lymph nodes from the bifurcation of the external and internal iliac vessels. The obturator artery and vein are often branching from the bifurcation area, where careful separation is necessary. The adipose tissues and lymph nodes in the base of the cardinal ligament are also removed. The base of the cardinal ligament takes drainage from the deep uterine vein into the internal iliac vein. This step enables greater appreciation of the anatomical structure of the cardinal ligament. Through these procedures, the lymphadenectomy for the dorsal side of the obturator nerve is completed. It is convenient to use monopolar or bipolar coagulation tools for lymphadenectomy. If the anesthesia is not deep enough, using monopolar energy close to the obturator nerve can lead to contraction movements in the patient's leg which can sometimes jolt the surgeon's movements. In order to avoid unexpected injury to the pelvic organs, the bipolar system appears to be safer than the monopolar system.

**Notes**

1. It is often said that the lymphadenectomy for the dorsal side of the obturator nerve is not necessary. However, if we may observe this region, there are a considerable number of small lymph nodes. Recently Ungar L. et al. reported very good prognosis (more than 90% 5-year survival rate without any adjuvant therapy) following the complete removal of lymph nodes within the base of the cardinal ligament as a mass of internal iliac blood vessel system (laterally extended parametrectomy) in case of lymph node positive patients. This report demonstrates the importance of the extent of lymphadenectomy for the survival of invasive cervical cancer patients. The removal of the adipose tissues by liposuction using a suction device reveals the network of small lymphatic channels, small blood vessels, and small lymph nodes with adipose tissues in the dorsal side of the obturator nerve. Using a bipolar coagulation tool, these vessels and the small lymph nodes with adipose tissues in the dorsal side of the obturator nerve are well treated. However, given the possibility of many variations of the branches from the internal iliac vein, such as the obturator vein and the deep uterine vein, careful separation of these structures is required.
2. Liposuction procedure was introduced by Fujiwara T. in 1983 [1] in Japan. The report of Heckels M. et al. [2, 3] is not the first on the use of liposuction for lymphadenectomy and radical hysterectomy.

### 6.2.18 Confirmation of the Base of the Cardinal Ligament (Figure 6.30)

By the removal of the adipose tissues with lymph nodes on the dorsal side of the obturator nerve, the internal iliac vein becomes well delineated in the obturator fossa. Moreover, venous drainage into the internal iliac vein from the uterine side is better appreciated. The base of the cardinal ligament is the draining portion of the deep uterine vein into the internal iliac vein.

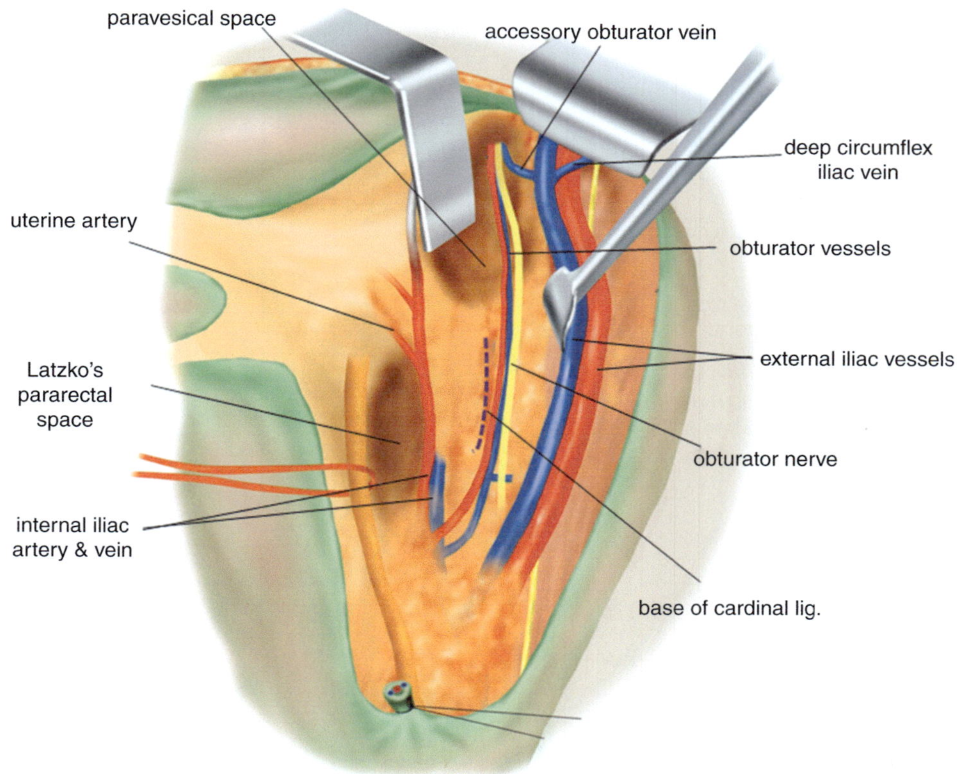


**Figure 6.30** Confirmation of the base of the cardinal ligament (a purple dotted line)

### 6.2.19 The Lymphadenectomy of the Common Iliac Nodes (Figures 6.31 and 6.32)

The connective tissues with lymph nodes at the bifurcation of the external and internal iliac vessels are already separated. The cranial side of the bifurcation is the common iliac artery and vein. Separating the ventral side of the connective tissues on the external iliac artery, the loose connective tissue between the iliopsoas muscle and the external iliac artery is also separated.

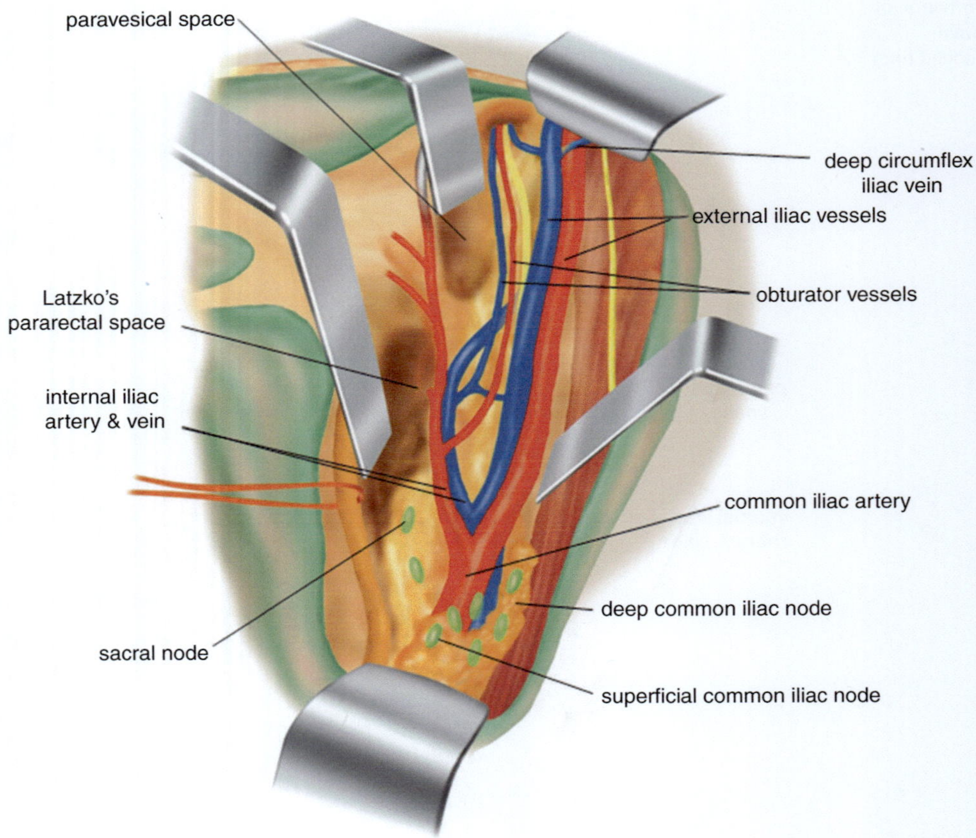


**Figure 6.31** Lymphadenectomy of the common iliac nodes [1]

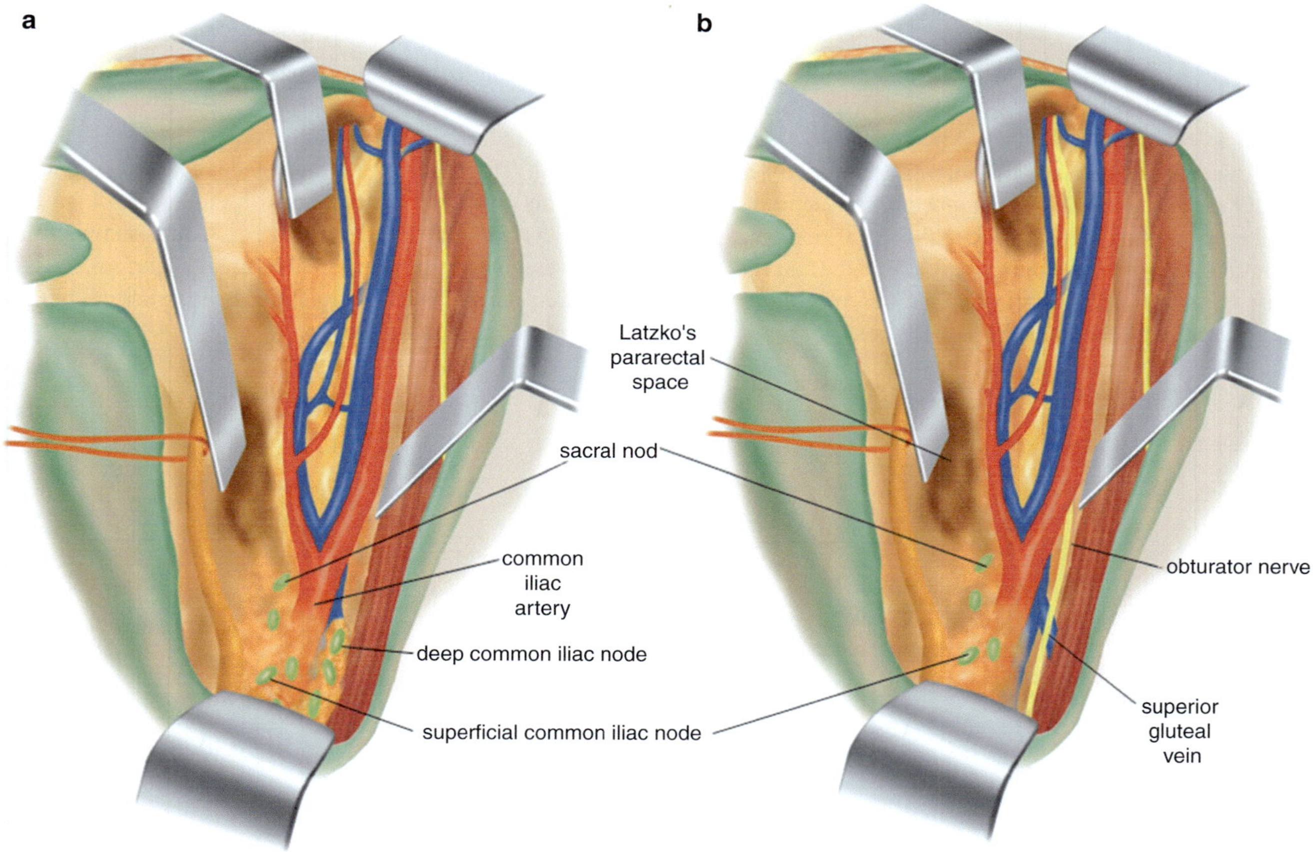


**Figure 6.32** Lymphadenectomy of the common iliac nodes [2]. (**a**) The anatomical location of the deep common iliac node. (**b**) The anatomical relationship between the obturator nerve of the cranial side and the superior gluteal vein

Separation is extended deep enough to visualize the obturator nerve and the superior gluteal vein. The adipose tissues and lymph nodes surrounding the obturator nerve are dissected between the common iliac artery/vein and the iliopsoas muscle by the level of the obturator nerve that disappears into the major psoas muscle cranially. The adipose tissues are separated from both the common iliac artery and vein as much as possible, and the deep common iliac nodes are removed (Figure 6.32a, b).

### 6.2.20 Lymphadenectomy of the Sacral Nodes (Figure 6.33a–c)

Separation of the connective tissue on the common iliac artery is extended medially along the internal iliac artery. The pararectal space has already been (Latzko's pararectal space) developed between the internal iliac artery and the lateral side of the rectum. The connective tissue in the pararectal space is separated as wide and deep as possible. Then the internal iliac vein running parallel to the internal iliac artery is appreciated. Connective tissues of the presacral space are separated toward the sacral bone. Then, the sacral node is included in the separated connective tissues (Figure 6.33a, b).

The cranial side of the separated adipo-connective tissues is divided. The divided adipo-connective tissues are separated from the sacral bone along with the internal iliac vein toward the foot/distal side (Figure 6.33c). Usually, small blood vessels are included in this area; therefore, careful separation using electrocoagulation device such as bipolar forceps or scissors is necessary.

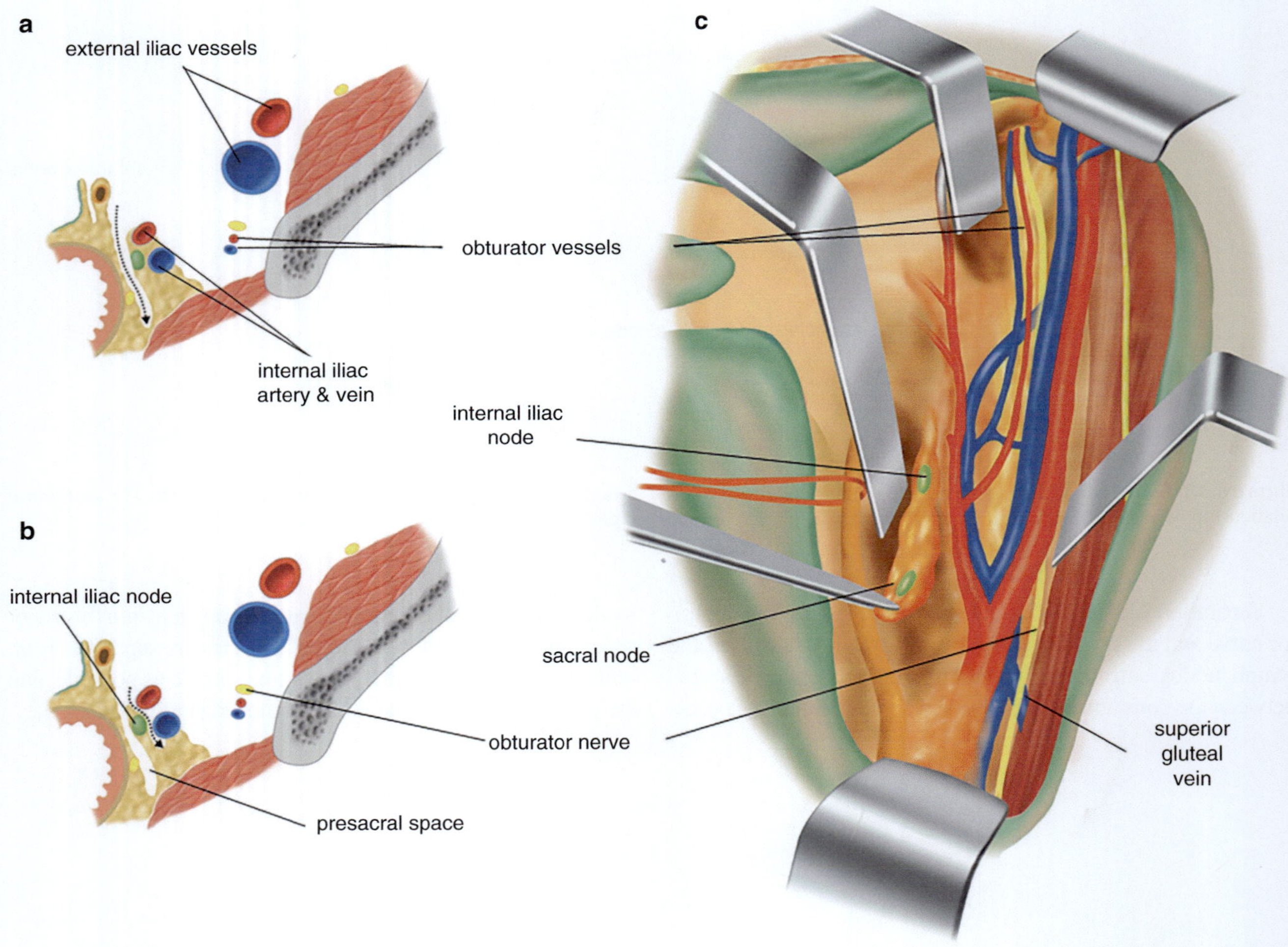


**Figure 6.33** Lymphadenectomy of the sacral node. (**a**) The connective tissue in the pararectal space is separated toward the presacral space (a dotted arrow line). (**b**) Connective tissues of the presacral space are separated toward the sacral bone. Then, the sacral node is included in the separated connective tissues. (**c**) The cranial side of the separated adipo-connective tissues is divided. The divided adipo-connective tissues are separated from the sacral bone along with the internal iliac vein toward the foot/distal side

### 6.2.21 Removal of the Common Iliac Nodes (Figure 6.34)

The cranial side of the common iliac lymphadenectomy is undertaken by separating the loose connective tissue layer from the bifurcation of the common iliac artery to the aorta. Ligating the cranial side of the adipo-connective tissues, the ventral side of the common iliac lymphadenectomy is carried out. Retract the psoas muscle laterally and the common iliac artery medially to develop the space between the common iliac artery/vein and the psoas muscle. The adipo-connective tissue in this area is removed from the common iliac artery/vein and obturator nerve, avoiding injury to the superior gluteal vein.

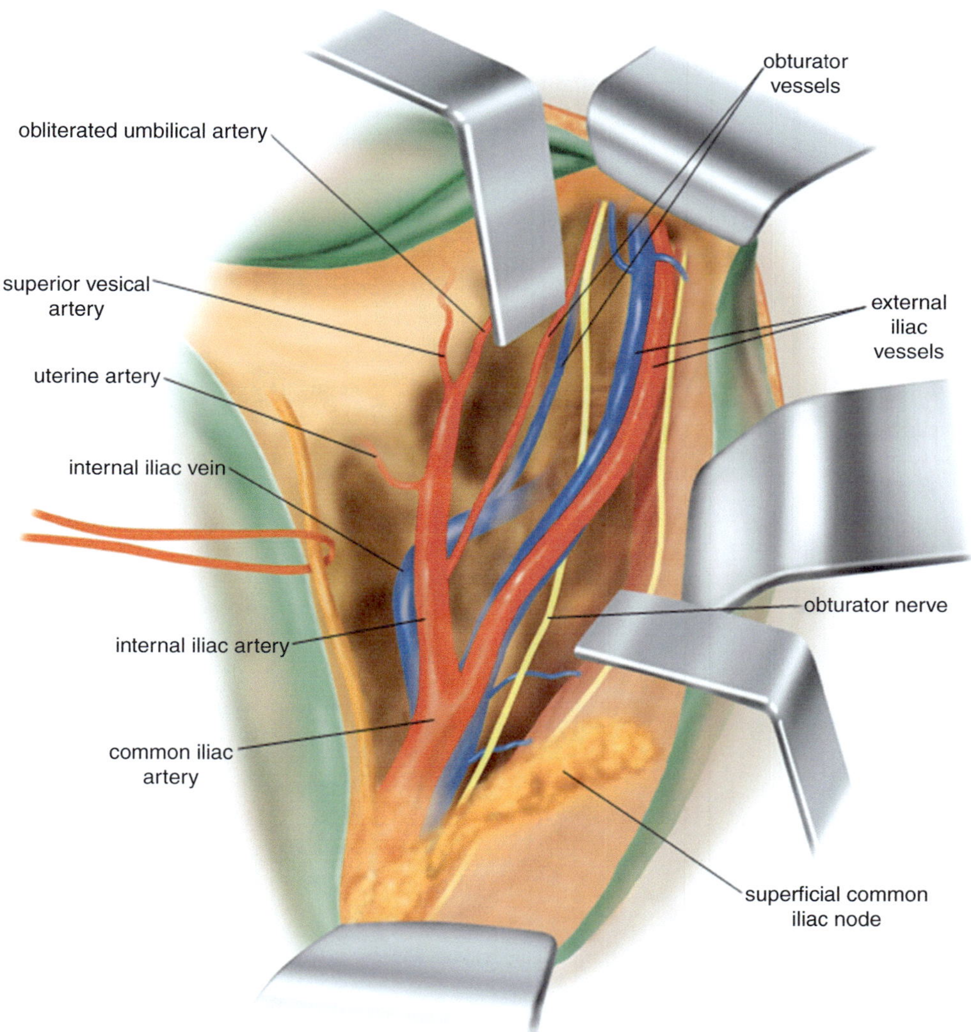


**Figure 6.34** Removal of the common iliac nodes

### 6.2.22 A View of the Pelvic Cavity After the Pelvic Lymphadenectomy (Figure 6.35)

After the pelvic lymphadenectomy, the majority of the artery and vein along the internal and external iliac artery/vein are exposed clearly. Lymphadenectomy should be undertaken thoroughly in the pelvic cavity. If pelvic lymph nodes are positive, lymphadenectomy is usually extended cranially to the level of the inferior mesenteric artery.

Thoroughness or completeness of lymphadenectomy is one of the most important prognostic factors and hence, should be undertaken carefully and as meticulously as possible.

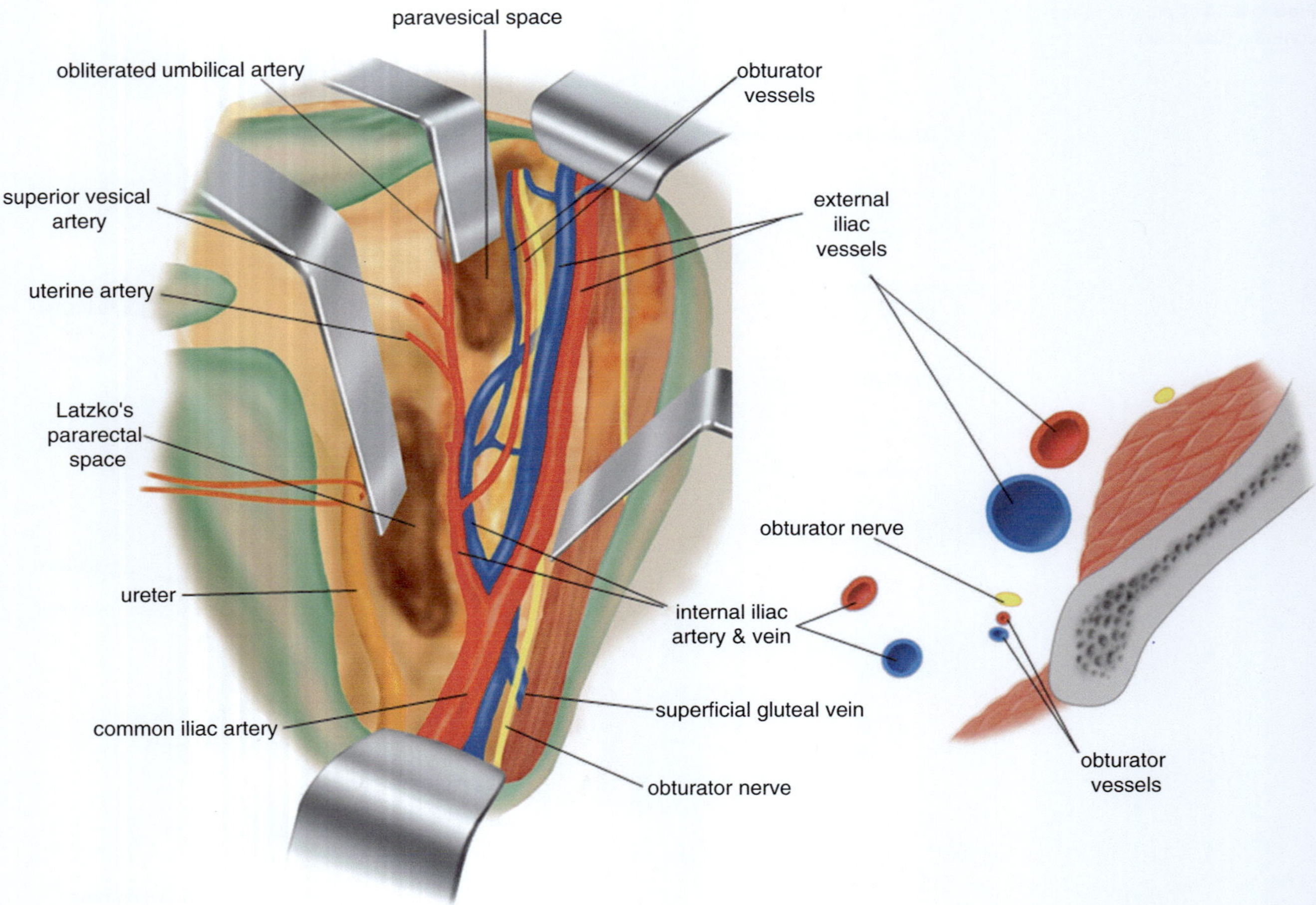


**Figure 6.35** A view of the pelvic cavity after the pelvic lymphadenectomy

## 6.3 Treatment of the Cardinal Ligament

### 6.3.1 A View of the Pelvis After the Lymphadenectomy (Figure 6.36)

After pelvic lymphadenectomy, both external and internal iliac blood vessels are almost skeletonized with a view of the obturator nerve and artery/vein in the obturator fossa. The paravesical space and pararectal space are well recognized.

**Figure 6.36** A view of the pelvis after the lymphadenectomy

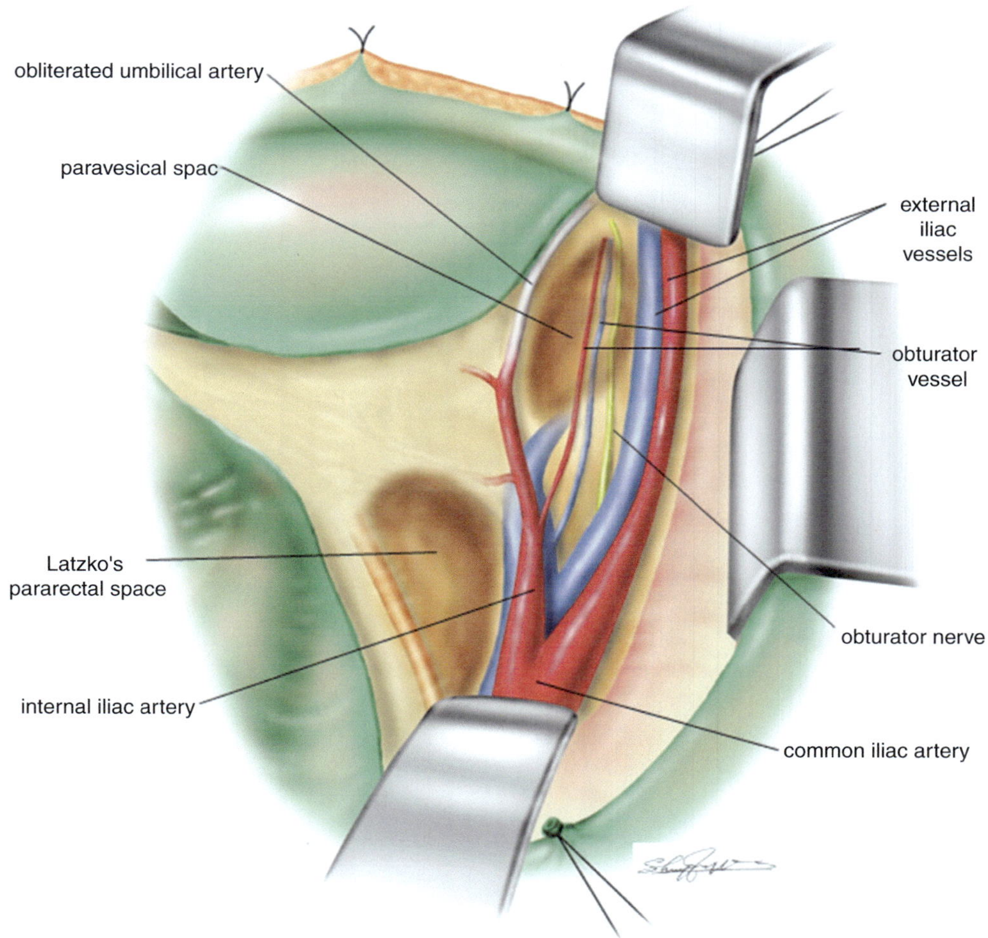

### 6.3.2 Separation of the Loose Connective Tissue Between the Uterine Artery and the Superior Vesical Artery (Figure 6.37)

In order to give tension to the uterine artery, the obliterated umbilical artery (bladder side of the internal iliac artery) is picked up with the forceps, and the loose connective tissue between the bladder and the obliterated umbilical artery is separated. The loose connective tissue layer between the uterine artery and the superior vesical artery is now appreciated. The connective tissue layer is separated to penetrate the paravesical space.

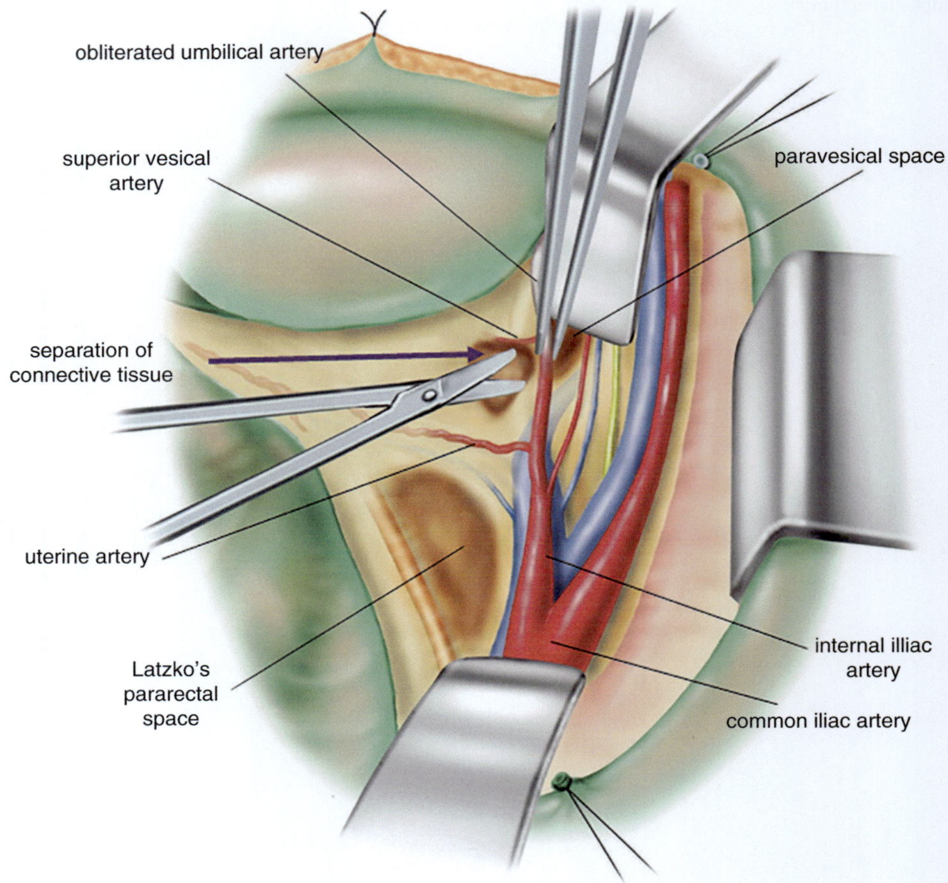


**Figure 6.37** Separation of the loose connective tissue between the uterine artery and the superior vesical artery (a purple arrow)

### 6.3.3 Development of the Paravesical Space and Confirmation of the Uterine Artery (Figure 6.38)

A long L-shaped retractor is inserted into the paravesical space through the divided connective tissue, to retract the structures to the upper-inguinal area, including the isolated obliterated umbilical artery. Then, the uterine artery from the internal iliac artery is stretched between its origin at the internal iliac artery and the sidewall of the uterus. This is a safer way to identify the uterine artery along its entire length.

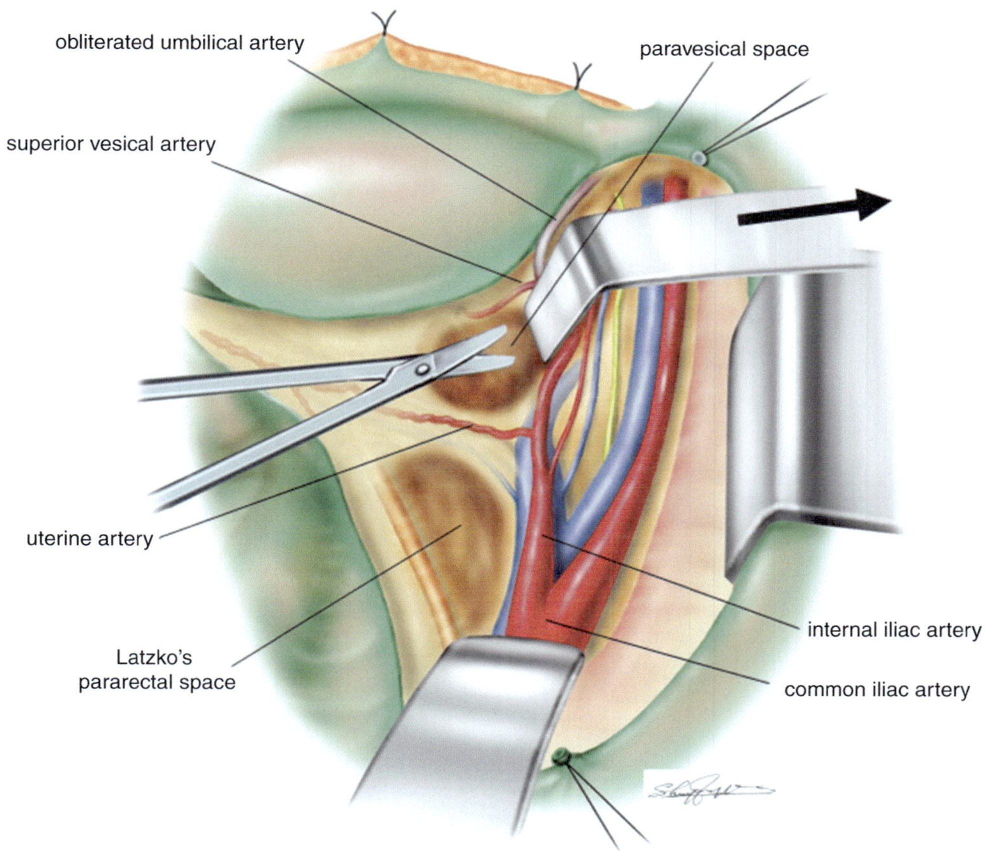


**Figure 6.38** Development of the paravesical space and confirmation of the uterine artery

### 6.3.4 Definition of the Cardinal Ligament (Figure 6.39)

Another long L-shaped retractor is inserted into the pararectal space pushing the rectum to the craniolateral side, in turn gradually expanding the pararectal space. The thick connective tissue bundle is created between the paravesical space and pararectal space. This is a gross feature of the cardinal ligament (a two-directional arrow in Figure 6.39). The cardinal ligament is a thick connective tissue bundle formed between the internal iliac blood vessels and the sidewall of the uterus/upper vagina. The uterine artery and the superficial uterine vein run along the most ventral side of the cardinal ligament.

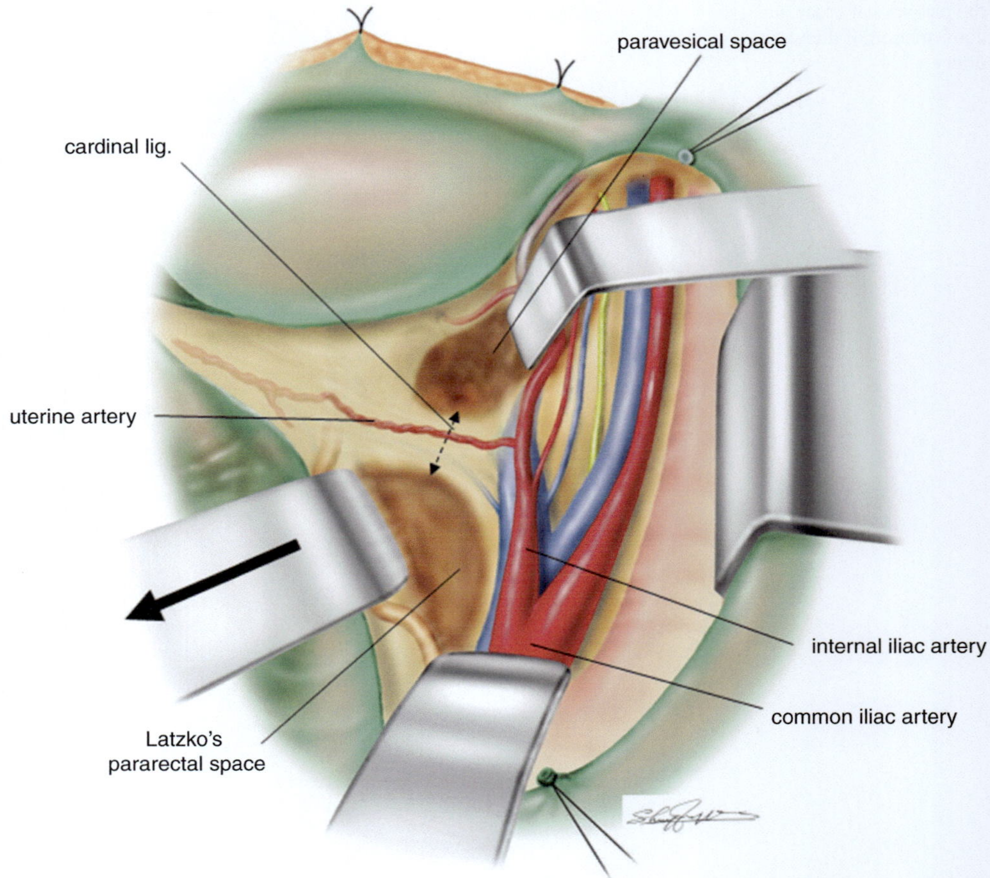


**Figure 6.39** Definition of the cardinal ligament (a dotted two-directional arrow)

> **Notes:**
> Do not insert the long L-shaped retractor too deep into the pelvic floor. There is a risk of the connective tissue of the pelvic floor being torn by the retractor, which can lead to considerable bleeding. The bleeding is usually difficult to manage and therefore, it is prudent to pay attention to the location of the retractor tip in the pararectal space.

### 6.3.5 Isolation and Division of the Uterine Artery (Figure 6.40)

The uterine artery originating from the internal iliac artery is appreciated on the most ventral side of the cardinal ligament. The uterine artery is easily isolated, doubly clamped, ligated, and divided between the two ligatures. The suture on the uterine side of the uterine artery is usually left longer to act as an anatomical landmark.

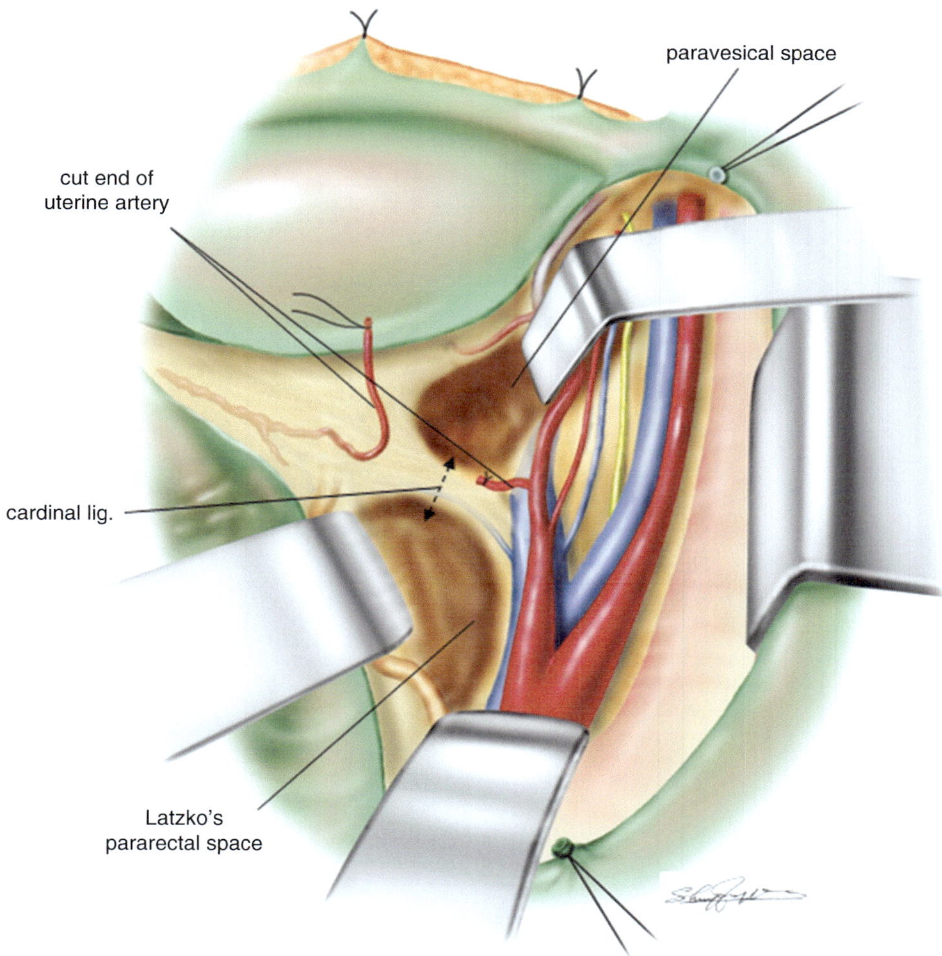


**Figure 6.40** Isolation and division of the uterine artery (a dotted two-directional arrow is the location of the cardinal ligament)

### 6.3.6 Separation of the Superficial Uterine Vein (Figure 6.41)

Careful separation of the cut-end of uterine side of the uterine artery from the connective tissue of the cardinal ligament usually reveals a vein running parallel to the uterine artery. This is the superficial uterine vein, which is fragile. Therefore, a careful approach is required in order to isolate it. If the vein does tear, an electric vessel sealing system such as monopolar or bipolar coagulation is effective. The superficial uterine vein is not always running parallel to the uterine artery. Rarely, it may run parallel to the ureter.

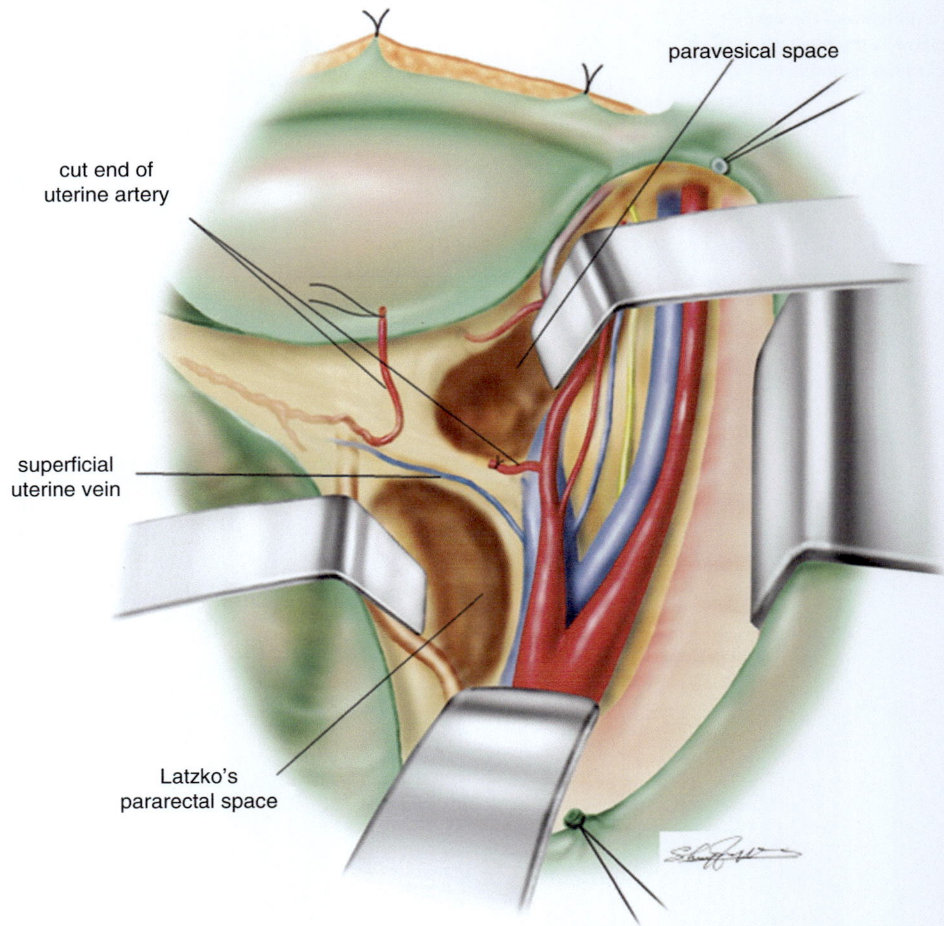


**Figure 6.41** Separation of the superficial uterine vein

### 6.3.7 Clamp, Divide, and Ligate the Superficial Uterine Vein (Figure 6.42)

The superficial uterine vein is isolated and doubly clamped by Pean forceps. Then the superficial uterine vein is divided between the two clamps and each clamp is replaced by ligature. The connective tissue of the cardinal ligament is separated toward the pelvic floor. A small vein or artery may be identified in the cardinal ligament. In such case, each small blood vessel should be sealed either by electrocautery or ligature. However, the deep uterine vein always resides in the dorsal part of the cardinal ligament. Therefore, careful separation of the connective tissue and lymph nodes in the cardinal ligament is required to identify the deep uterine vein.

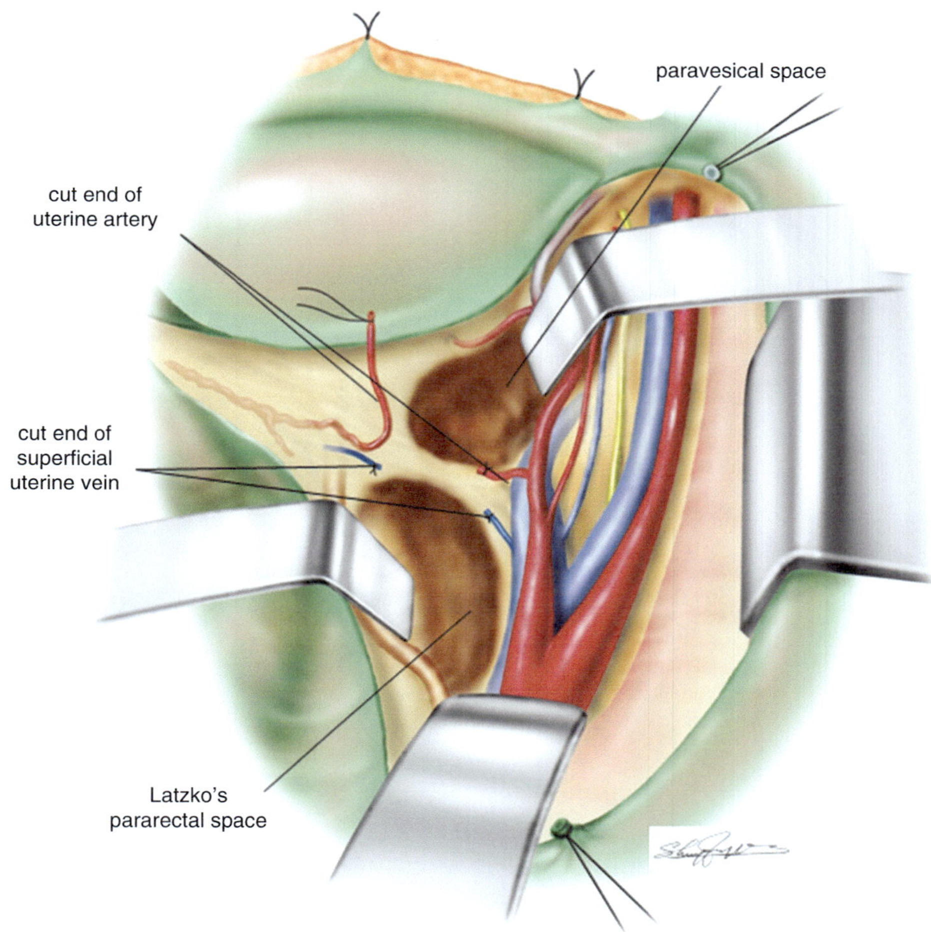


**Figure 6.42** Clamp, divide, and ligate the superficial uterine vein

### 6.3.8 Separation of the Deep Uterine Vein (Figure 6.43)

Careful separation of the connective tissue and lymph nodes in the cardinal ligament can reveal a vein running from the uterine sidewall to the internal iliac vein. This is the deep uterine vein. The connective tissue and adipose tissue surrounding the deep uterine vein should be divided as much as possible. This is very important for the isolation of the deep uterine vein.

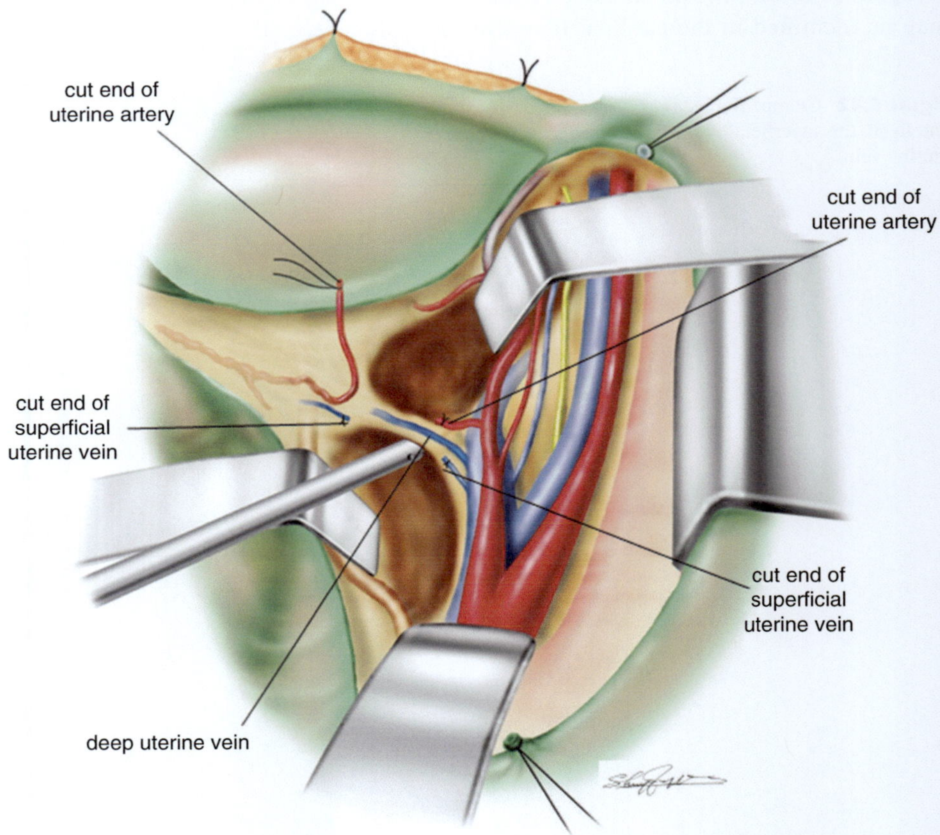


**Figure 6.43** Separation of the deep uterine vein

### 6.3.9 Clamp, Divide, and Ligate the Deep Uterine Vein (Figure 6.44)

In the dorsal part of the deep uterine vein, a white-yellow bundle is usually appreciated parallel to the deep uterine vein. This is one of the branches of the pelvic splanchnic nerve. After isolation, the deep uterine vein is doubly clamped by Pean forceps. The deep uterine vein is then divided between the two clamps. Each clamp is replaced by ligature. Cleaning up the connective tissue and the adipose tissue in the base of the cardinal ligament (draining portion of the deep uterine vein into the internal iliac vein) is a very important step to perform a safe radical hysterectomy.

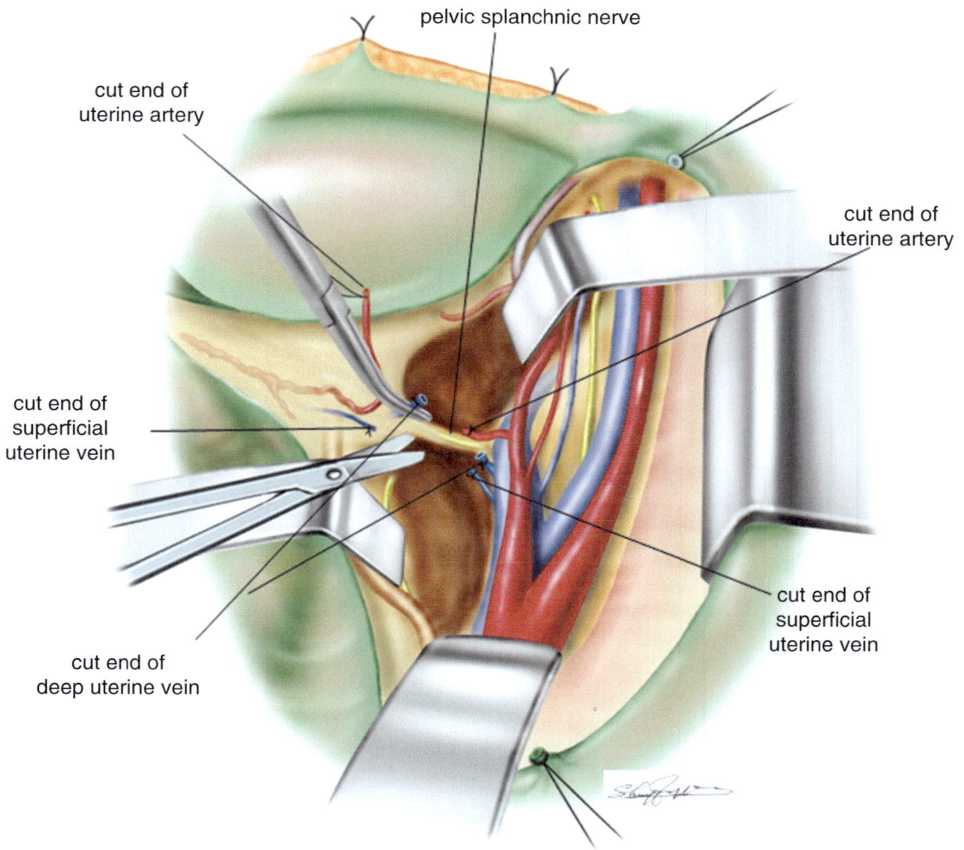


**Figure 6.44** Clamp, divide, and ligate the deep uterine vein

**Notes:**
If damage to the deep uterine vein occurs, a considerable amount of bleeding can be expected. However, if the deep uterine vein is already isolated, it is possible to clamp the damaged portion of the deep uterine vein and manage the bleeding safely.

### 6.3.10 Confirmation and Division of the Pelvic Splanchnic Nerve (Figure 6.45)

The pelvic splanchnic nerve merges with the hypogastric nerve to form the inferior hypogastric plexus bilaterally at the level of the sidewall of the cervix/upper vagina. During Okabayashi's radical hysterectomy, one of the branches of the pelvic splanchnic nerve is often divided. Since the nerve is usually accompanied by a small blood vessel, it is better to clamp the pelvic splanchnic nerve using Pean forceps and divide between the two clamps. Each clamp is replaced by ligature. A loose connective tissue layer in the dorsal part is easily separated and the two spaces (the paravesical space and the pararectal space) are connected with the base of the pelvic floor.

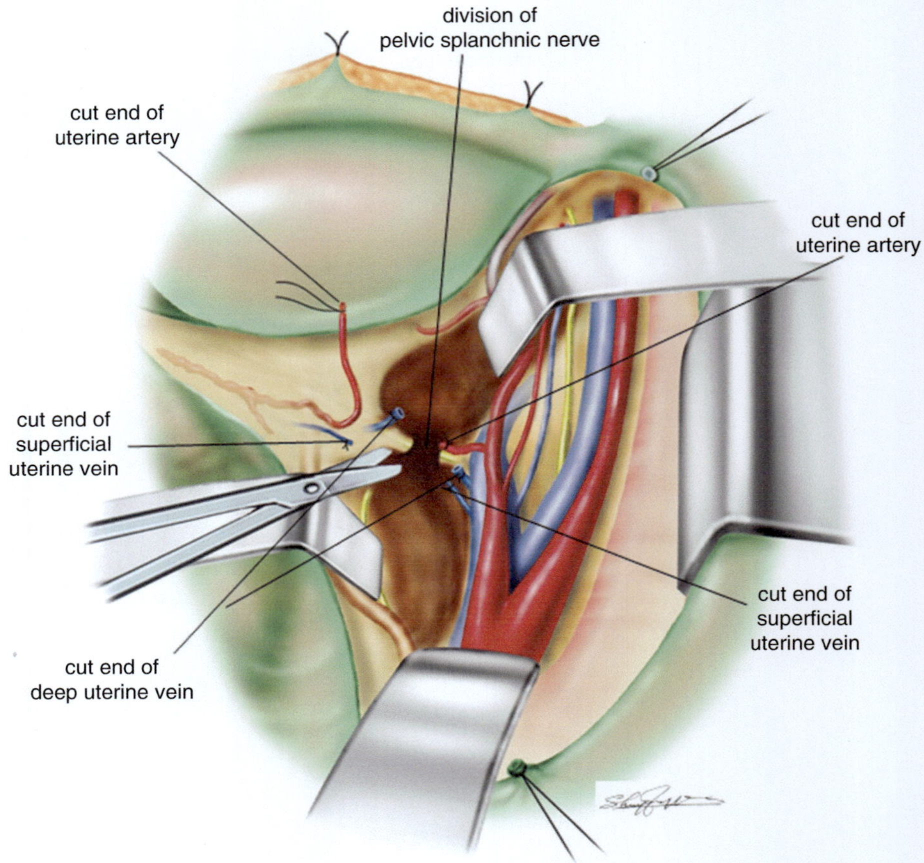


**Figure 6.45** Confirmation and division of the pelvic splanchnic nerve

**Notes:**
By the division of the cardinal ligament, the middle part of the three uterine supportive tissues is divided at a level close to the internal iliac vein.

## 6.4 Development of the Rectovaginal Space and Division of the Uterosacral Ligament

### 6.4.1 Separation and Division of the Peritoneum of the Douglas' Pouch (Figure 6.46)

The uterus is drawn toward the pubic arch and the rectum with its peritoneal surface is stretched by hand toward the cranial side. The peritoneum between the uterus and the rectum is lifted from the bottom of the Pouch of Douglas. An incision is made on the elevated peritoneum and carried with scissors across the dorsal side (back) of the cervix. This step connects both sides of the retroperitoneal space of the broad ligament. The rectum is then gently freed from the cervical/vaginal wall with scissors or with a finger. With the uterus held over to the pubic arch and the rectum stretched toward the cranial side by hand, a loose connective tissue layer between the rectum and the cervix/vagina is appreciated. This is the landmark of the rectovaginal space.

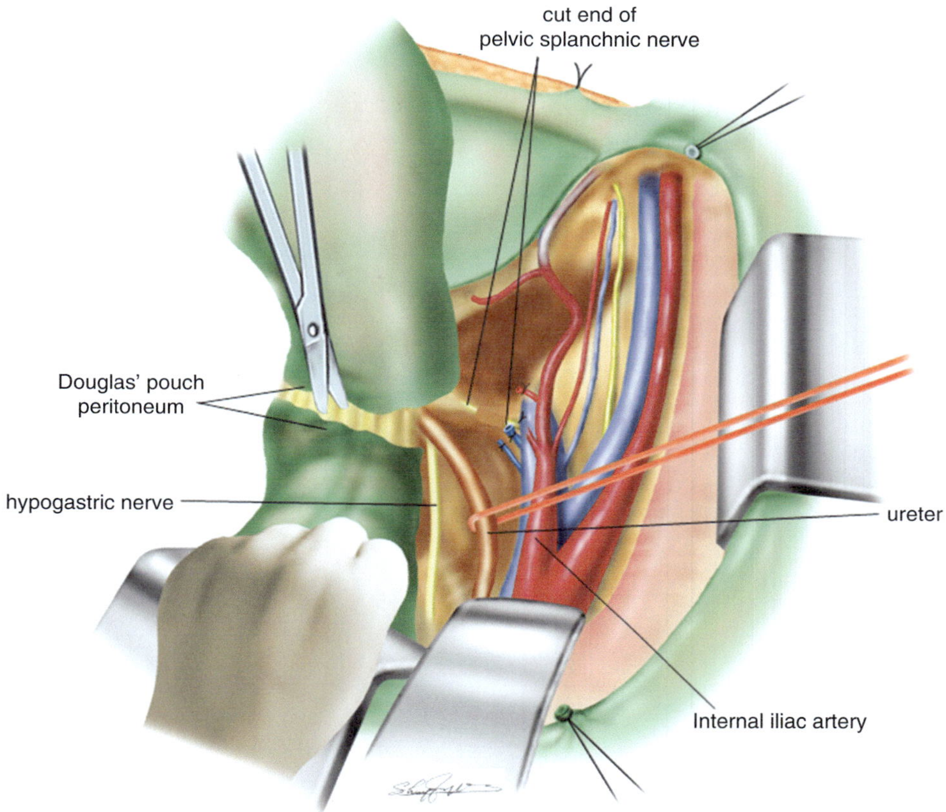


**Figure 6.46** Separation and division of the peritoneum of the Douglas' pouch

### 6.4.2 **Development of the Rectovaginal Space** (Figure 6.47)

If there is no infectious adhesion or cancer invasion, the loose connective tissue layer between the rectum and the vagina is easily separated and can develop the rectovaginal space. Pressing the tips of scissors against the cervical fascia, the rectum is bluntly detached from the cervix/upper part of the vagina. The separation should be carried in the correct plane. There is risk of injury to the rectum, if the plane is developed too close to the surface of the rectum. At this stage, the bilateral thick connective tissue bundles (uterosacral ligament) become defined between the rectovaginal space and the retroperitoneal space of the broad ligament.

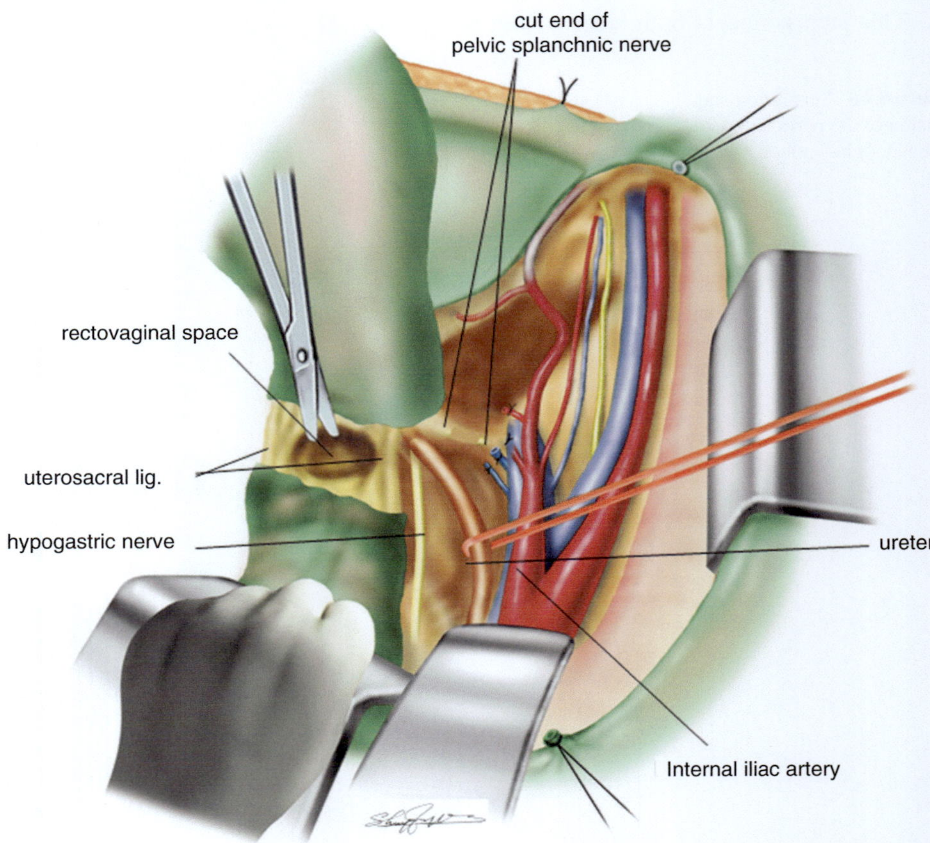


**Figure 6.47** Development of the rectovaginal space

### 6.4.3 **Division of the Uterosacral Ligament** (Figure 6.48)

The uterosacral ligament on either side is stretched forward and dissected at its base at the rectal sidewall. Hypogastric nerve is often divided by this procedure.

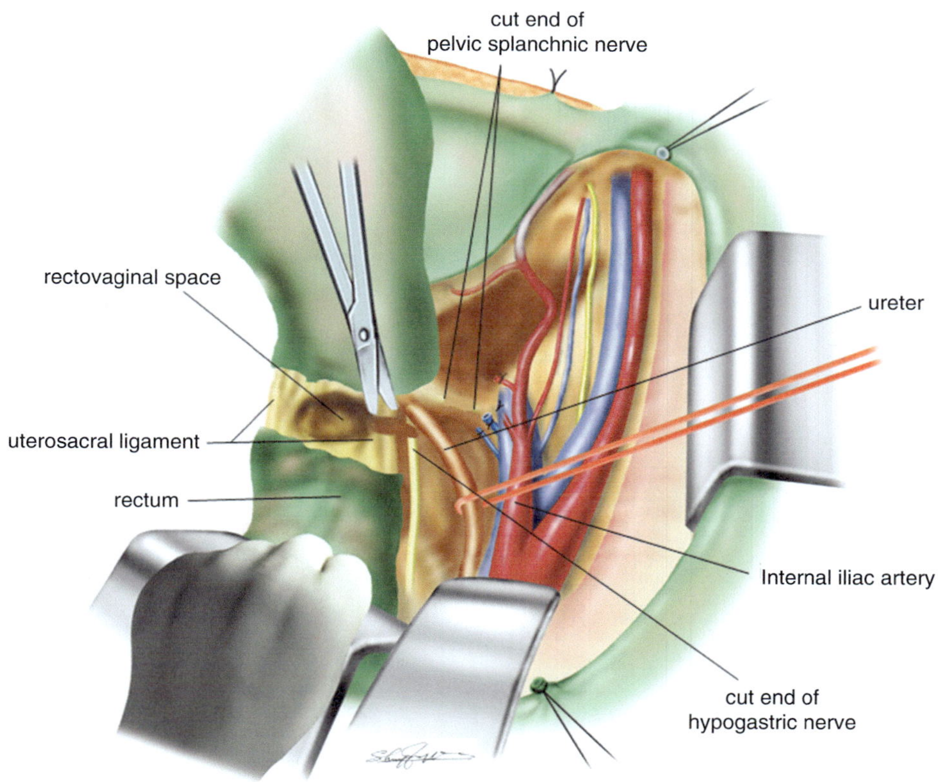


**Figure 6.48** Division of the uterosacral ligament

### 6.4.4 Further Division of the Uterosacral Ligament and Development of the Okabayashi's Pararectal Space (Figure 6.49)

Further division of connective tissue of the uterosacral ligament toward the base of the pelvis reveals a space filled with cobweb-like connective tissues between the rectal sidewall and the connective tissue layer in which the hypogastric nerve is included. This space is the Okabayashi's pararectal space.

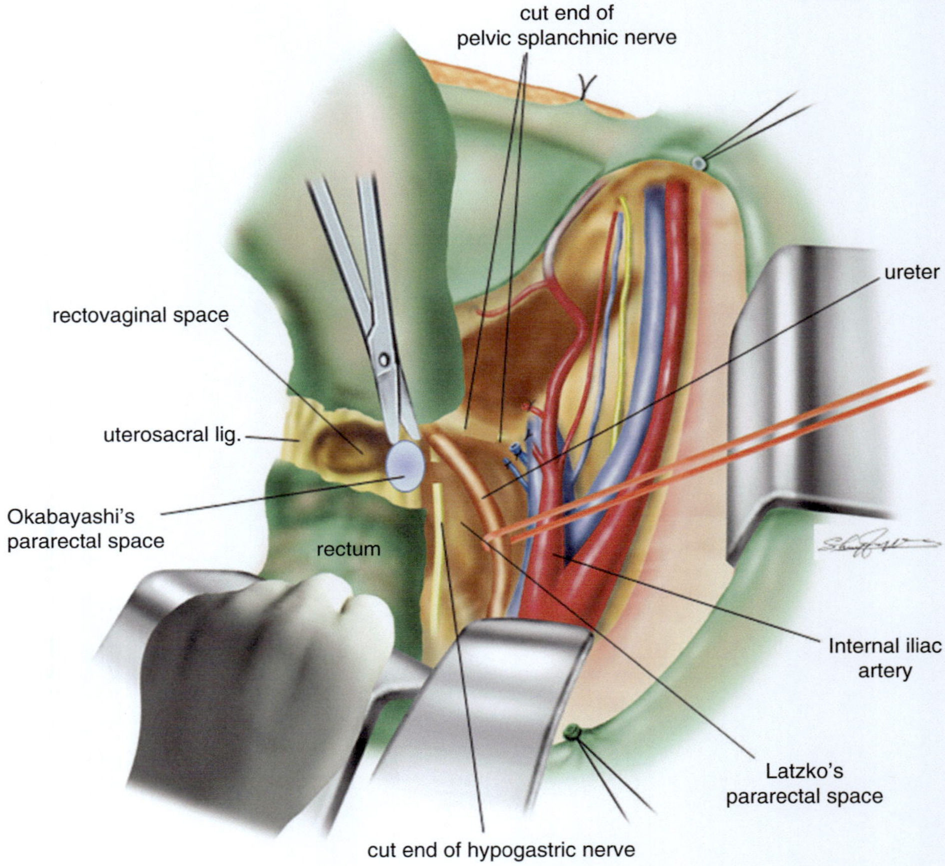


**Figure 6.49** Entrance to Okabayashi's pararectal space (circle filled with blue color)

**Notes:**
Ureter is already reflected laterally from this connective tissue layer toward the pelvic sidewall.

### 6.4.5 Development of the Pararectal Space (Figure 6.50)

Okabayashi's pararectal space is very close to the rectum, and so it is necessary to expand the space toward the pelvic sidewall. During the process of expanding the pararectal space, the hypogastric nerve is usually divided. With this step, Okabayashi's pararectal space connects with Latzko's pararectal space. The pararectal space is surrounded by the rectal sidewall (uterine side), the internal iliac blood vessels (pelvic sidewall), the sacral bone (cranial side), and blood vessels and connective tissue of the cardinal ligament (inguinal side). The pararectal space is filled with the loose connective tissues to the base of the pelvis. The development of the pararectal space can be done using fingers inserted between the rectum and the internal iliac artery/vein. The direction of insertion is toward the pelvic axis.

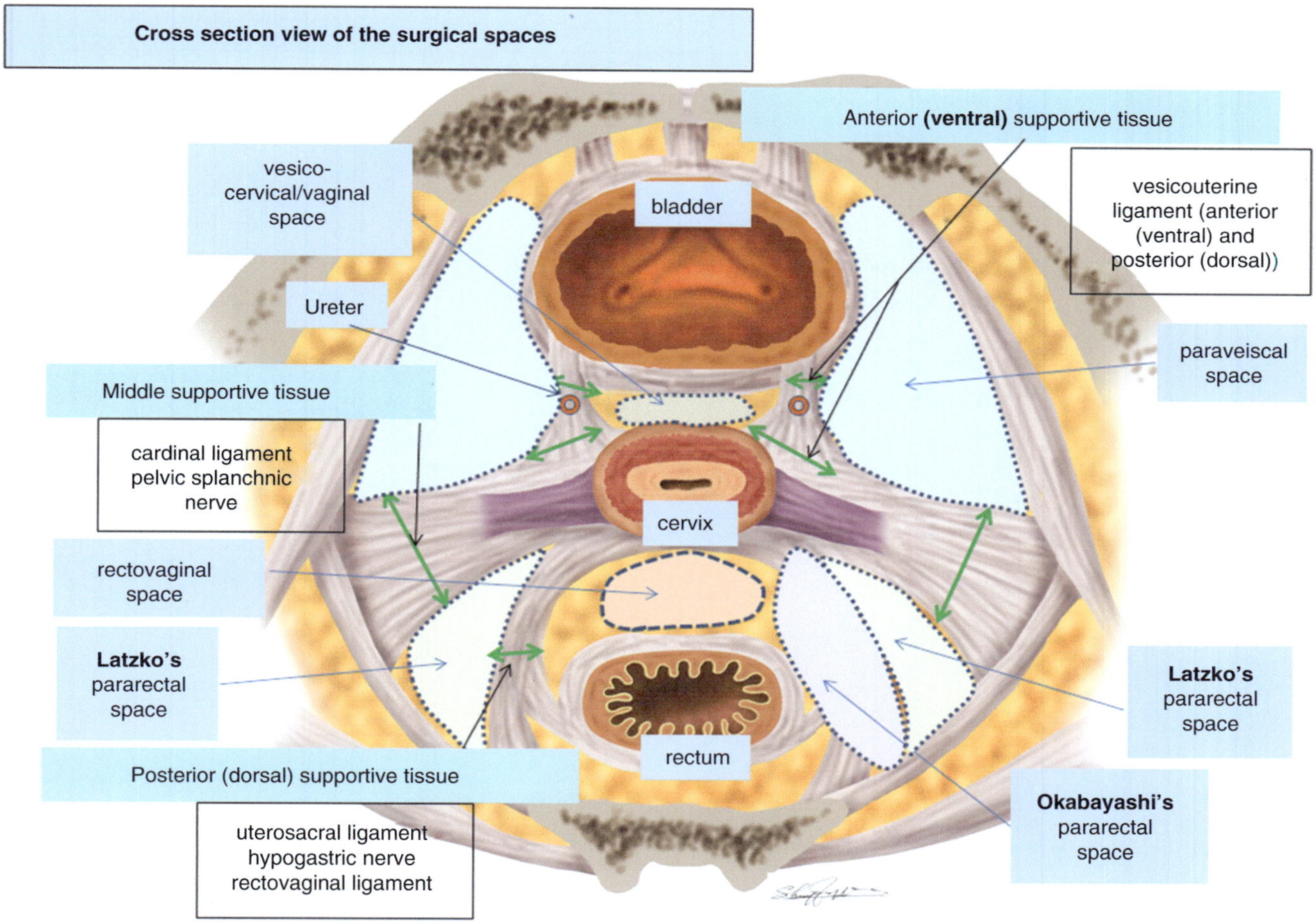


**Figure 6.50** The relationship between the surgically developable spaces and the supportive tissues of the female pelvic organ. The surgically developable spaces are the paravesical space, vesicovaginal space, rectovaginal space, and pararectal space. The pararectal space developed very close to the rectal sidewall is named Okabayashi's pararectal space. The next space from the Okabayashi's pararectal space to the internal iliac vessels is named Latzko's pararectal space

## 6.5 Separation of the Urinary Bladder and the Vesicouterine Ligament

### 6.5.1 Separation of the Urinary Bladder from the Cervical Fascia (Figure 6.51)

Picking up the bladder itself with the peritoneum, the bladder is separated from the center of the cervical fascia to the level of the trigone of the urinary bladder. Connective tissue bundles become defined on both sides of the cervix. The connective tissue bundle contains the ureter, the uterine artery, and several blood vessels. This is the vesicouterine ligament.

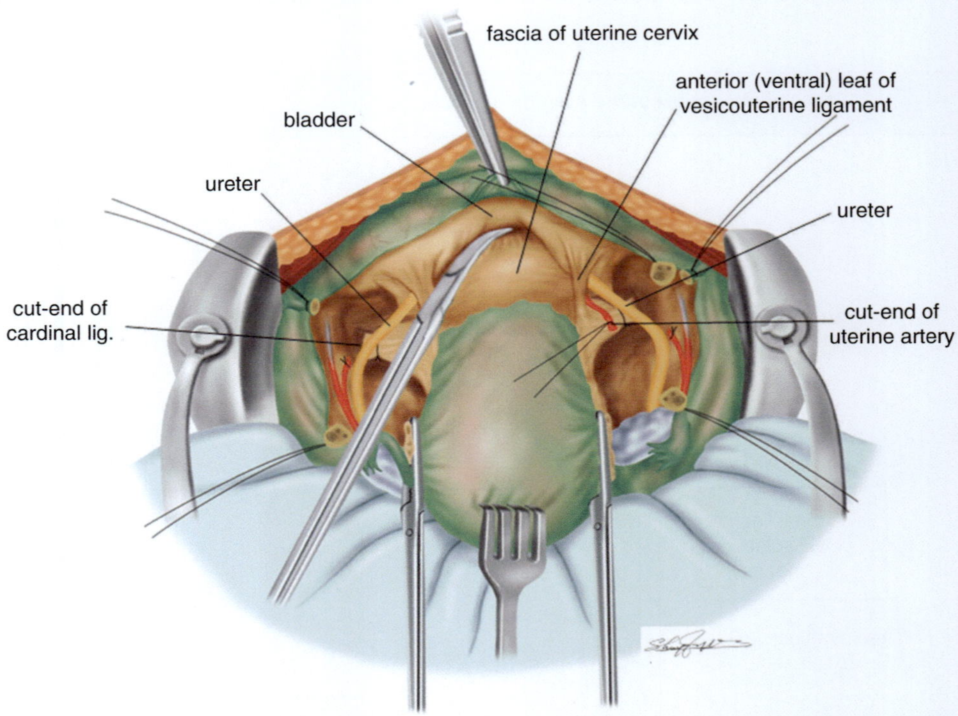


**Figure 6.51** Separation of the urinary bladder from the cervical fascia

### 6.5.2 Anatomy of the Vesicouterine Ligament (Figure 6.52)

Since the ureter is running in the vesicouterine ligament, separation of the connective tissue of the vesicouterine ligament is essential during radical hysterectomy. At first, it is necessary to separate the ventral part of the ureter. However, the detailed anatomy of the vesicouterine ligament was unclear for more than 100 years, until it was clarified in 2007. The illustration below is a transparent view of the ureter and the blood vessels in the vesicouterine ligament by Shingo Fujii.

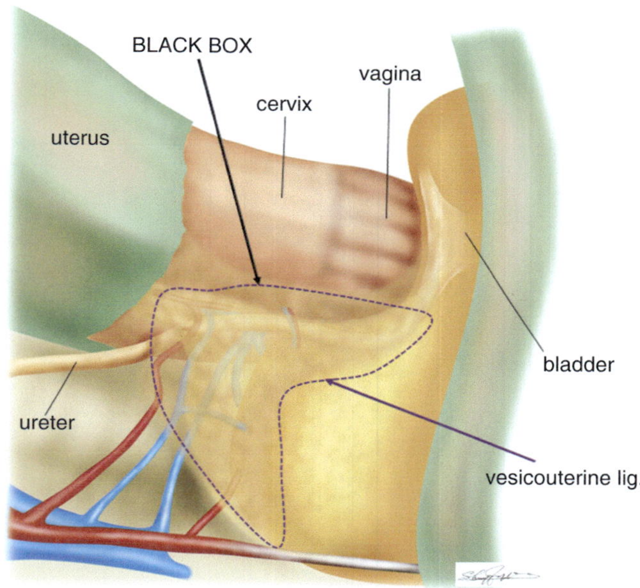


**Figure 6.52** Anatomy of the vesicouterine ligament. The surrounded area with a purple dotted line is showing the anatomical location of the vesicouterine ligament and its detailed anatomy was a black box for more than 100 years. The inserting line of the ureter to the urinary bladder and the existing blood vessels in the vesicouterine ligament are illustrated faintly in the figure

### 6.5.3 Anatomy of the Anterior (Ventral) Leaf of the Vesicouterine Ligament (Figure 6.53)

Figure 6.53 illustrates the cut-ends of the blood vessels which reside in the anterior (ventral) leaf of the vesicouterine ligament and the blood vessels in the posterior (dorsal) leaf of the vesicouterine ligament (shown as a transparent view). After the separation of the anterior (ventral) leaf of the vesicouterine ligament, it is possible to roll the ureter laterally from the surface of the posterior (dorsal) leaf of the vesicouterine ligament.

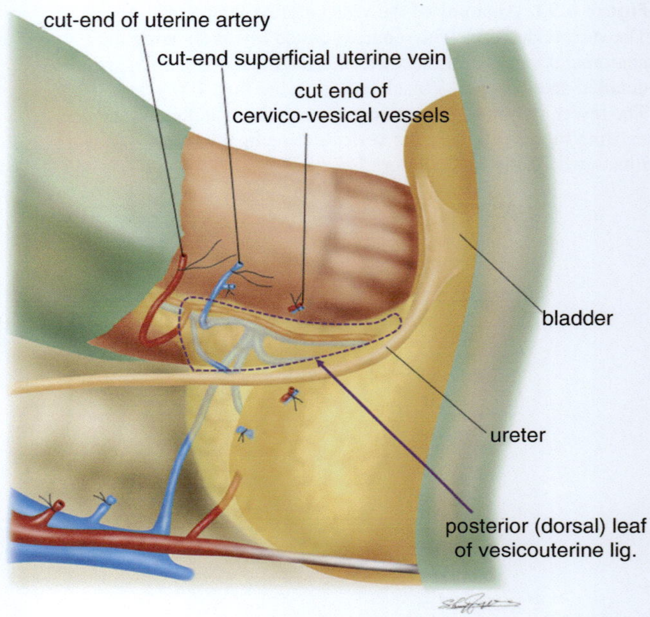


**Figure 6.53** The divided blood vessels in the anterior (ventral) leaf of the vesicouterine ligament is illustrated with a transparent view of the blood vessels in the posterior (dorsal) leaf of the vesicouterine ligament (a surrounded area with a purple dotted line)

### 6.5.4 Anatomy of the Posterior(Dorsal) Leaf of the Vesicouterine Ligament (Figure 6.54)

By mobilizing the ureter toward the inguinal side, the surface of the posterior (dorsal) leaf of the vesicouterine ligament is exposed as the connective tissue triangle formed by the upper cervix/vagina and the ureter/the cranioventral side of the urinary bladder. Figure 6.54 shows a transparent view of the blood vessels in the posterior (dorsal) leaf of the vesicouterine ligament.

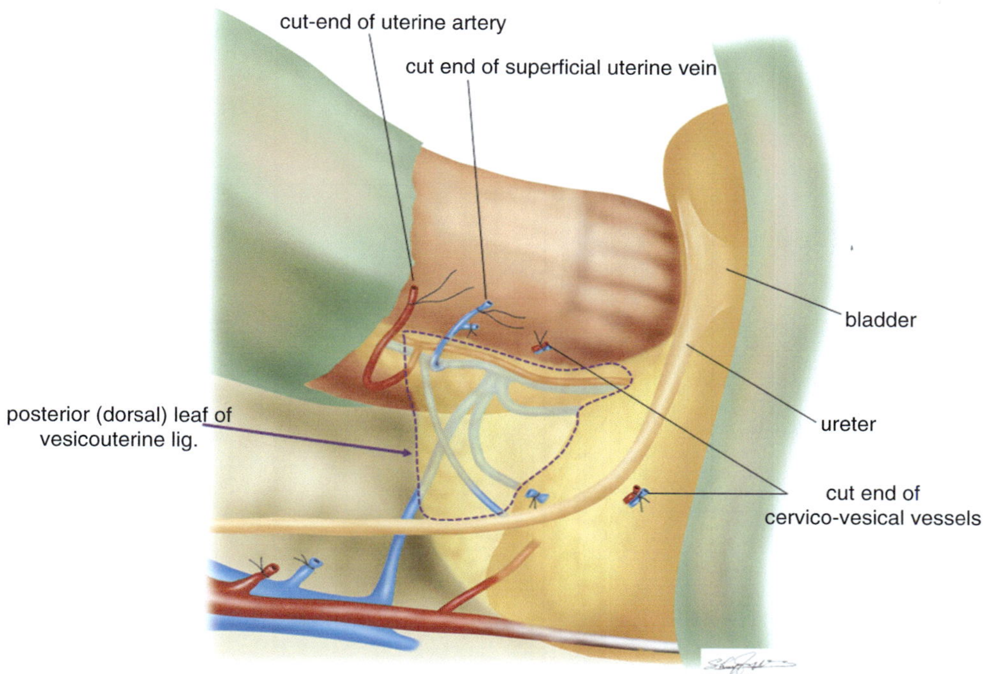


**Figure 6.54** Exposed figure of the posterior (dorsal) leaf of the vesicouterine ligament (a surrounded area with a dotted purple line) is showing a transparent view of the each blocd vessel in the ligament

### 6.5.5 Cross-Sectional Pelvic View of the Blood Vessels in the Vesicouterine Ligament with Each Surgical Step

#### 6.5.5.1 Division of the Uterine Artery and the Superficial Uterine Vein (Figure 6.55)

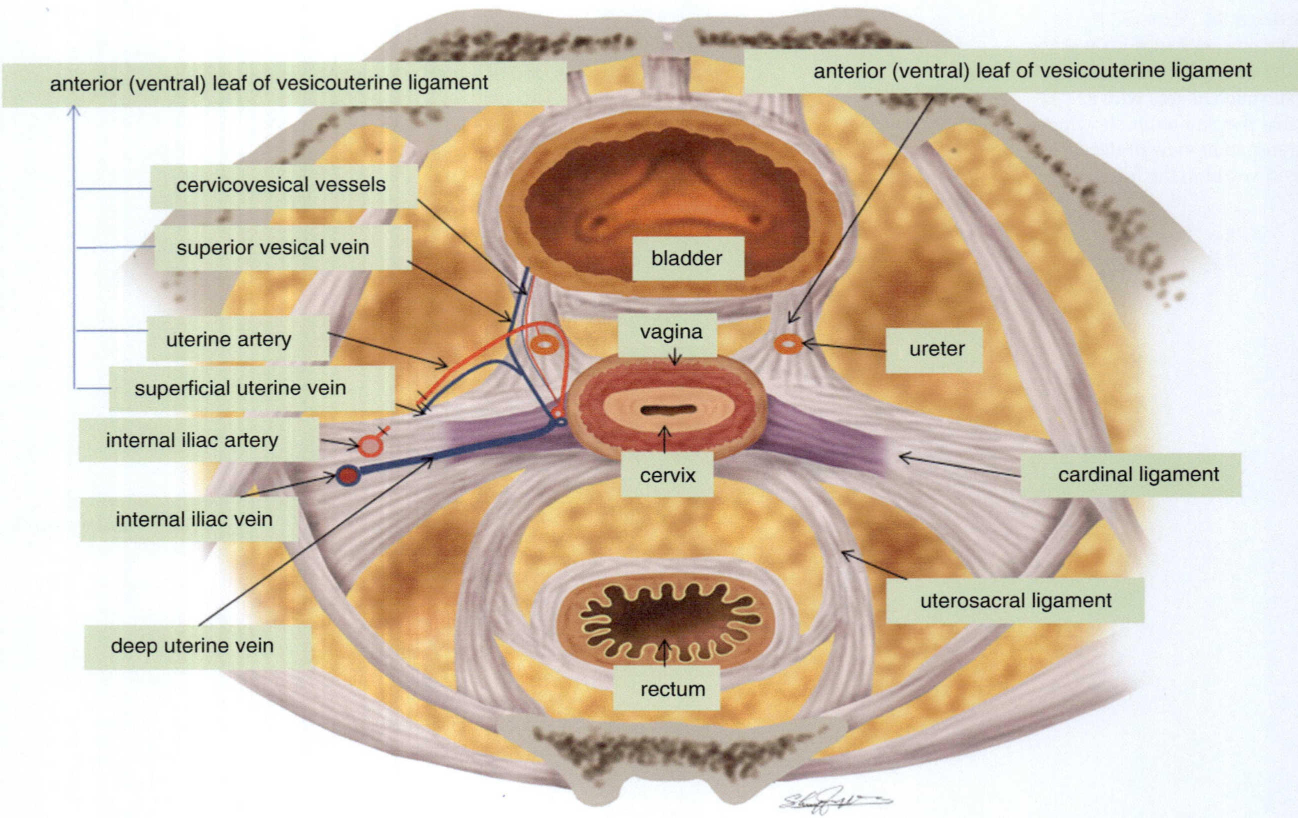


**Figure 6.55** Cross-sectional view of the blood vessels in the vesicouterine ligament and the cardinal ligament in the left side of the pelvic cavity. The uterine artery and the superficial uterine vein are divided

### 6.5.5.2 Division of the Deep Uterine Vein (Figure 6.56)

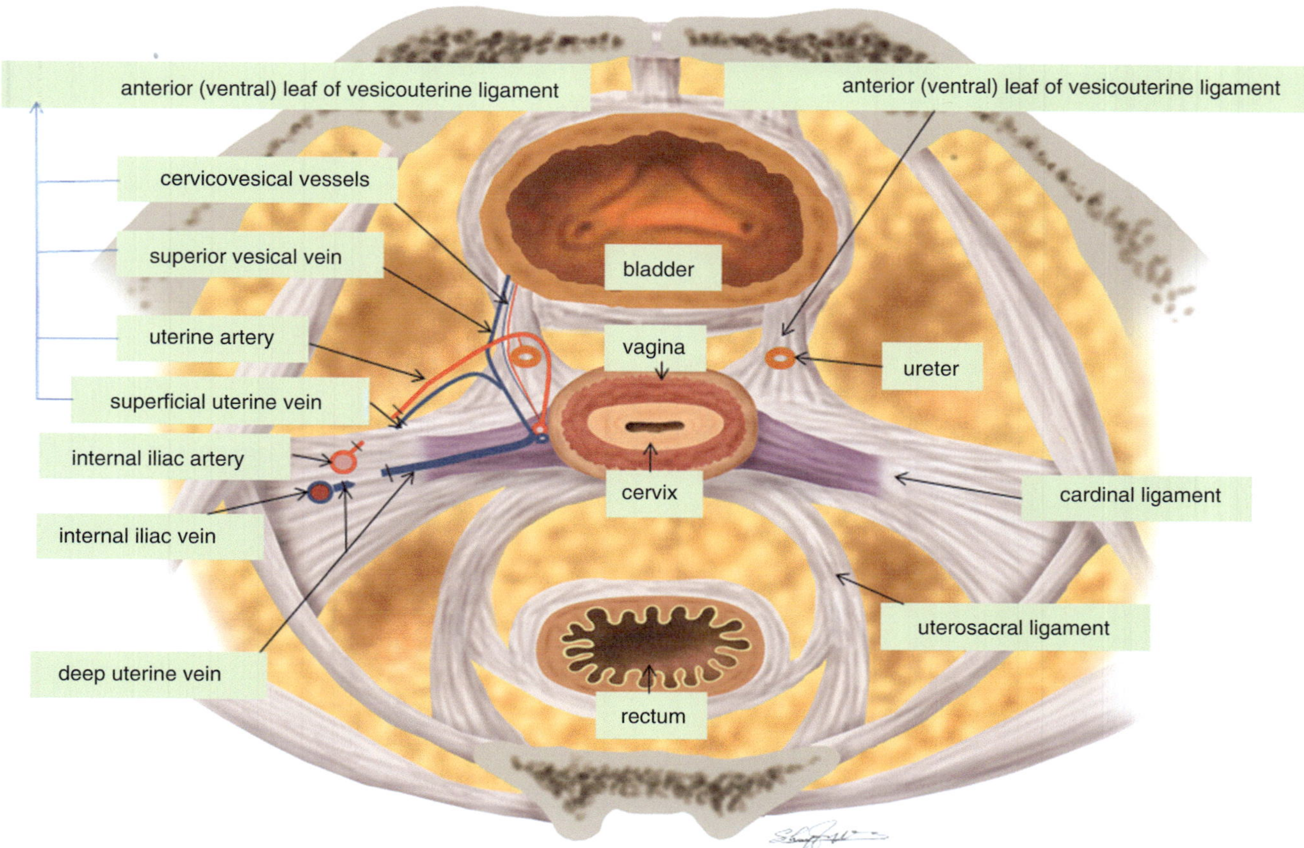


**Figure 6.56** The deep uterine vein is divided

#### 6.5.5.3 Division of the Superior Vesical Vein That Drains into the Superficial Vein in the Anterior (Ventral) Leaf of the Vesicouterine Ligament (Figure 6.57)

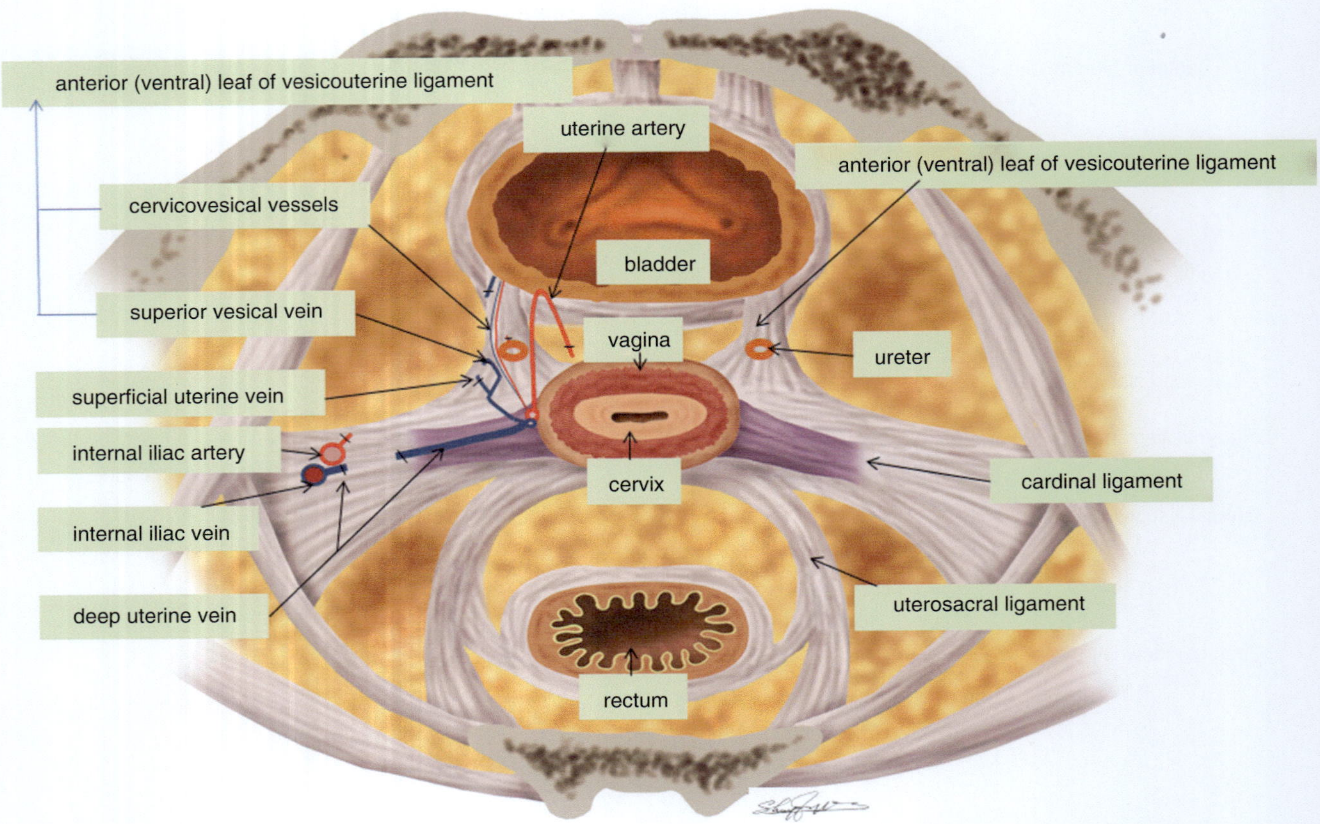


**Figure 6.57** The superior vesical vein is divided

### 6.5.5.4 Division of the Cervicovesical Vessels in the Anterior (Ventral) Leaf of the Vesicouterine Ligament (Figure 6.58)

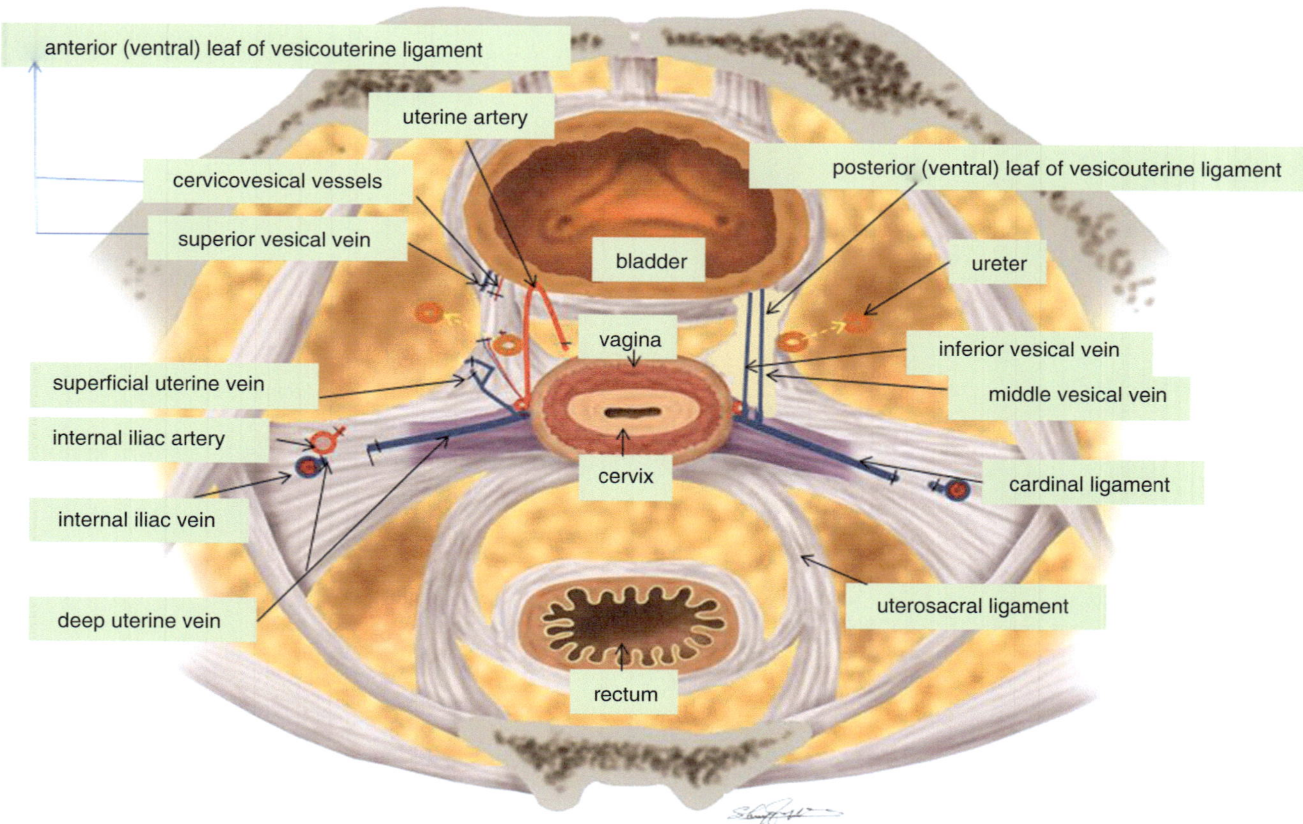


**Figure 6.58** The cervicovesical vessels in the anterior (ventral) leaf of the vesicouterine ligament are divided. In the right side of this figure, the veins in the posterior (dorsal) leaf of the vesicouterine ligament are illustrated between the urinary bladder and the deep uterine vein

### 6.5.5.5 Division of Vesical Veins in the Posterior(Dorsal) Leaf of the Vesicouterine Ligament (Arrow in the Right Side) (Figure 6.59)

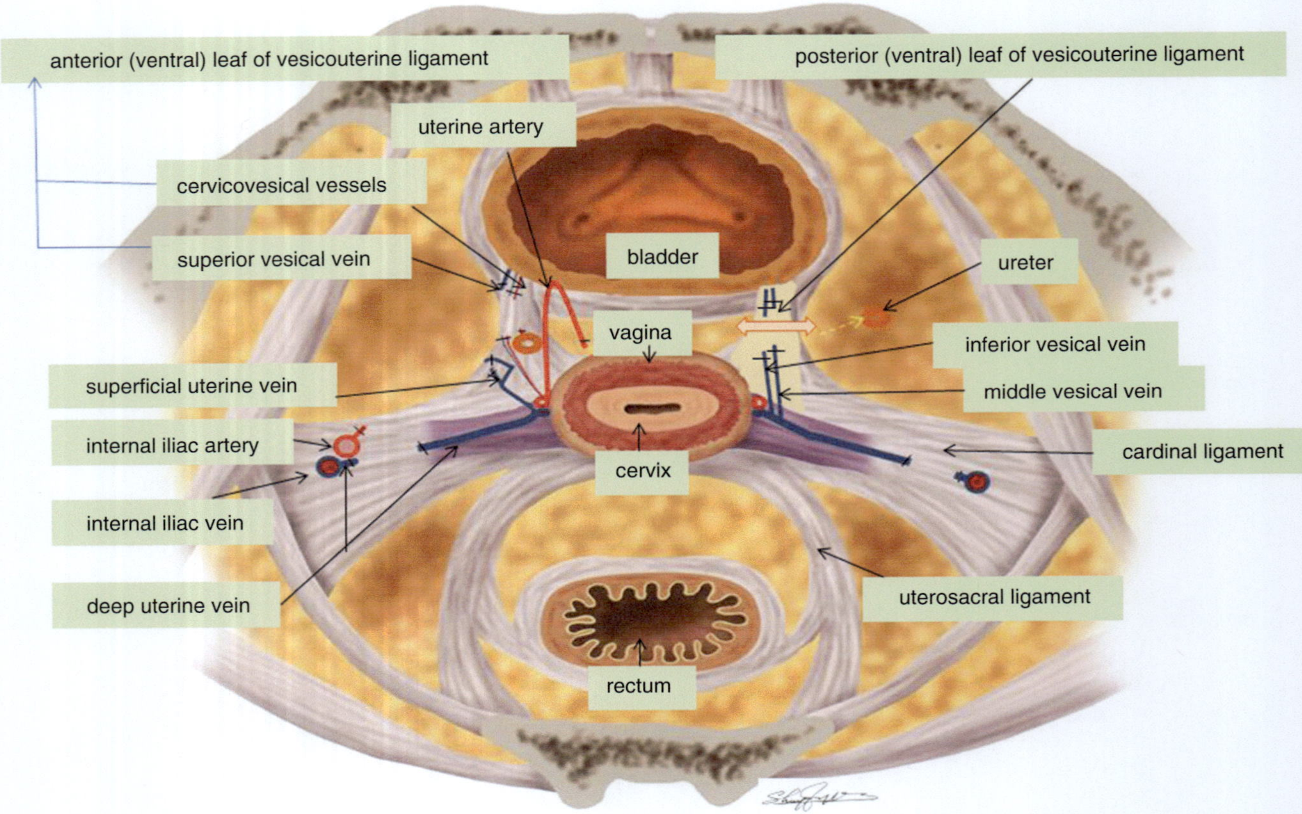


**Figure 6.59** The vesical veins that drain into the deep uterine vein in the posterior (dorsal) leaf of the vesicouterine ligament are divided (right side)

## 6.5.6 Lateral(Right) Side View of the Treatment of the Anterior (Ventral) Leaf of the Vesicouterine Ligament with Each Surgical Step

### 6.5.6.1 Separation of the Uterine Artery and Superficial Uterine Vein from the Ventral Surface of the Ureter

### 6.5.6.2 Isolation of the Ureteral Branch of the Uterine Artery (Figure 6.60)

The cut-end of the uterine artery at the uterine side is lifted with forceps. The connective tissue between the ureter and the uterine artery is carefully divided. The ureteral branch of the uterine artery is often appreciated. It is usually better to clamp, cut, and ligate the ureteral branch. However, if the ureteral branch of the uterine artery is not well developed, the vessel sealing system such as monopolar or bipolar device is enough to seal the ureteral branch. Nevertheless, excessive electrocoagulation near the ureter can lead a heat-induced necrosis to the ureter (delayed onset: postoperative 7–14 days) and lead to fistula formation. Therefore, every possible care should be taken when using electrical energy during the separation of the ureter in the vesicouterine ligament.

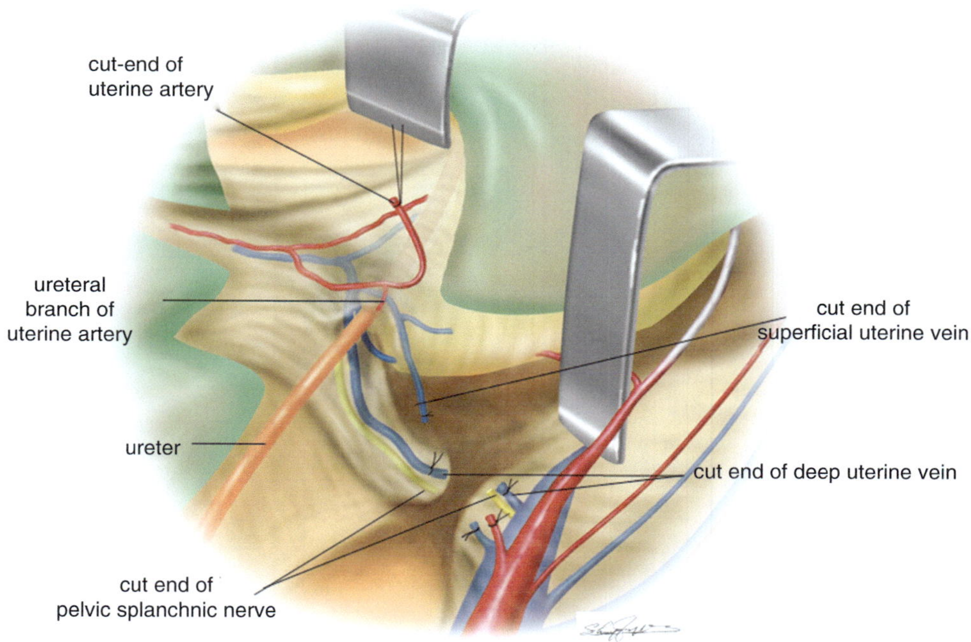


**Figure 6.60** Isolation of the ureteral branch of the uterine artery

#### 6.5.6.3 Division of the Ureteral Branch of the Uterine Artery (Figure 6.61)

The identified ureteral branch of the uterine artery is usually clamped, cut, and ligated. Following this step, the uterine artery is completely separated from the ventral surface of the ureter. In addition, the superficial uterine vein is often found on the ventral surface of the ureter, which should also be separated from the ventral surface of the ureter.

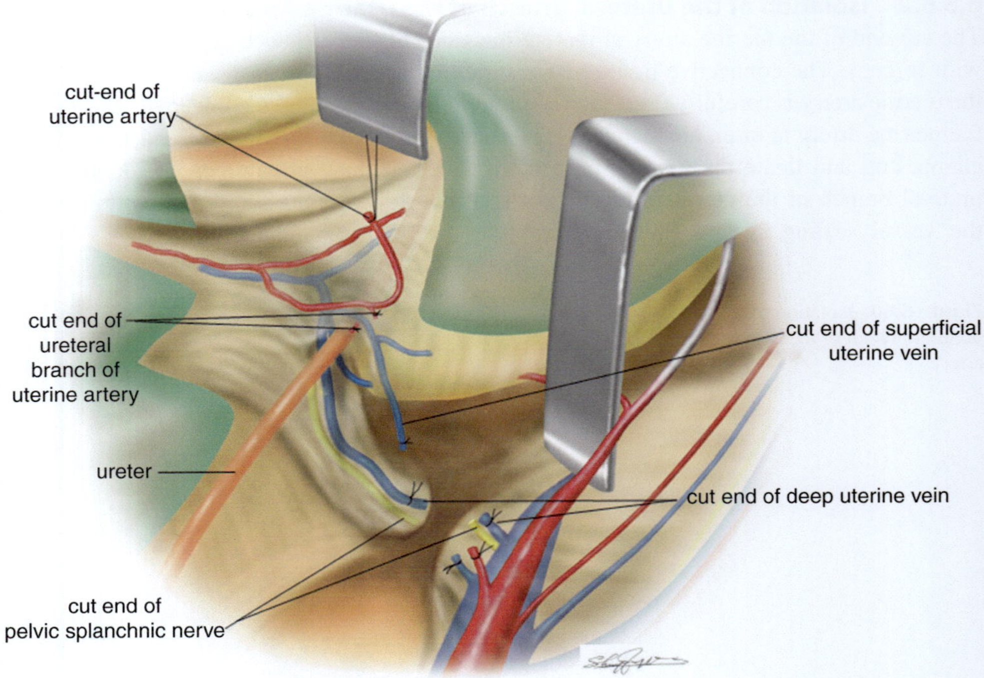


**Figure 6.61** Division of the ureteral branch of the uterine artery

#### 6.5.6.4 Separation of the Superficial Uterine Vein from the Surface of the Ureter and Confirmation of the Superior Vesical Vein That Drains into the Superficial Uterine Vein (Figure 6.62)

The cut-end of the superficial uterine vein is lifted and separated gently from the ventral surface of the ureter. This allows a connecting vein from the urinary bladder to the superficial uterine vein to be identified between the ureter and the urinary bladder. This vein drains blood from the urinary bladder to the superficial uterine vein and is located in the most superior (ventral) portion of the urinary bladder. It is therefore named as the superior vesical vein.

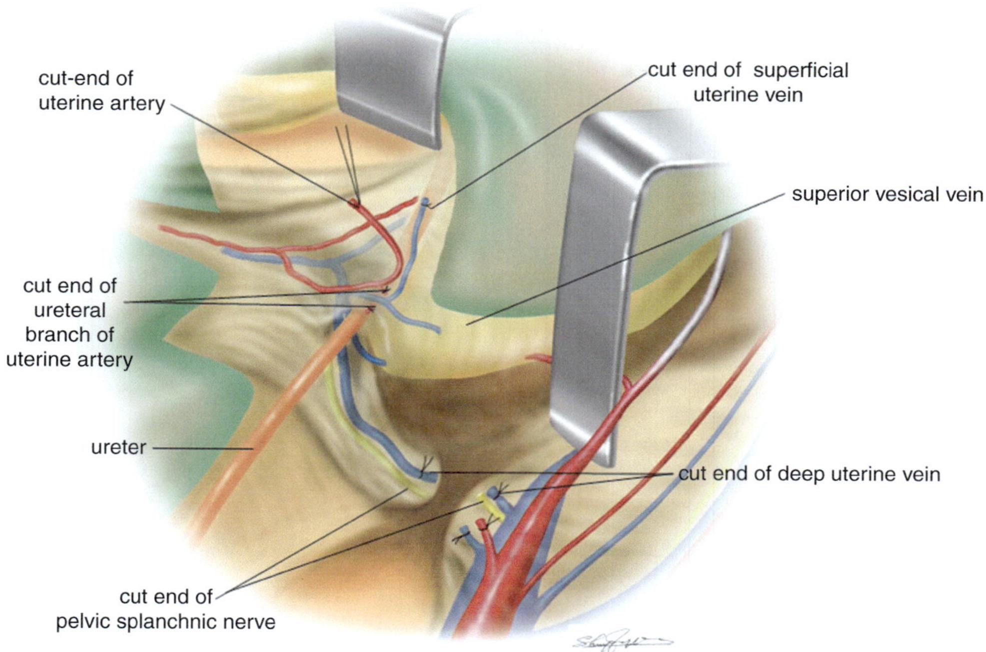


**Figure 6.62** Separation of the superficial uterine vein from the surface of the ureter and confirmation of the superior vesical vein that drains into the superficial uterine vein

#### 6.5.6.5 Isolation and Division of the Superior Vesical Vein That Drains into the Superficial Uterine Vein (Figure 6.63)

The superior vesical vein is carefully isolated, clamped, divided, and ligated. At the end of this step, the uterine side of uterine artery with the superficial uterine vein is completely separated from the ventral surface of the ureter.

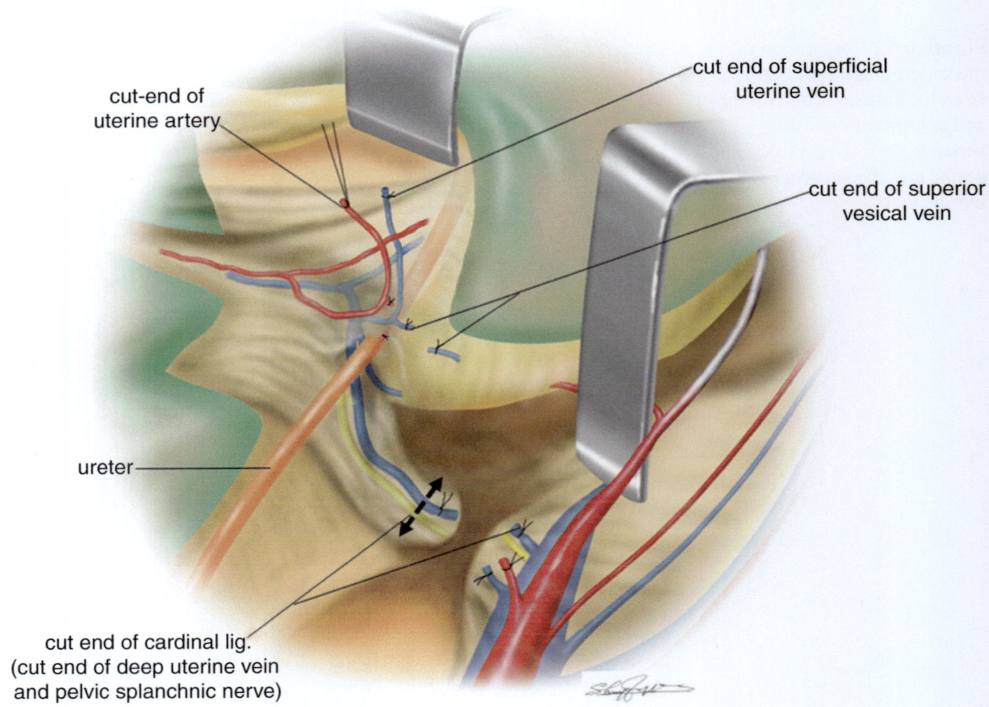


**Figure 6.63** Isolation and division of the superior vesical vein that drains into the superficial uterine vein

**Notes:**
This is the most difficult step during the separation of the anterior (ventral) leaf of the vesicouterine ligament. The superficial uterine vein as well as the superior vesical vein is very fragile and bleeds easily.

#### 6.5.6.6 Separation of the Cut-Ends of the Uterine Artery and the Superficial Uterine Vein from the Ventral Surface of the Ureter (Figure 6.64)

The separation of both the uterine artery and the superficial uterine vein from the ventral surface of the ureter can reduce hemorrhage and is the most important step prior to further dissection of the anterior (ventral) leaf of the vesicouterine ligament.

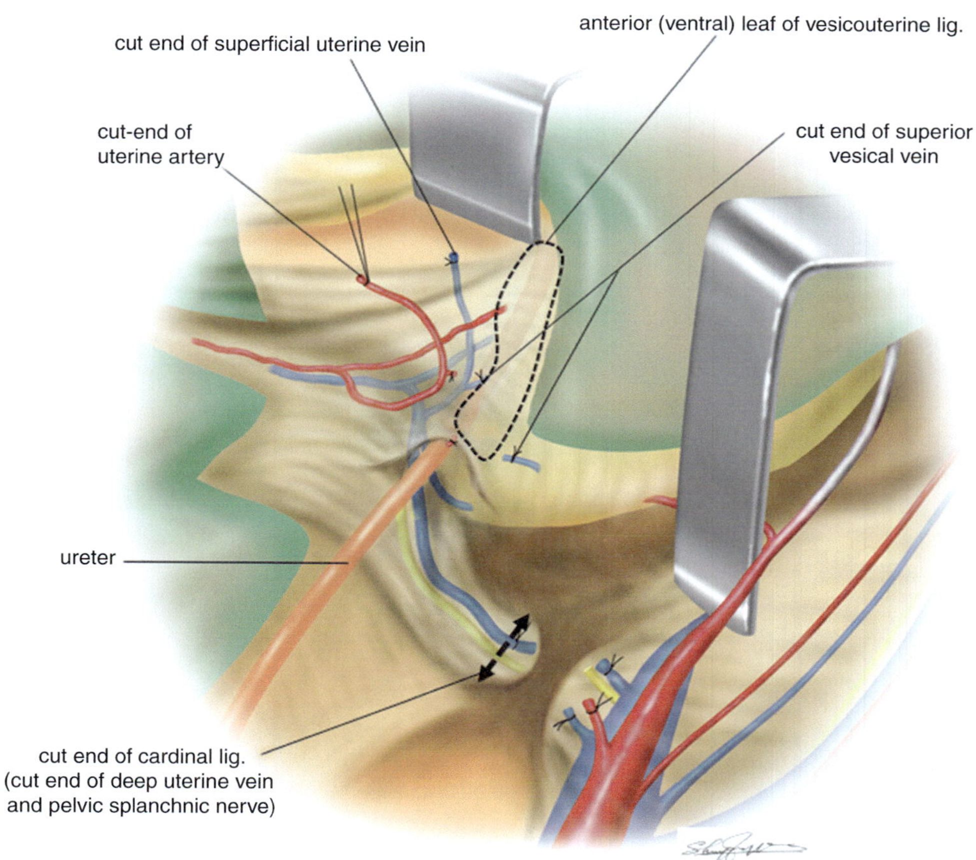


**Figure 6.64** Separation of the cut-ends of the uterine artery and the superficial uterine vein from the ventral surface of the ureter (a surrounded area with a dotted line is the location of the anterior (ventral) leaf of the vesicouterine ligament)

### 6.5.6.7 Confirmation of the Anterior (Ventral) Leaf of the Vesicouterine Ligament and the Ureter Tunnel (Figure 6.65)

With the completion of the separation of the uterine artery and the superficial uterine vein from the ventral surface of the ureter, the anterior (ventral) leaf of the vesicouterine ligament and the so-called ureteral tunnel are appreciated.

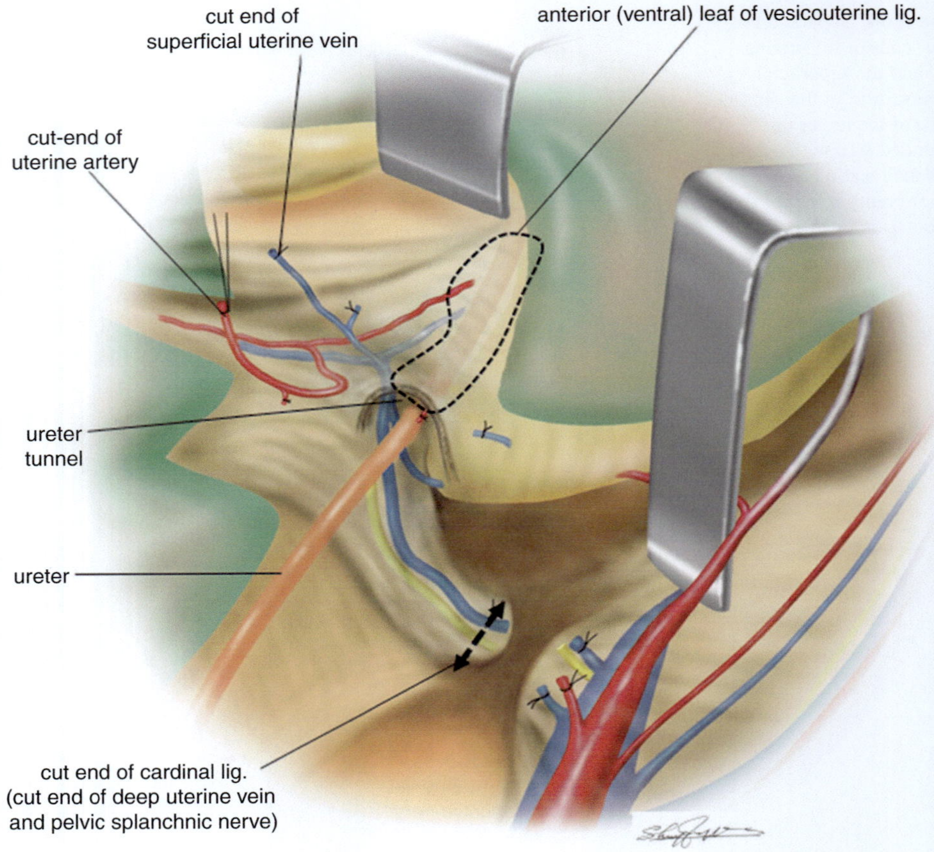


**Figure 6.65** By the traction of both cut-ends of the uterine artery and the superficial uterine vein to the uterine side, the whole surface of the anterior (ventral) leaf of the vesicouterine ligament (an area surrounded by a dotted line) is revealed. The entrance of the ureter tunnel is the cranial side of the ligament. Two-directional arrow line is showing the location of the cut-end of the cardinal ligament

## 6.5.7 Step-by-Step Separation of the Anterior (Ventral) Leaf of the Vesicouterine Ligament

### 6.5.7.1 Separation of the Connective Tissues in the Anterior (Ventral) Leaf of the Vesicouterine Ligament (Figure 6.66)

Instead of the development of the ureter tunnel described in Chaps. 4 and 5, the connective tissue of the ventral side of the ureter is carefully separated and divided from the entrance of the tunnel toward the urinary bladder at the point of ureteric insertion. From the entrance of the ureteric tunnel 1–1.5 cm apart, a pair of small blood vessels that cross the ureter from the bladder to the cervix are appreciated in the anterior (ventral) leaf of the vesicouterine ligament. As the blood vessels run between the bladder and the cervix, these are named as the cervicovesical vessels.

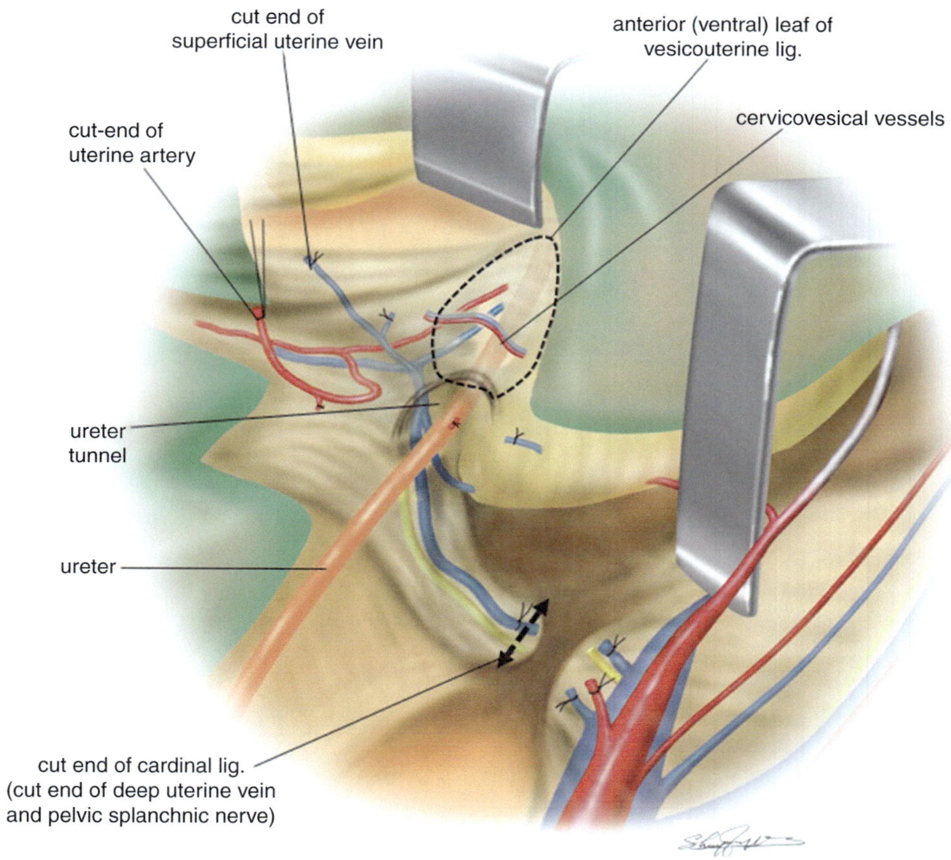


**Figure 6.66** Separation of the connective tissue in the anterior (ventral) leaf of the vesicouterine ligament (an area surrounded by a dotted line) reveals the blood vessels that run between the bladder and the cervix (cervicovesical vessels)

#### 6.5.7.2 Division of the Cervicovesical Vessels (Figure 6.67)

The connective tissue is separated from the ventral surface of the ureter, in order to isolate the cervicovesical vessels. The isolated cervicovesical vessels are doubly clamped, divided, and ligated. After the division of the cervicovesical vessels, the connective tissues surrounding the ureter are easily separated from the anterior (ventral) leaf of the vesicouterine ligament because other blood vessels are usually not identified in the anterior (ventral) leaf of the vesicouterine ligament. By separating the connective tissues from the anterior (ventral) leaf of the vesicouterine ligament, the ureter is completely freed from its attachment to the posterior (dorsal) leaf of the vesicouterine ligament.

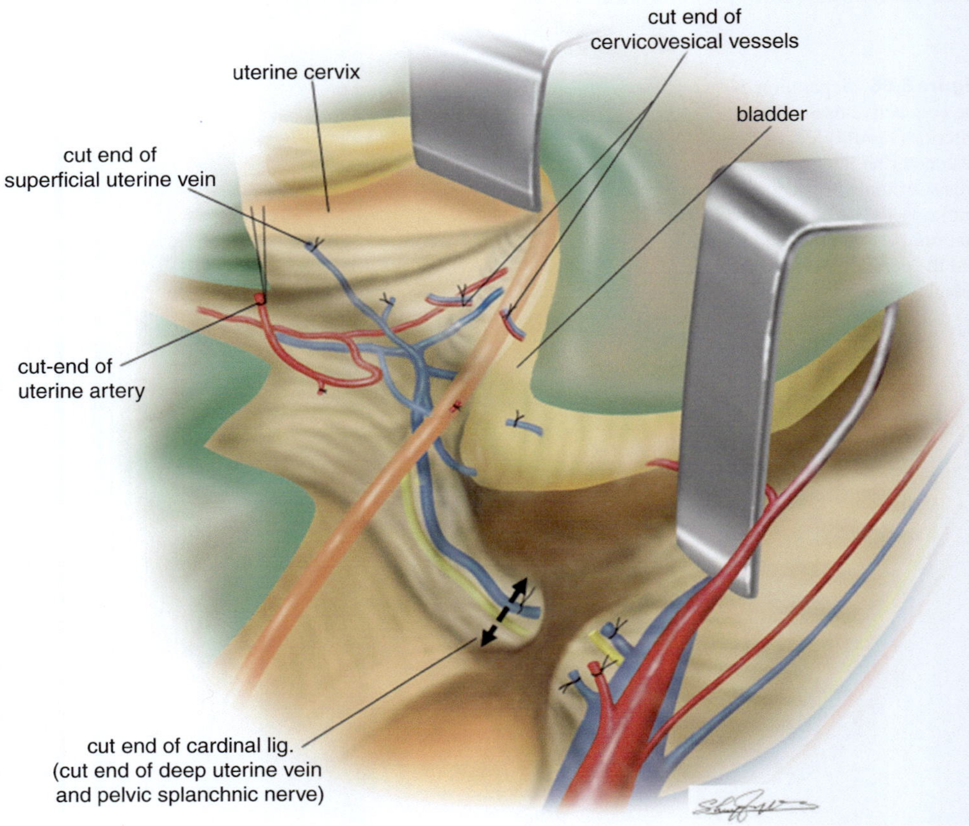


**Figure 6.67** Division of the cervicovesical vessels

#### 6.5.7.3 Mobilization of the Ureter to the Symphysis Side and Confirmation of the Posterior (Dorsal) Leaf of the Vesicouterine Ligament (Figure 6.68)

The connective tissue can be easily separated from the dorsal side of the ureter, in order to detach the ureter from the ventral side of the posterior (dorsal) leaf of the vesicouterine ligament. The ureter is separated at its junction to the urinary bladder to allow the ureter to be mobilized with the urinary bladder to the symphysis side in order to reveal the ventral side of the posterior (dorsal) leaf of the vesicouterine ligament as wide as possible. By these steps, the anterior (ventral) leaf of the vesicouterine ligament is completely separated with minimal blood loss.

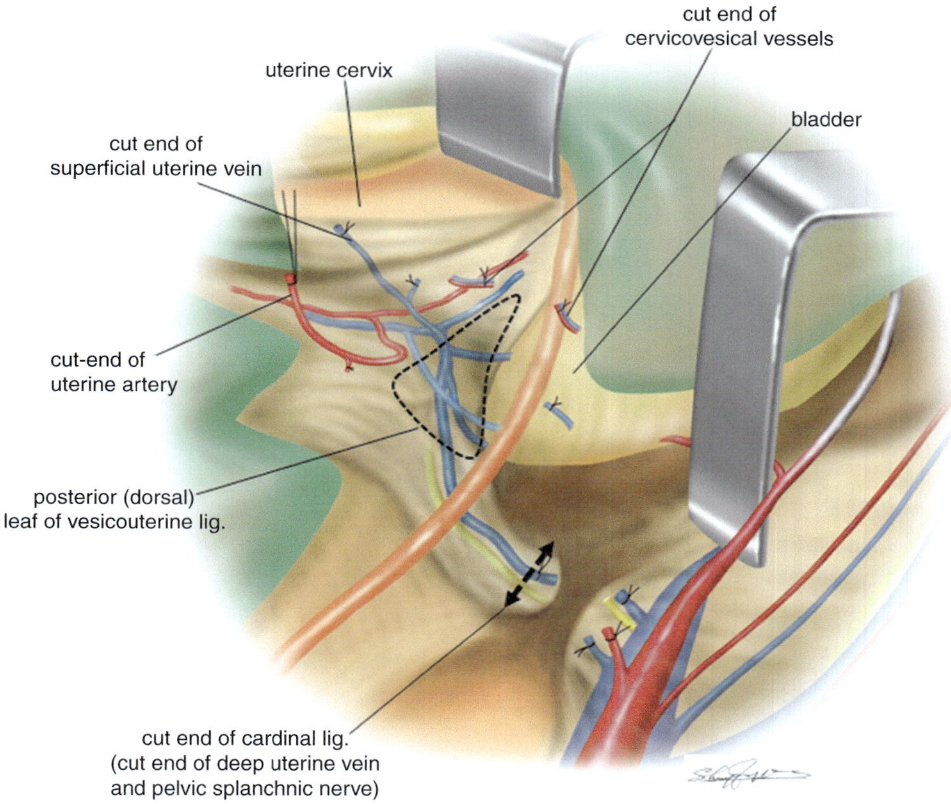


**Figure 6.68** Mobilization of the ureter to the symphysis side and confirmation of the posterior (dorsal) leaf of the vesicouterine ligament (an area surrounded by a dotted line)

## 6.6 Treatment of the Posterior (Dorsal) Leaf of the Vesicouterine Ligament

### 6.6.1 Step-by-Step Separation of the Posterior (Dorsal) Leaf of the Vesicouterine Ligament

#### 6.6.1.1 Treatment of a Vein Between the Ureter and the Cervix (Figure 6.69)

By mobilizing the ureter with the urinary bladder to the symphysis side, the posterior (dorsal) leaf of the vesicouterine ligament is appreciated. In the cranial side of the posterior (dorsal) leaf of the vesicouterine ligament, a vein running from the ureter to the cervix is appreciated. The vein is isolated from the connective tissue and doubly clamped, divided, and ligated. Following this step, there is increased mobility of the ureter with the urinary bladder, facilitating the shift of the ureter toward the symphysis side.

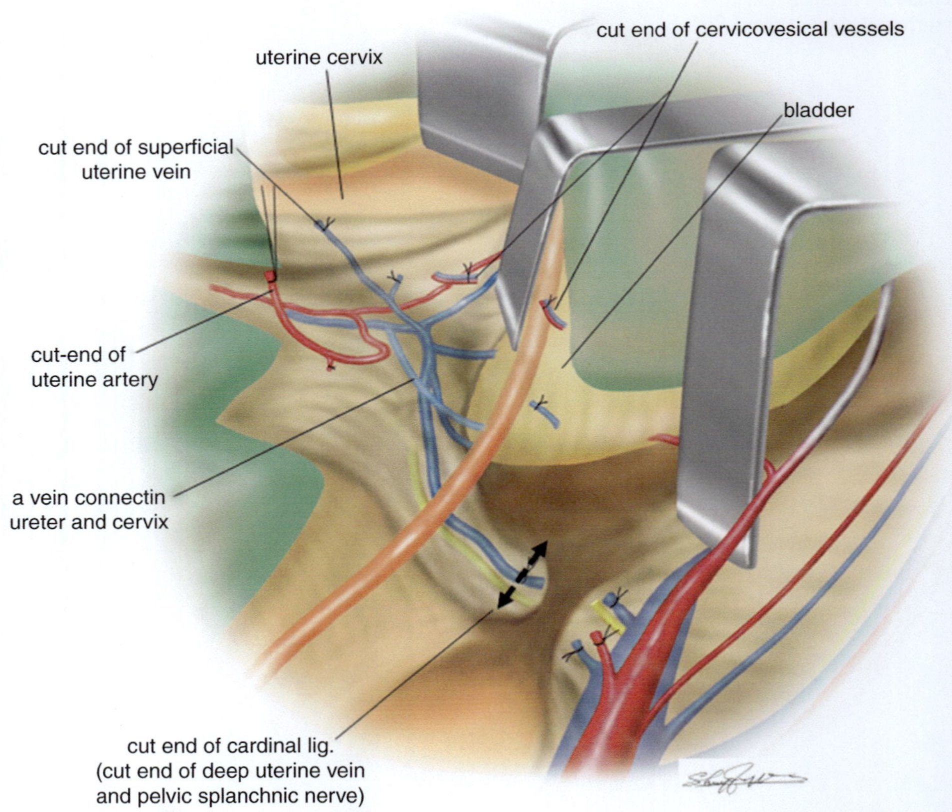


**Figure 6.69** Mobilization of the ureter and the urinary bladder toward the symphysis side reveals the posterior (dorsal) leaf of the vesicouterine ligament. In the cranial side of the posterior (dorsal) leaf of the vesicouterine ligament, a vein running from the ureter to the cervix is usually observed. The vein is divided (not shown in this figure)

#### 6.6.1.2 Confirmation of the Posterior (Dorsal) Leaf of the Vesicouterine Ligament by the Mobilization of the Ureter with the Urinary Bladder Toward the Symphysis Side and the Separation of the Cut-End of the Cardinal Ligament from the Pelvic Sidewall and the Sidewall of the Rectum (Figure 6.70)

The cut-end of cardinal ligament (with the deep uterine vein and one of the branches of the pelvic splanchnic nerve) is then clamped with Pean forceps. The connective tissue on the dorsal side of the cardinal ligament should be separated from the pelvic wall and the sidewall of the rectum.

After the division of the vein connecting the ureter and the cervix, the ureter and the urinary bladder are pulled toward the symphysis side, using two L-shaped forceps. This also lifts up the cut-end of cardinal ligament (with the deep uterine vein and one of the branches of the pelvic splanchnic nerve) cranially. This traction allows the connective tissue of the posterior (dorsal) leaf of the vesicouterine ligament to be stretched and well defined between the cranial side of the bladder and the uterine side of the cardinal ligament. Providing tension to the connective tissue between the cardinal ligament and the urinary bladder is very important for the separation of the posterior (dorsal) leaf of the vesicouterine ligament. In the connective tissue of posterior (dorsal) leaf of the vesicouterine ligament, veins pass from the urinary bladder into the deep uterine vein in the cardinal ligament. The tension given to the connective tissue is helpful to identify the veins in the posterior (dorsal) leaf of the vesicouterine ligament.

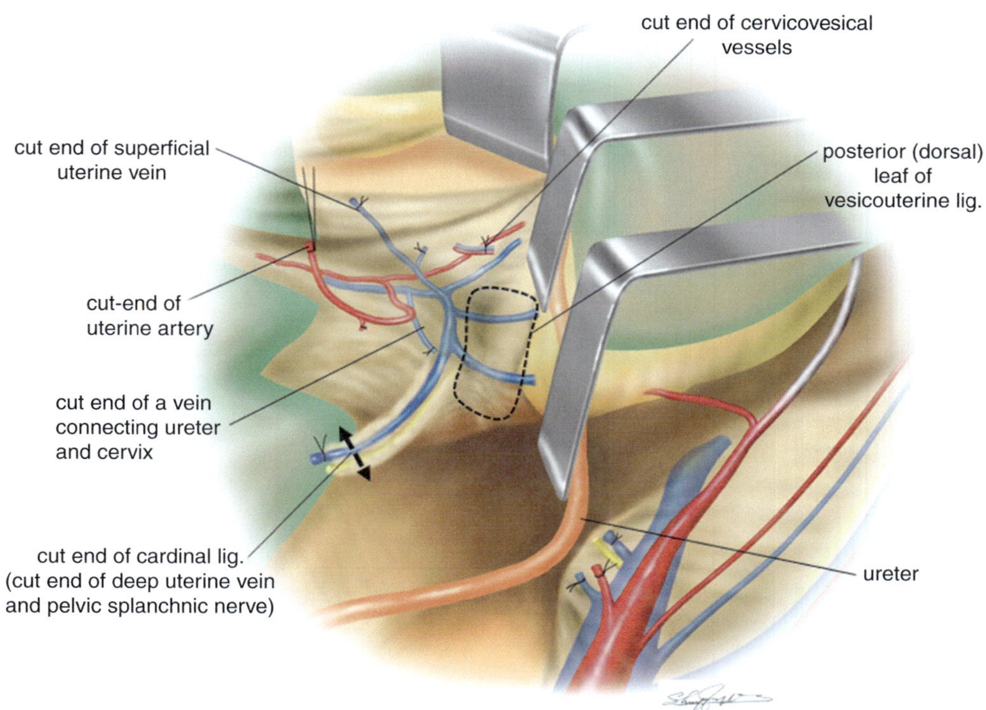


**Figure 6.70** Pulling down the ureter and the urinary bladder toward the symphysis side and lifting up the cut-end of the cardinal ligament toward the cranial side, give tension to the posterior (dorsal) leaf of the vesicouterine ligament for the recognition of the vesical veins connecting with the deep uterine vein in the ligament (an area surrounded by a dotted line)

#### 6.6.1.3 Isolation of the Middle Vesical Vein (Figure 6.71)

The connective tissue in the posterior (dorsal) leaf of the vesicouterine ligament is carefully separated. In the cranial portion of the posterior (dorsal) leaf of the vesicouterine ligament, the middle vesical vein that runs from the urinary bladder into the deep uterine vein in the cardinal ligament is appreciated. The middle vesical vein is isolated.

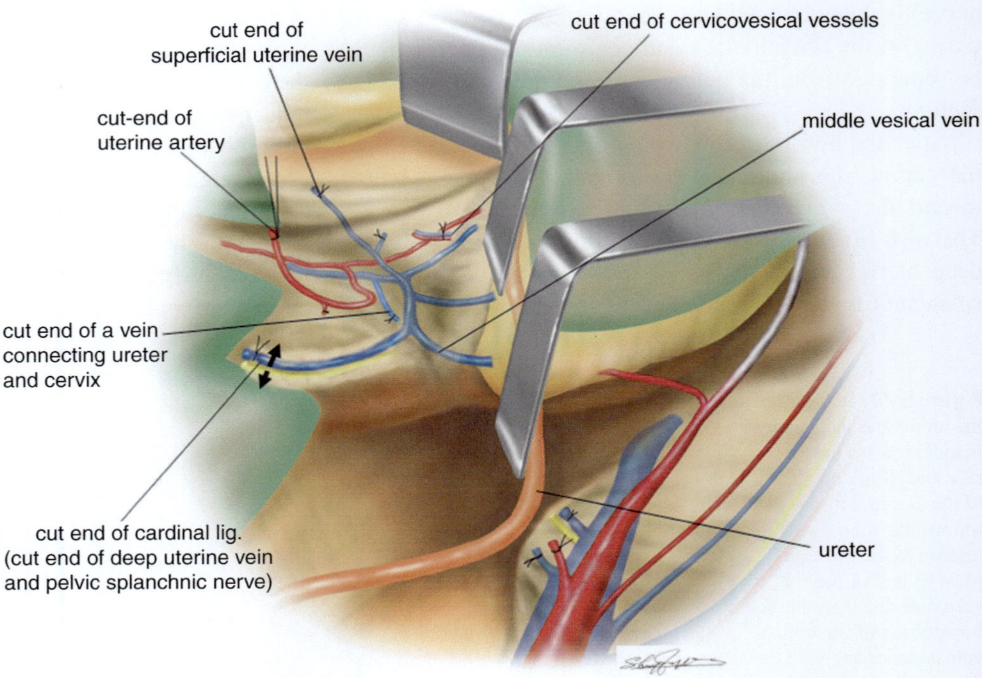


**Figure 6.71** Isolation of the middle vesical vein

#### 6.6.1.4 Division of the Middle Vesical Vein and Isolation of the Inferior Vesical Vein (Figure 6.72)

The middle vesical vein is doubly clamped, divided, and ligated.

In addition, a vein (the inferior vesical vein) that runs parallel to the cervix from the posterior aspect of the urinary bladder and drains into the deep uterine vein is isolated.

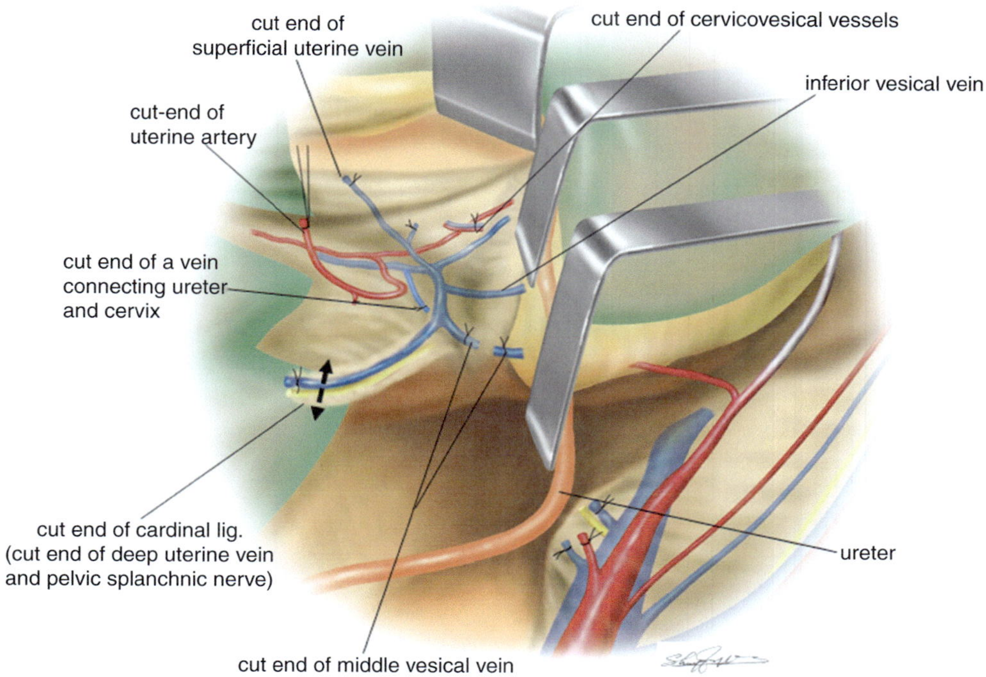


**Figure 6.72** Division of the middle vesical vein and isolation of the inferior vesical vein

#### 6.6.1.5 Division of the Inferior Vesical Vein (Figure 6.73)

The inferior vesical vein is doubly clamped, ligated, and divided. Usually, by the division of the inferior vesical vein, the urinary bladder with the ureter is completely separated from the lateral cervix and the upper vagina. In the sidewall of the cervix and upper vagina, the blood vessels from the vagina (paracolpium) can be identified.

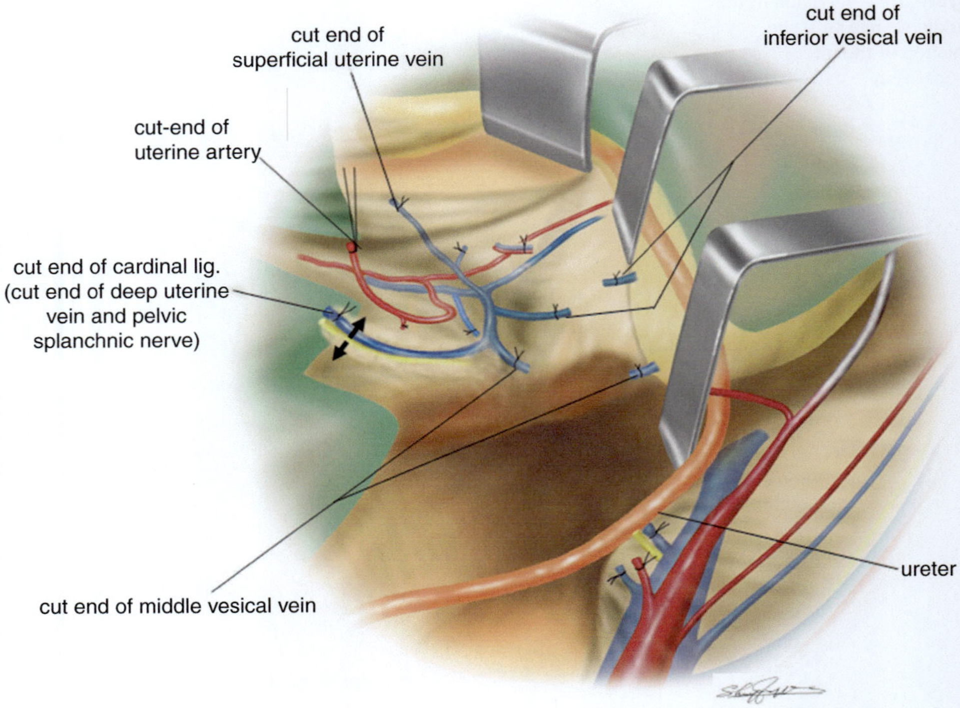


**Figure 6.73** Division of the inferior vesical vein

#### 6.6.1.6 A View After the Division of the Posterior (Dorsal) Leaf of the Vesicouterine Ligament (Figure 6.74)

The division of the posterior (dorsal) leaf of the vesicouterine ligament enables the separation of the ureter with the urinary bladder from the cervix and the upper vagina. The picture formed between the cranial side of the urinary bladder with ureter and the lateral side of the cervix/upper vagina resembles that of an open book. The complete separation of the posterior (dorsal) leaf of the vesicouterine ligament frees the urinary bladder with ureter from the vaginal wall.

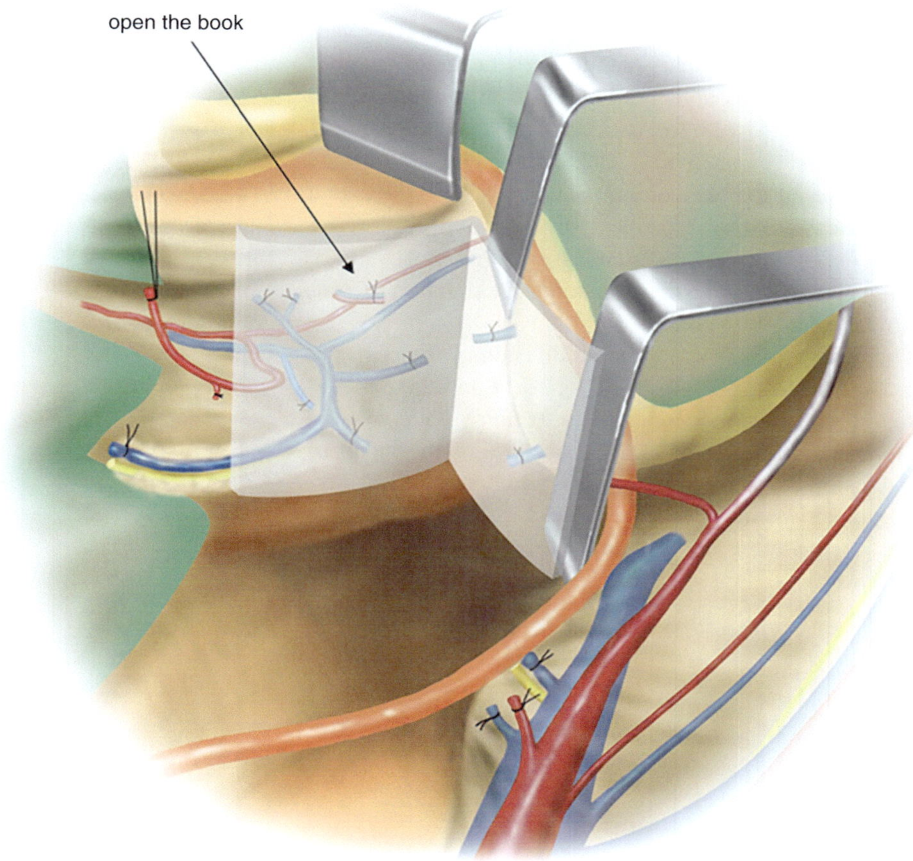


**Figure 6.74** Complete division of the posterior (dorsal) leaf of the vesicouterine ligament creates the situation of the urinary bladder with ureter free from the vaginal wall with the paracolpium (vaginal blood vessels). The anatomical structure formed by the cranial side of the urinary bladder with ureter and by the lateral side of the cervix/ upper vagina resembles that of an open book

#### 6.6.1.7 An Advantage of the Division of the Posterior (Dorsal) Leaf of the Vesicouterine Ligament

The division of the posterior (dorsal) leaf of the vesicouterine ligament means the division of the vesical veins that drain into the deep uterine vein. As a result, the urinary bladder with the ureter becomes detached from the blood vessels of the uterus and the vagina. Moreover, if the urinary bladder can be separated from the ventral vaginal wall (the connective tissue between the trigone of the urinary bladder and the ventral vaginal wall), the urinary bladder with the ureter becomes free from the uterus and the vagina. In this situation, the uterus is connected with the vagina by the remaining vaginal blood vessels (paracolpium) bilaterally. The appropriate division level of the paracolpium is dependent on the extent of the disease. The independent division of the posterior (dorsal) leaf of the vesicouterine ligament has an advantage of being able to tailor the division of the paracolpium according to the extent of the disease.

The concept of the independent division of the posterior (dorsal) leaf of the vesicouterine ligament and the paracolpium did not exist in the radical hysterectomy undertaken in Western countries. The surgical procedure of the independent division of the posterior (Dorsal) leaf of the vesicouterine ligament was introduced by Hidekazu Okabayashi. This is one of the most novel points of Okabayashi's radical hysterectomy.

**Notes**

1. The connective and adipose tissues are not always the same during the step-by-step separation of the posterior (dorsal) leaf of the vesicouterine ligament. Sometimes, isolation and separation of each vessel can be complicated by adhesions. In such cases, the classic approach of Okabayashi' radical hysterectomy that describes penetrating/piercing Okabayashi's paravaginal space using scissors or Pean forceps permits the separation of the posterior (dorsal) leaf of the vesicouterine ligament from the vaginal blood vessels (paracolpium), giving you an alternative route (described in Chaps. 4 and 5).
2. The removal of the adipose tissue in the paravesical space, especially in the dorsal portion of the posterior (dorsal) leaf of the vesicouterine ligament and that of the urinary bladder, helps the identification of the blood vessels in the posterior (dorsal) leaf of the vesicouterine ligament.

#### 6.6.1.8 Separation of the Cut-End of the Cardinal Ligament (the Deep Uterine Vein and the Pelvic Splanchnic Nerve) from the Lateral Surface of the Rectum (Figure 6.75)

The cut-end of the cardinal ligament (the deep uterine vein with the pelvic splanchnic nerve) is lifted and separated from the connective tissues of the lateral surface of the rectum at the level where the pelvic splanchnic nerve merges with the hypogastric nerve. This merging point is the inferior hypogastric plexus.

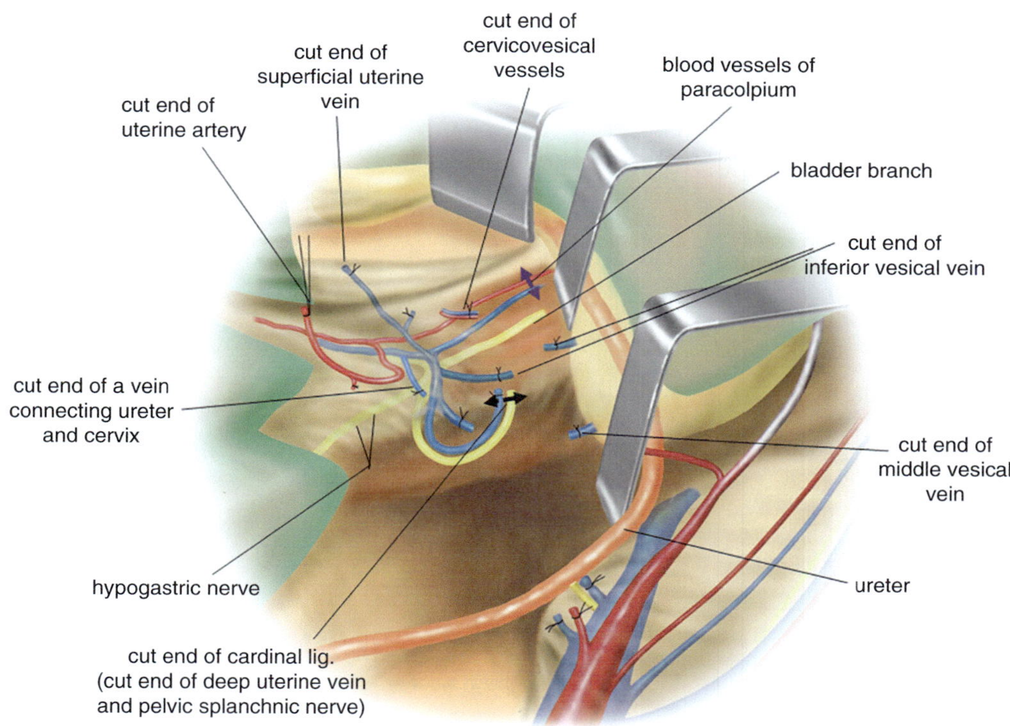


**Figure 6.75** Separation of the cut-end of the cardinal ligament (the deep uterine vein and the pelvic splanchnic nerve) from the lateral surface of the rectum. A purple two-directional arrow is indicating the blood vessels of the paracolpium

### 6.6.2 Division of the Rectovaginal Ligament

#### 6.6.2.1 Cranial Side View (Figure 6.76)

Draw the uterus to the ventral/pubic bone side and stretch the rectum toward cranial portion by the hand. This helps delineate the connective tissue bundle between the rectum and the vagina bilaterally. This bundle is the rectovaginal ligament. The rectovaginal ligament is divided using monopolar or bipolar electrocautery. Division of the rectovaginal ligament frees the dorsal side of the vaginal wall. Therefore, the length of the vaginal cuff can be tailored to the desired length, depending on extent of disease.

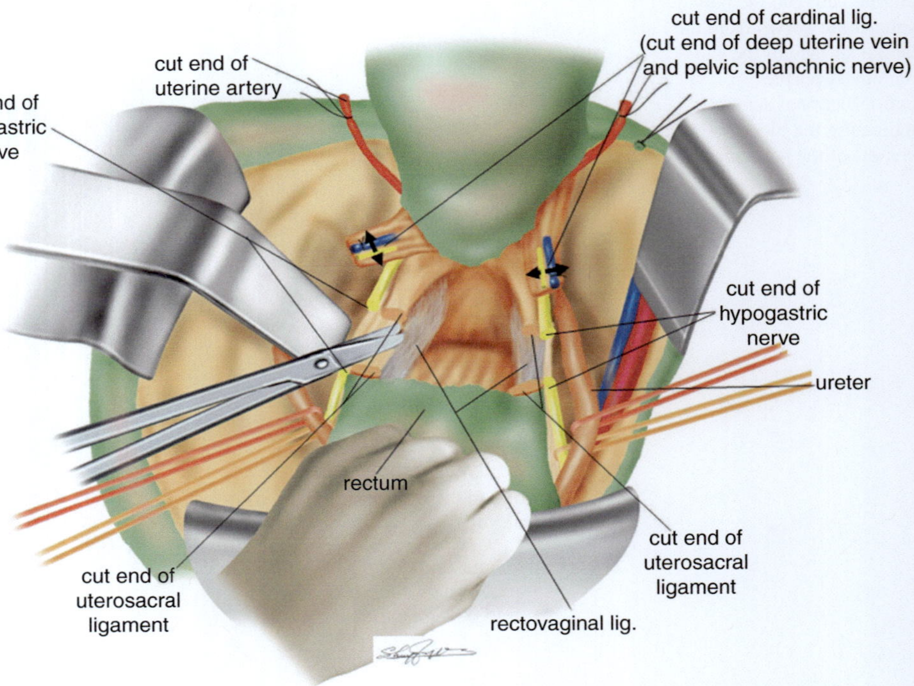


**Figure 6.76** A cranial side view of the division of the rectovaginal ligament. The hypogastric nerve is usually divided at the time of the development of Okabayashi's pararectal space, the connective tissue bundle between the rectum and the upper vagina is the rectovaginal ligament. This ligament is divided

#### 6.6.2.2 Pelvic Side View (Figure 6.77)

Figure 6.77 demonstrates the division of the rectovaginal ligament visualized laterally from the pelvic side.

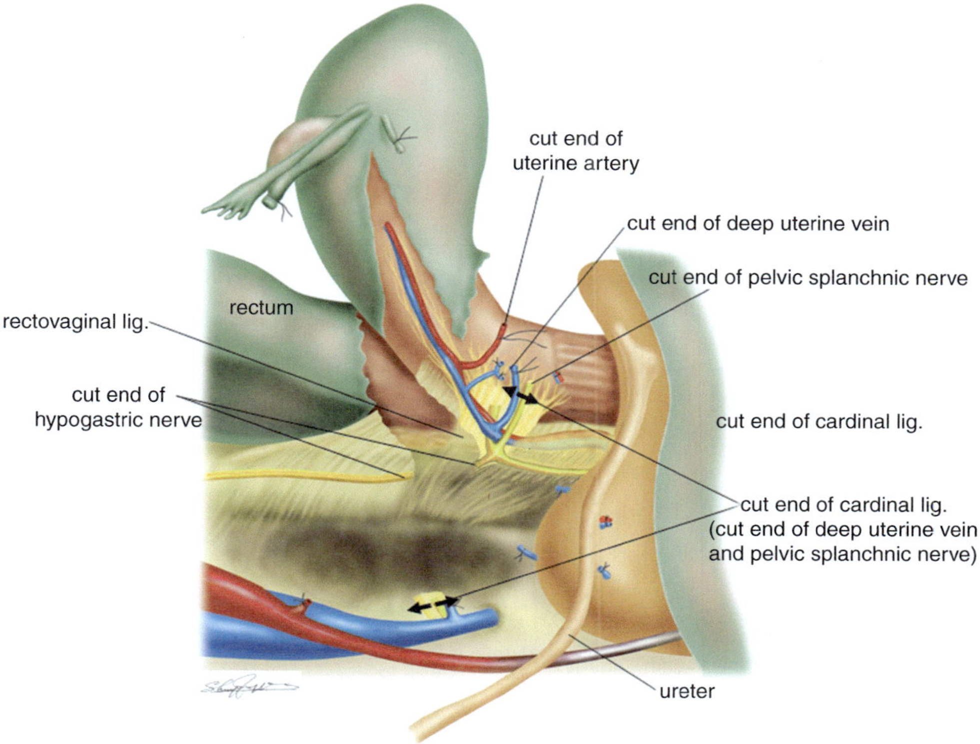


**Figure 6.77** The location of the rectovaginal ligament is illustrated as the pelvic side view

### 6.6.3 Further Division of the Rectovaginal Ligament (Figure 6.78)

Traction of the uterus toward the cranial side stretches the bladder branch of the inferior hypogastric plexus in the uterine side. During the division of the rectovaginal ligament the bladder branch from the inferior hypogastric plexus is likely to be sacrificed.

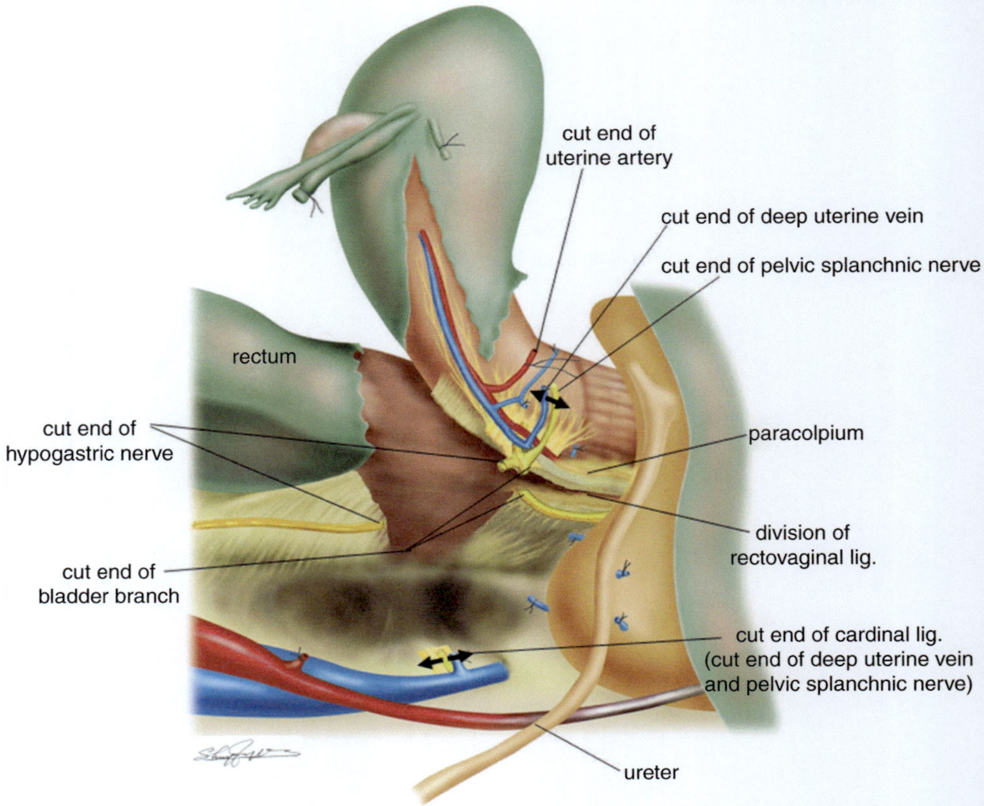


**Figure 6.78** The further direction of the division of the rectovaginal ligament is illustrated. The bladder branch from the hypogastric plexus is usually damaged or divided during the process of the division of the rectovaginal ligament

### 6.6.4 Division of the Paracolpium (Vaginal Blood Vessels) (Figure 6.79)

The division of the rectovaginal ligament can separate the vaginal blood vessels (the paracolpium) from the connective tissue of the rectal sidewall. The division is extended caudally to obtain vaginal length deemed appropriate by the extent of cervical disease. At the designated level, the blood vessels of the paracolpium are clamped, cut, and ligated.

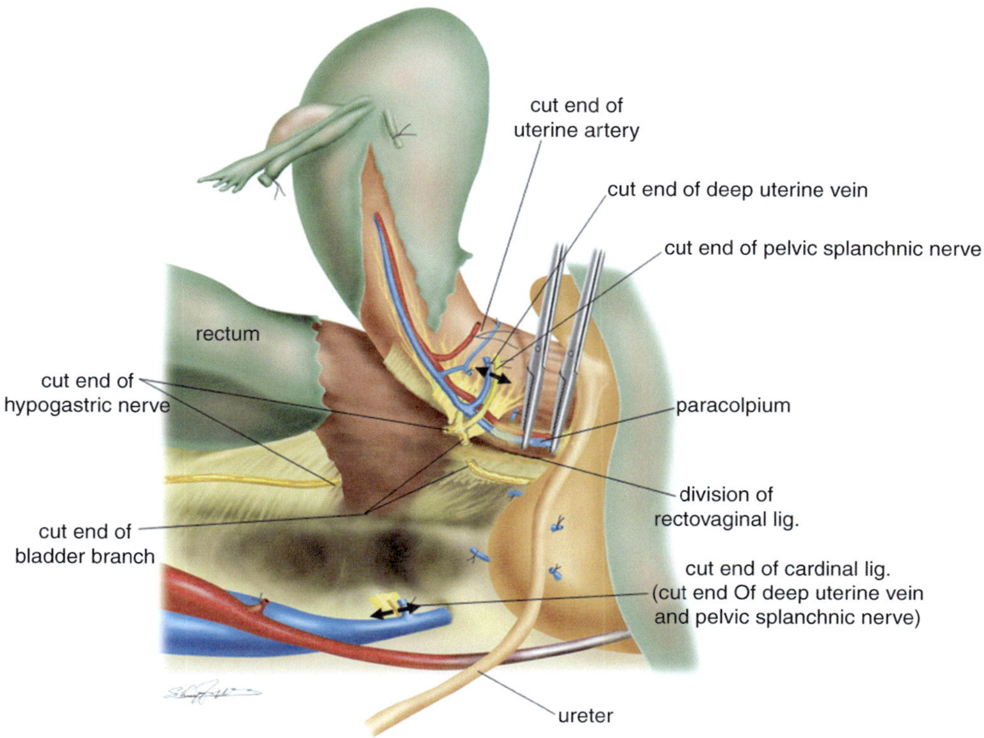


**Figure 6.79** Clamp the paracolpium (vaginal blood vessels) and divide between the two forceps

### 6.6.5 **Incision to the Vaginal Wall** (Figure 6.80)

The division of the paracolpium leads to the detachment of the uterus from all structures except the vagina. Once the paracolpium is divided bilaterally, the length of the vaginal cuff is confirmed. The incision is then made in the ventral wall of the vagina.

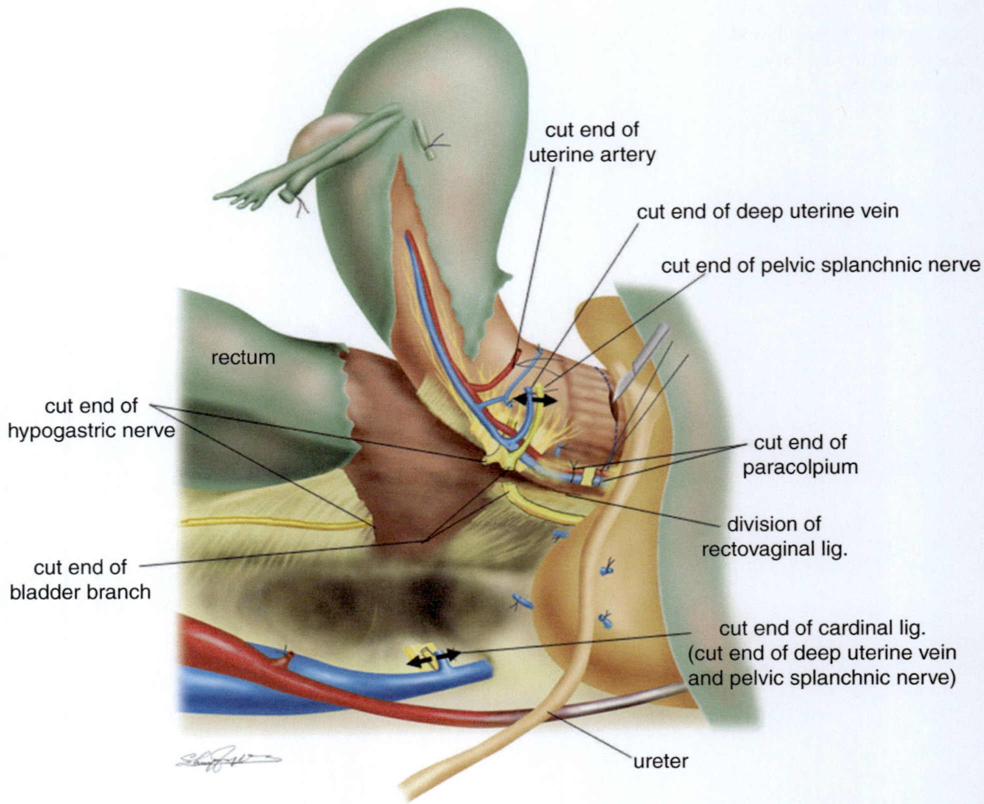


**Figure 6.80** Incision to the vaginal wall

### 6.6.6 Amputation of the Vaginal Wall and Closure of the Vaginal Cuff (Figure 6.81)

Figure 6.81 is a ventral side view of the extirpation of the uterus. Long L-shaped forceps is applied to the uterine side of the vagina at the level of vaginal length that is deemed appropriate for the disease state. Long L-shaped forceps can be used to secure the length of the vaginal cuff and for the confinement of cancer cells and fluid from the upper vagina. At the time of opening of the vaginal wall, the accumulated fluid and cancer cells are pushed down the vagina by placing a gauze in the vagina. At the division of the vaginal wall, long Kocher forceps is applied to the foot side of the divided vaginal wall. After extirpation of the uterus, each long Kocher forceps is replaced by ligature. Two to three interrupted stitches are taken from the ventral vaginal edge to the dorsal vaginal edge and the vaginal cuff is closed by ligature.

**Figure 6.81** Amputation of the vaginal wall

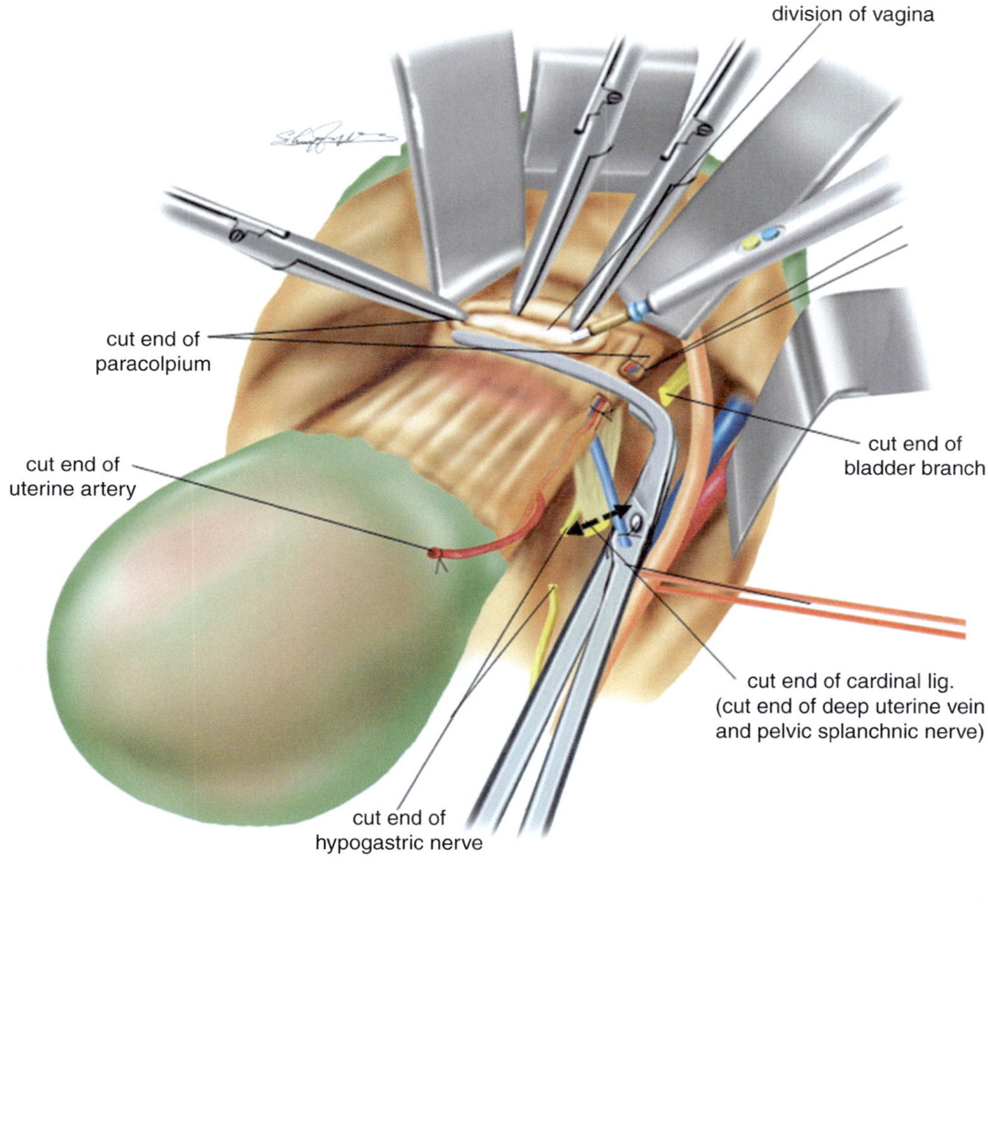

### 6.6.7 Partial Suture to the Pelvic Peritoneum and Insertion of Drains into the Retroperitoneal Space (Figure 6.82)

Careful observation of the pelvic cavity is undertaken to identify bleeding and ensure hemostasis. The pelvic cavity is then washed with saline water. Partial closure of the visceral peritoneum is undertaken between the peritoneum of the cranial side of the urinary bladder and the peritoneum of the Pouch of Douglas. The peritoneum of the ventral side of the pararectal space is not closed in order to facilitate absorption of lymph fluid by the surface of the peritoneum secondary to lymphadenectomy. Pelvic drains are inserted transabdominally into the retroperitoneal space bilaterally. The drainage tubes are usually removed if bleeding is not observed for 2 days.

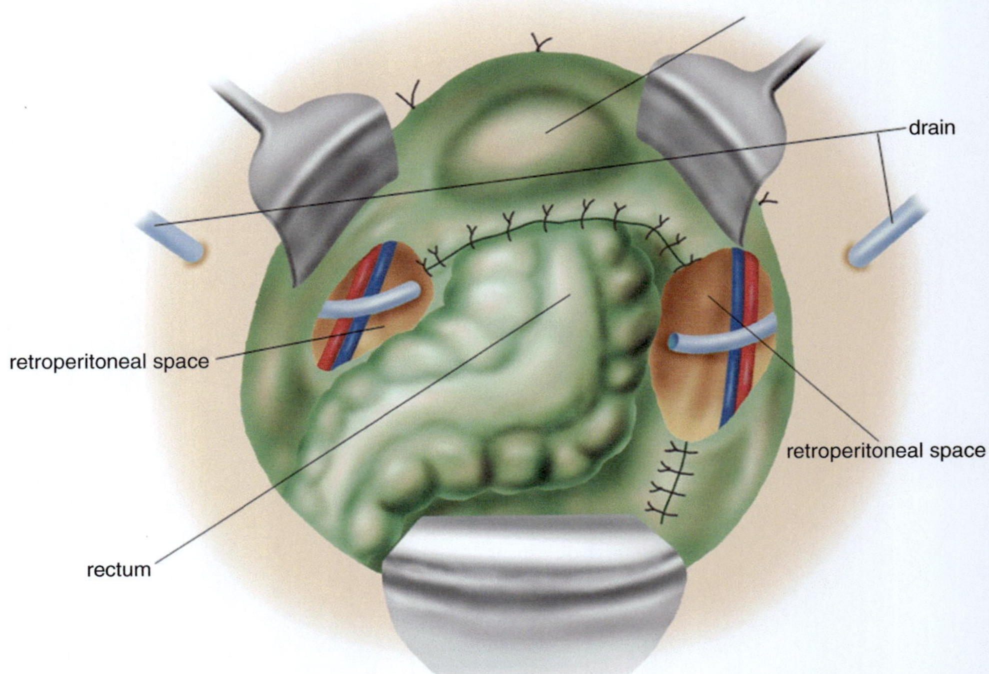


**Figure 6.82** Partial suture to the pelvic peritoneum and insertion of drains into the retroperitoneal space

### 6.6.8 Closure of the Abdominal Cavity (Figure 6.83)

Following closure of the ventral abdominal peritoneum and the fascia, interrupted skin suture is undertaken. Cosmetic sutures are popular now. Using a vaginal speculum, the packed gauze is removed from the vagina and the vaginal stump suture is checked. The surgery is now finished.

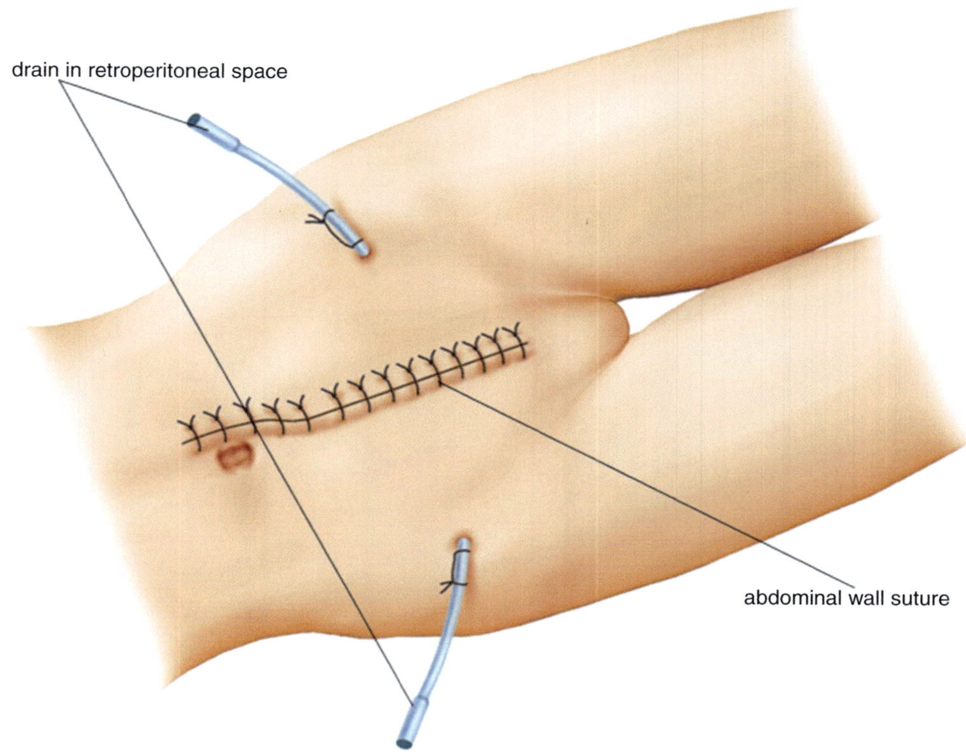


**Figure 6.83** Closure of the abdominal cavity

## References

1. Fujiwara T. Surgery for cervical cancer (in Japanese). Tokyo: Igakushoin; 1983.
2. Höckel M, Konerding MA, Heussel CP. Liposuction-assisted nerve-sparing extended radical hysterectomy: oncologic rationale, surgical anatomy, and feasibility study. Am J Obstet Gynecol. 1998;178:971–6.
3. Horn LC, Fischer U, Höckel M. Occult tumor cells in surgical specimens from cases of early cervical cancer treated by liposuction-assisted nerve-sparing radical hysterectomy. Int J Gynecol Cancer. 2001;11:159–63.

# 7 What Is Nerve-Sparing Radical Hysterectomy?

## 7.1 Severe Bladder Dysfunction/Colorectal Motility Disorders Are Common Complications of Radical Hysterectomy (Figure 7.1)

Since Wertheim introduced radical hysterectomy in 1911 [1], his method became the standard procedure for the surgical treatment of cervical cancer in Western Countries. However, in Japan, Takayama and Okabayashi at Kyoto Imperial University thought that Wertheim's method is not radical enough for invasive cervical cancers. They pursued to create a "better" surgery and Okabayashi established an anatomy oriented method to accomplish more radical surgery than that of Wertheim's method in 1921 [2]. However, postoperatively both methods have often been associated with severe bladder dysfunction and colorectal motility disorders that adversely impacted the patient's quality of life.

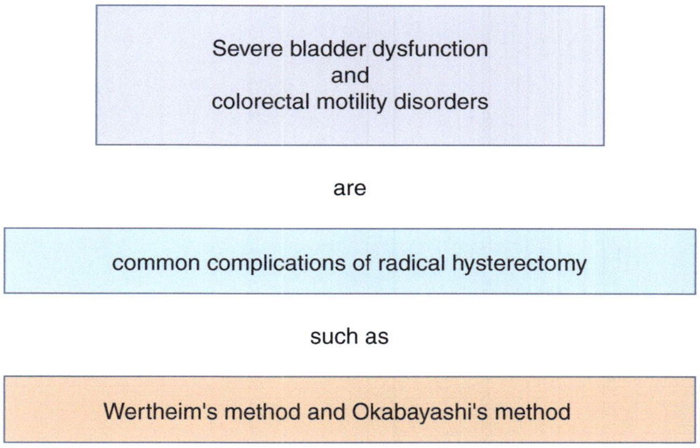


**Figure 7.1** Common complications of radical hysterectomy

---

**Electronic supplementary material** The online version of this chapter (https://doi.org/10.1007/978-981-13-8098-3_7) contains supplementary material, which is available to authorized users.


S. Fujii, K. Sekiyama, *Precise Neurovascular Anatomy for Radical Hysterectomy*, https://doi.org/10.1007/978-981-13-8098-3_7

### 7.1.1 Nerve Supply to the Uterus, Rectum, and Urinary Bladder (Figure 7.2)

The uterus, vagina, urinary bladder, and rectum are innervated by a motor and sensory autonomic nerve supply (sympathetic and parasympathetic origin). The sympathetic fibers come from T10-L2 to form the inferior hypogastric nerve. The parasympathetic fibers come from S2, 3 and 4 at the pelvic wall to form the pelvic splanchnic nerve. These fibers merge and construct the inferior hypogastric plexus that has branches to the uterus and to the urinary bladder [3–6].

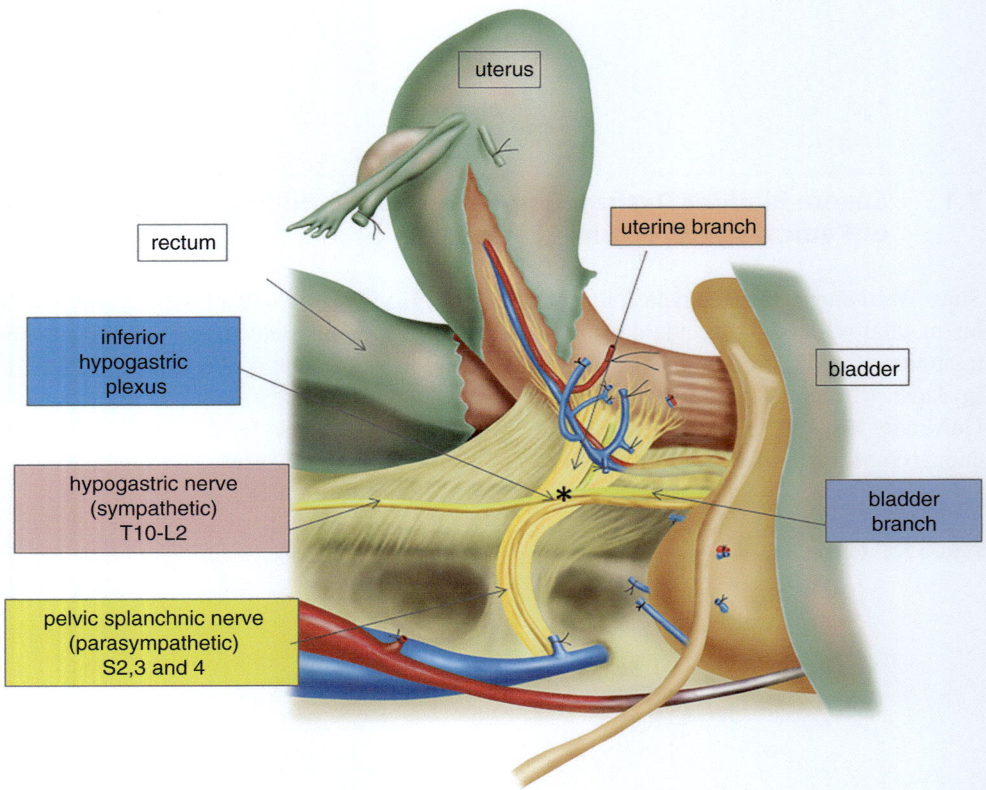


**Figure 7.2** Nerve supply to the uterus, rectum, and urinary bladder

### 7.1.2 Locations of Nerve Damages During Radical Hysterectomy (Figure 7.3)

During radical hysterectomy, such as Wertheim's method and Okabayashi's method, surgical procedures to the uterosacral ligament and the rectovaginal ligament can lead to injury of the hypogastric nerve [7, 8]. The surgical procedures to the paracolpium (vaginal blood vessels) can give rise to damage to the bladder branch of the inferior hypogastric plexus [7, 8]. During Okabayashi's method, the treatment to the deep uterine vein in the cardinal ligament can injure the pelvic splanchnic nerve. In contrast, Wertheim's method usually does not divide the deep uterine vein (cardinal ligament). Therefore, it appears unlikely to injure the pelvic splanchnic nerve. However, instead of dividing the cardinal ligament, Wertheim's method divides the paracervical tissues including the parametrial tissues and the paracolpium. During the division of the paracervical tissues, Wertheim's method increases the possibility of injury to the bladder branch from the inferior hypogastric plexus.

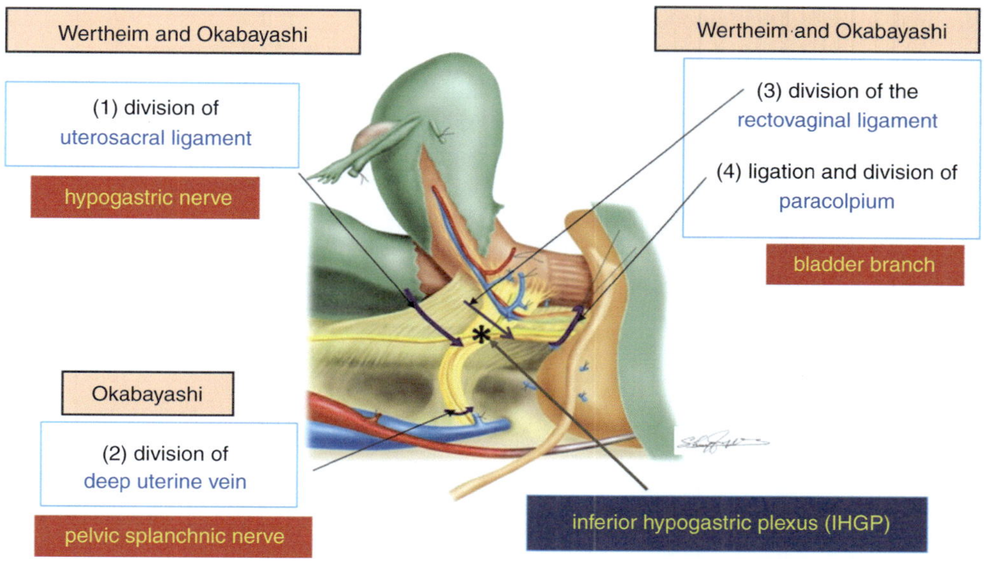


**Figure 7.3** Locations of nerve damages during radical hysterectomy

### 7.1.3 Efforts on Nerve-Sparing Radical Hysterectomy (Figure 7.4)

Japanese doctor Takashi Kobayashi at Tokyo University is a pioneer of the nerve-sparing radical hysterectomy. Modifying Okabayashi's radical hysterectomy Kobayashi tried to preserve nerve functions during radical hysterectomy. In 1961, Kobayashi [9] described the concept for the improvement of postoperative bladder function by preserving the pelvic splanchnic nerve by the separation of the vascular part (the deep uterine vein) from the dorsal hard bundle (the pelvic splanchnic nerve) during the division of the cardinal ligament. Sakamoto [10, 11] and Kuwabara [12] succeeded in these concepts. Then, in 1983, Fujiwara [13] at Kitano Hospital described the importance of the preservation of the hypogastric nerve with the pelvic splanchnic nerve and the bladder branch by the division of only the uterine branch from the inferior hypogastric plexus. Since then, many Japanese as well as Western countries' doctors started to undertake a nerve-sparing radical hysterectomy and published many papers on nerve-sparing radical hysterectomy [14–25]. Nevertheless, almost all published papers on nerve-sparing radical hysterectomy could not clearly show the surgical anatomy of the inferior hypogastric plexus with the bladder branch and the uterine branch. Publications using Wertheim or Piver Type III surgery show mainly the process of isolation of the inferior hypogastric nerve, and there is usually no clear description on the pelvic splanchnic nerve or the bladder branch from the inferior hypogastric plexus [14–20]. The reason is clear because Wertheim and Piver Type III surgeries neither reveal nor isolate the deep uterine vein beneath which the pelvic splanchnic nerve resides. Moreover, although these surgeries divide the anterior (ventral) leaf of the vesicouterine ligament, the concept of separation and division of the posterior (dorsal) leaf of the vesicouterine ligament, beneath which the bladder branch resides, is lacking. In contrast, Japanese doctors usually perform Okabayashi's radical hysterectomy [26]. Okabayashi's radical hysterectomy separates and divides the posterior (dorsal leaf of the vesicouterine ligament. Therefore, the publications from Japan have described both inferior hypogastric nerve and pelvic splanchnic nerve, and provided more information on the inferior hypogastric plexus [21–25]. In 2007, Fujii et al. [3] published a clear description of the surgical anatomy of the cross-shaped inferior hypogastric plexus (Figures 7.4, 7.5, and 7.6) and reported how to divide the uterine branch alone from the plexus. If the uterine branch is solely divided, the urinary bladder function is preserved following surgery. This publication stimulated and generated great interest in many doctors as a result of which nerve-sparing radical hysterectomy became very popular [27–29].

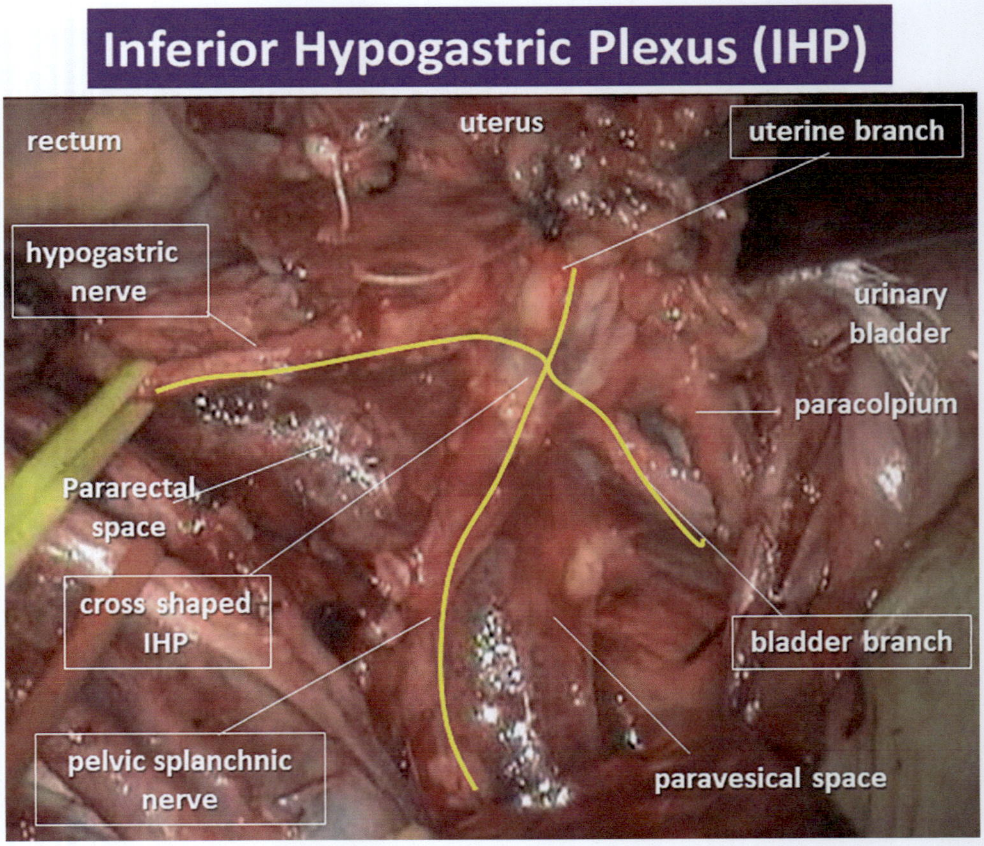


**Figure 7.4** Inferior hypogastric plexus: a photo of the cross-shaped inferior hypogastric nerve composed by the hypogastric nerve, pelvic splanchnic nerve, bladder branch and uterine branch during nerve-sparing radical hysterectomy

### 7.1.4 Principle of Nerve-Sparing Radical Hysterectomy (Figure 7.5)

The principle of nerve-sparing radical hysterectomy is very simple. Firstly, identification of the inferior hypogastric nerve, confirmation of the cross-shaped inferior hypogastric plexus and the branches to the uterus (uterine branch)/the urinary bladder (bladder branch) is required before the uterine branch can be isolated and divided.

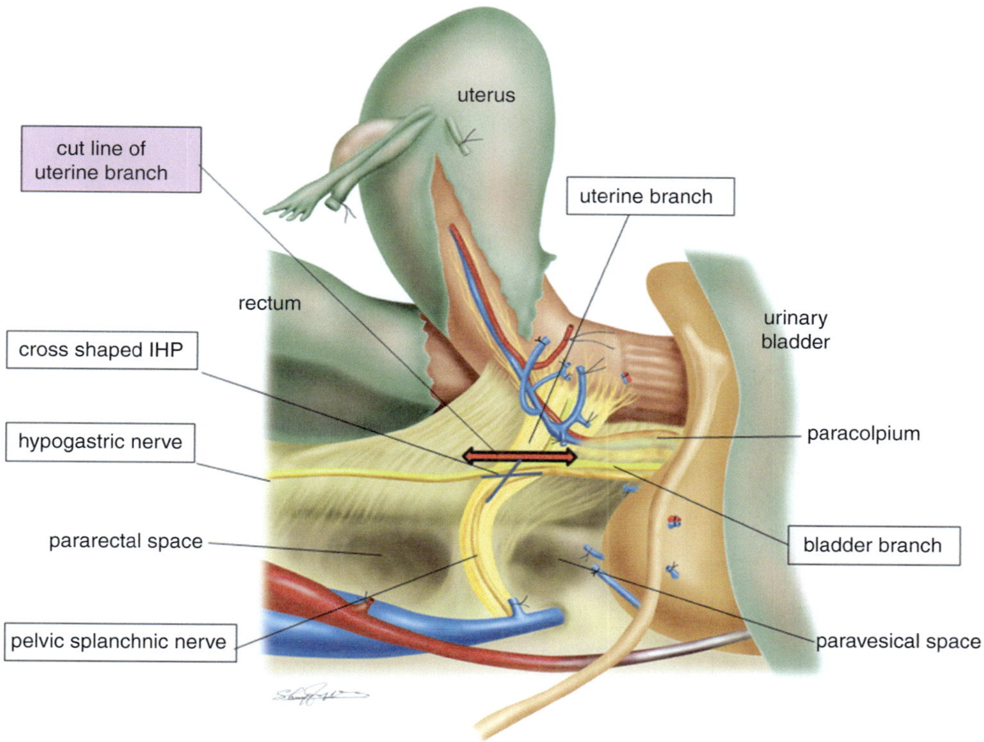


**Figure 7.5** The principle of nerve sparing radical hysterectomy: the division of solely the uterine branch from the inferior hypogastric nerve is illustrated as a red line with two-directional arrow

### 7.1.5 The Description of Anatomy for Nerve-Sparing Radical Hysterectomy (Figure 7.6)

By solely dividing the uterine branch, the cross-shaped inferior hypogastric plexus changes into a T-shaped one composed of hypogastric nerve, the pelvic splanchnic nerve, and the bladder branch. The preservation of the T-shaped inferior hypogastric plexus is the goal of nerve-sparing radical hysterectomy. This provides the outcome of satisfactory urinary function for patients.

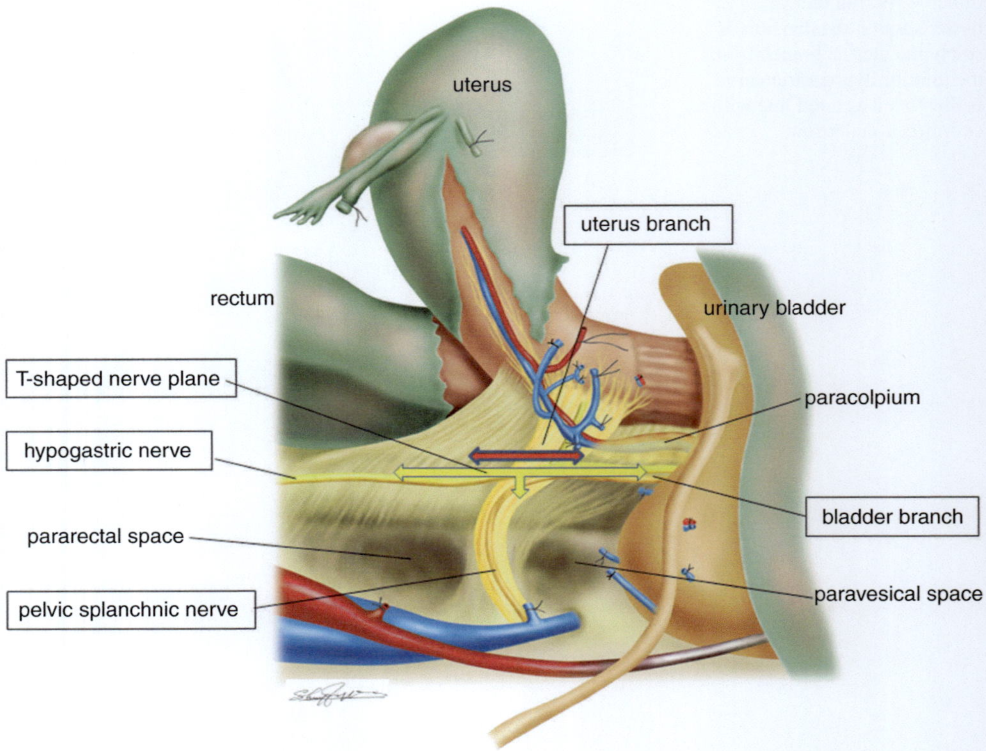


**Figure 7.6** By the division of solely the uterine branch (shown as a red line with two-directional arrow), the cross-shaped inferior hypogastric plexus changes into a T-shaped one (shown as a yellow T-shaped line with three-directional arrow)

### 7.1.6 Indication of Nerve-Sparing Radical Hysterectomy (Figure 7.7)

The nerve-sparing radical hysterectomy separates and preserves medially one tissue's layer (containing the pelvic nerve plane) more than that of the classical radical hysterectomy. Therefore, the indication of nerve-sparing radical hysterectomy should be reserved for patients with FIGO IB stage disease. In case of stage IB2 disease, if invasion is strongly suspected, the preservation of the nerve is not recommended. For patients with FIGO IIB stage disease, nerve-sparing procedures should not be selected because the location of the inferior hypogastric plexus is usually very close to the invasive foci of IIB lesion. In such cases, if the invasion is confined to only one side of the parametrium, nerve-sparing surgery on the opposite side is feasible. The preservation of unilateral T-shaped inferior hypogastric plexus can also result in satisfactory bladder function. However, it is very important to confirm the extension of the cancer lesion very carefully. In case of younger patients with an invasive lesion in the cardinal ligament on either side, total extirpation of the cardinal ligament with internal iliac blood vessel system (TEIIBS) or lateral extended parametrectomy (LEP) is the choice of surgery. However if the opposite side does not contain invasive disease, unilateral nerve-sparing radical hysterectomy can be a surgical option for that side. If we can preserve T-shaped nerve plane in either side of the rectum, urinary function is preserved in the patient.

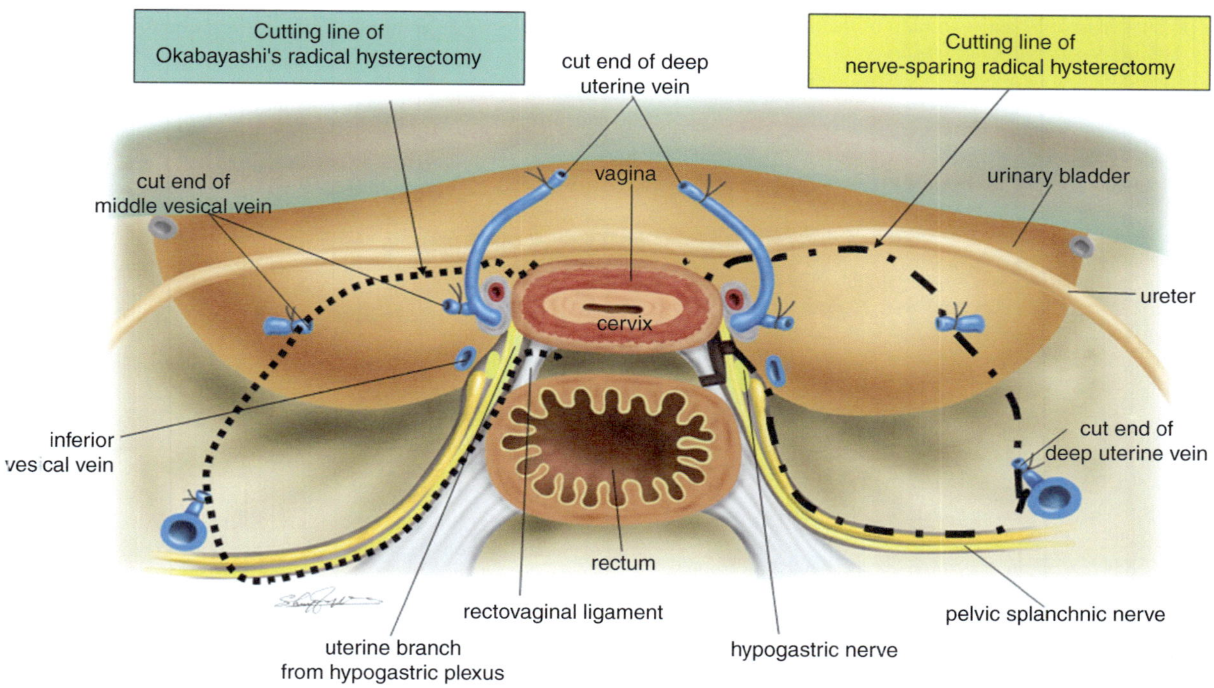


**Figure 7.7** On a cross section of the pelvis at the level of the cervix in the vagina, the cutting line of Okabayashi's radical hysterectomy is illustrated as a dotted line (left side of the pelvis). A dotted line using two different lengths in the right side of the pelvis is showing the cutting line of nerve-sparing radical hysterectomy

## References


1. Wertheim E. Die erweiterte abdominale Operation bei Carcinoma colli Uteri (auf Grund von 500 Fallen). Berlin: Urban & Schwarzenberg; 1911.
2. Okabayashi H. Radical abdominal hysterectomy for cancer of the cervix uteri, modification of the Takayama operation. Surg Gynecol Obstet. 1921;33:335–41.
3. Fujii S, Takakura K, Matsumura N, Higuchi T, Yura S, Mandai M, Baba T, Yoshioka S. Anatomic identification and functional outcomes of the nerve sparing Okabayashi radical hysterectomy. Gynecol Oncol. 2007;107:4–13.
4. Maas CP, Trimbos JB, DeRuiter MC, van de Velde CJ, Kenter GG. Nerve sparing radical hysterectomy: latest developments and historical perspective. Crit Rev Oncol Hematol. 2003;48:271–9.
5. Dursun P, Ayhan A, Kuscu E. Nerve-sparing radical hysterectomy for cervical carcinoma. Crit Rev Oncol Hematol. 2009;70:195–205.
6. Rob L, Halaska M, Robova H. Nerve-sparing and individually tailored surgery for cervical cancer. Lancet Oncol. 2010;11:292–301.
7. Fujii S. Original film of the Okabayashi's radical hysterectomy by Okabayashi himself in 1932, and two films of the precise anatomy necessary for nerve-sparing Okabayashi's radical hysterectomy clarified by Shingo Fujii. Int J Gynecol Cancer. 2008;18:383–5.
8. Fujii S. Anatomic identification of nerve-sparing radical hysterectomy: a step-by-step procedure. Gynecol Oncol. 2008;111:S33–41.
9. Kobayashi T. Abdominal radical hysterectomy with pelvic lymphadenectomy for cancer of the cervix (in Japanese). Tokyo: Nanzando; 1961.
10. Sakamoto S. Radical hysterectomy with pelvic lymphadenectomy—the Tokyo method. In: Coppleson M, editor. Gynecologic oncology. 2nd ed. Edinburg: Churchill Livingstone; 1992. p. 1257–68.
11. Sakamoto S, Takizawa K. An improved radical hysterectomy with fewer urological complications and with no loss of therapeutic results for invasive cervical cancer. Baillieres Clin Obstet Gynaecol. 1988;2:953–62.
12. Kuwabara Y, Suzuki M, Hashimoto M, Furugen Y, Yoshida K, Mitsuhashi N. New method to prevent bladder dysfunction after radical hysterectomy for uterine cervical cancer. J Obstet Gynaecol Res. 2000;26:1–8.
13. Fujiwara T. Surgery for cervical cancer (in Japanese). Tokyo: Igakushoin; 1983.
14. Possover M, Stöber S, Plaul K, Schneider A. Identification and preservation of the motoric innervation of the bladder in radical hysterectomy type III. Gynecol Oncol. 2000;79:154–7.
15. Trimbos JB, Maas CP, Deruiter MC, Peters AA, Kenter GG. A nerve-sparing radical hysterectomy: guidelines and feasibility in Western patients. Int J Gynecol Cancer. 2001;11:180–6.
16. Barton DP, Butler-Manuel SA, Buttery LD, A'Hern RP, Polak JM. A nerve-sparing radical hysterectomy: guidelines and feasibility in Western patients. Int J Gynecol Cancer. 2002;12:319.
17. Possover M. Technical modification of the nerve-sparing laparoscopy-assisted vaginal radical hysterectomy type 3 for better reproducibility of this procedure. Gynecol Oncol. 2003;90:245–7.
18. Raspagliesi F, Ditto A, Fontanelli R, Solima E, Hanozet F, Zanaboni F, Kusamura S. Nerve-sparing radical hysterectomy: a surgical technique for preserving the autonomic hypogastric nerve. Gynecol Oncol. 2004;93:307–14.
19. Maas CP, Kenter GG, Trimbos JB, Deruiter MC. Anatomical basis for nerve-sparing radical hysterectomy: immunohistochemical study of the pelvic autonomic nerves. Acta Obstet Gynecol Scand. 2005;84:868–74.
20. Raspagliesi F, Ditto A, Fontanelli R, Zanaboni F, Solima E, Spatti G, Hanozet F, Vecchione F, Rossi G, Kusamura S. Type II versus type III nerve-sparing radical hysterectomy: comparison of lower urinary tract dysfunctions. Gynecol Oncol. 2006;102:256–62.
21. Murakami G, Yabuki Y, Kato T. A nerve-sparing radical hysterectomy: guidelines and feasibility in Western patients. Int J Gynecol Cancer. 2002;12:319–21.
22. Kato T, Murakami G, Yabuki Y. A new perspective on nerve-sparing radical hysterectomy: nerve topography and over-preservation of the cardinal ligament. Jpn J Clin Oncol. 2003;33:589–91.
23. Sakuragi N, Todo Y, Kudo M, Yamamoto R, Sato T. A systematic nerve-sparing radical hysterectomy technique in invasive cervical cancer for preserving postsurgical bladder function. Int J Gynecol Cancer. 2005;15:389–97.
24. Katahira A, Niikura H, Kaiho Y, Nakagawa H, Kurokawa K, Arai Y, Yaegashi N. Intraoperative electrical stimulation of the pelvic splanchnic nerves during nerve-sparing radical hysterectomy. Gynecol Oncol. 2005;98:462–6.
25. Kato K, Suzuka K, Osaki T, Tanaka N. Unilateral or bilateral nerve-sparing radical hysterectomy: a surgical technique to preserve the pelvic autonomic nerves while increasing radicality. Int J Gynecol Cancer. 2007;17:1172–8.
26. Okabayashi H. Abdominale systematische Panhysterektomie fur Karzinoma des Uterus. Jpn J Obstet Gynecol. 1928;11:136–53.
27. Magrina JF, Pawlina W, Kho RM, Magtibay PM. Robotic nerve-sparing radical hysterectomy: feasibility and technique. Gynecol Oncol. 2011;121:605–9.
28. Narducci F, Collinet P, Merlot B, Lambaudie E, Boulanger L, Lefebvre-Kuntz D, Nickers P, Taieb S, Houvenaeghel G, Leblanc E. Benefit of robot-assisted laparoscopy in nerve-sparing radical hysterectomy: urinary morbidity in early cervical cancer. Surg Endosc. 2013;27:1237–42.
29. Sakuragi N. Nerve-sparing radical hysterectomy: time for a new standard of care for cervical cancer? J Gynecol Oncol. 2015;26:81–2.

# 8 Step-by-Step Nerve-Sparing Radical Hysterectomy with Pelvic Lymphadenectomy

## 8.1 The Surgical Process of the Step-by-Step Nerve-Sparing Radical Hysterectomy Is Listed in the Following Pages

However, each surgical procedure until the division of the deep uterine vein in the cardinal ligament is the same as that of the step-by-step radical hysterectomy without nerve-sparing radical hysterectomy as described in Chap. 5. Therefore, the detailed surgical procedure necessary for nerve-sparing radical hysterectomy shall start from the division of the cardinal ligament.

## 8.2 The Following Are Described in Chap. 6

1. Open the abdominal cavity
2. Exposure of the pelvic cavity
3. Visual and manual examination of the spread of the disease and operability
4. Traction of the uterus
5. Ligation and division of the round ligament (open the connective tissue of the broad ligament)
6. Ligation and division of suspensory ligament of ovary (ovarian vessels) and confirmation of the ureter
7. Tentative development of the pararectal space
8. Division of the peritoneum of the Douglas' pouch
9. Separation of the peritoneum of the vesicouterine pouch
10. Pelvic lymphadenectomy

## 8.3 Contents in Chap. 8

1. Treatment of the cardinal ligament
2. Treatment of the hypogastric nerve
3. Development of the rectovaginal space and division of the uterosacral ligament
4. Separation of the urinary bladder and anatomy of the vesicouterine ligament
5. Treatment of the anterior(ventral) leaf of the vesicouterine ligament
6. Treatment of the posterior (dorsal) leaf of the vesicouterine ligament
7. Confirmation of the inferior hypogastric plexus
8. The concept of the pelvic nerve plane
9. Separation of the rectovaginal ligament
10. Separation of the bladder branch from the paracolpium
11. Separation of the uterine branch from the inferior hypogastric plexus
12. Division of the uterine branch
13. Separation of the rectovaginal ligament preserving T-shaped nerve plane
14. Clamp of the paracolpium
15. Ligation and division of the paracolpium
16. Incise the vaginal wall for amputation of the vagina
17. Removal of the uterus preserving T-shaped nerve plan
18. Closure of the vaginal cuff
19. Partial suture to the pelvic peritoneum and insertion of drains into the retroperitoneal space
20. Closure of the abdominal wall
21. Treatment after the operation

**Electronic supplementary material** The online version of this chapter (https://doi.org/10.1007/978-981-13-8098-3_8) contains supplementary material, which is available to authorized users.



S. Fujii, K. Sekiyama, *Precise Neurovascular Anatomy for Radical Hysterectomy*,
https://doi.org/10.1007/978-981-13-8098-3_8

## 8.4 Treatment of the Cardinal Ligament

### 8.4.1 A View of Pelvis After the Lymphadenectomy (Figure 8.1)

After pelvic lymphadenectomy, both the external and internal iliac blood vessels are almost skeletonized with a view of the obturator nerve and artery/vein in the obturator fossa. The paravesical space and Latzko's pararectal space are well recognized.

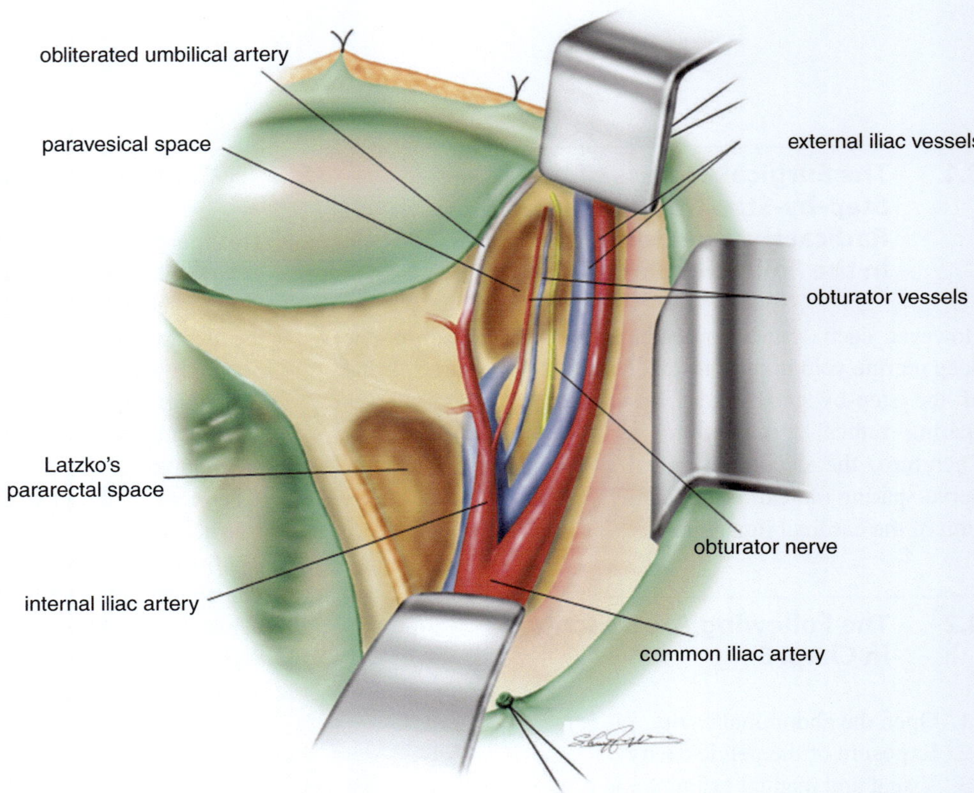


**Figure 8.1** A view of pelvis after the lymphadenectomy

### 8.4.2 Separation of the Loose Connective Tissue Between the Uterine Artery and Superior Vesical Artery (Figure 8.2)

In order to give tension to the uterine artery, the obliterated umbilical artery (bladder side of the internal iliac artery) is picked up with the forceps, and the loose connective tissue between the urinary bladder and the obliterated umbilical artery is separated. The loose connective tissue layer between the uterine artery and the superior vesical artery is separated. The connective tissue layer is separated and penetrated, to enter the paravesical space.

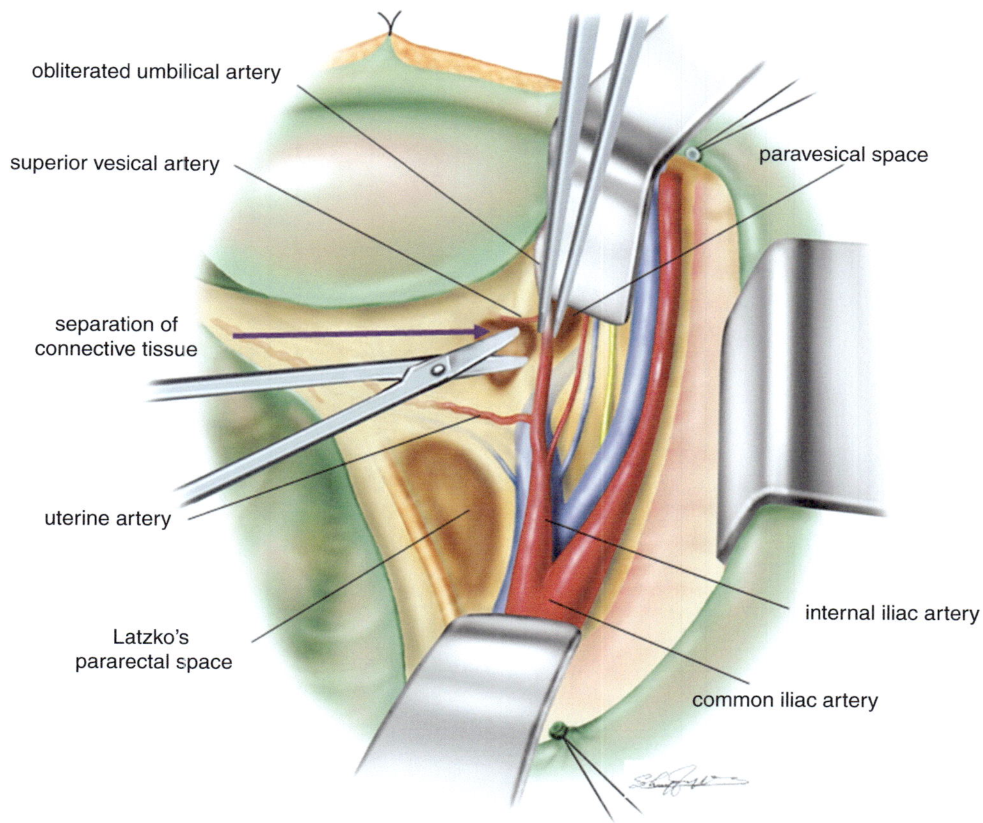


**Figure 8.2** Separation of the loose connective tissue between the uterine artery and superior vesical artery

### 8.4.3 Development of the Paravesical Space and Confirmation of the Uterine Artery (Figure 8.3)

A long L-shaped retractor is inserted through the penetrated connective tissue and into the paravesical space to retract the tissue (including the isolated obliterated umbilical artery) toward the inguinal side. The uterine artery from the internal iliac artery is stretched between its origin of the internal iliac artery and the side wall of the uterus. This is a safer way to expose the uterine artery along its whole length.

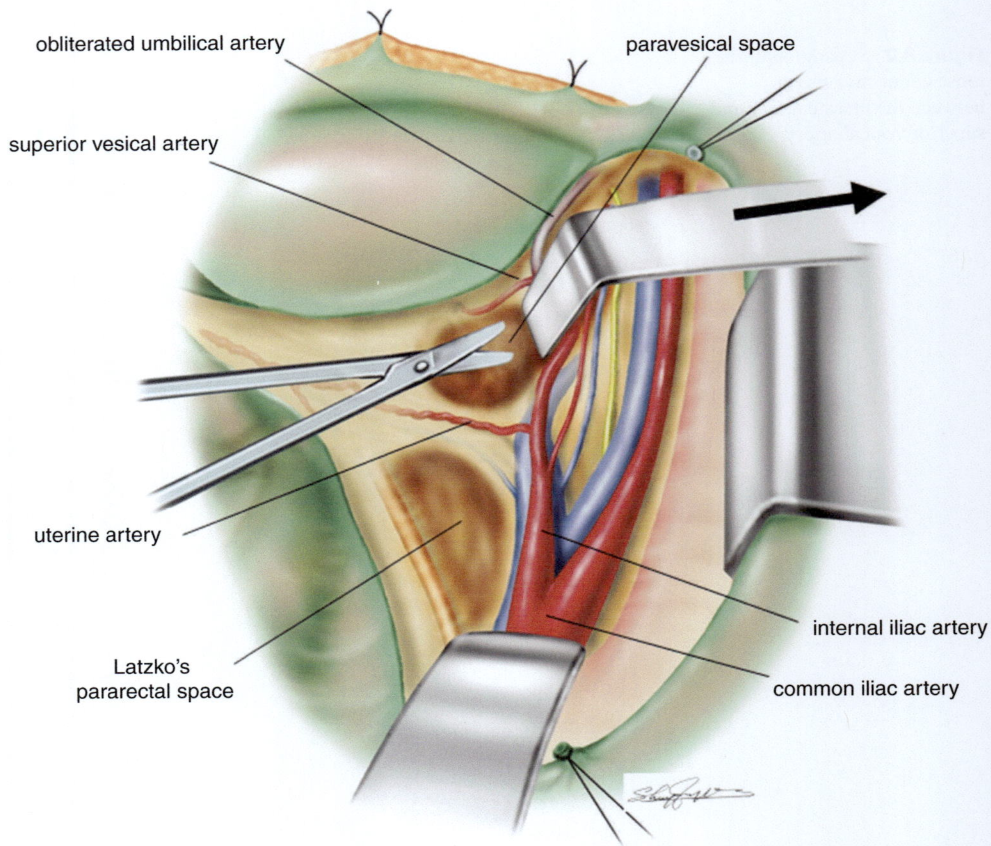


**Figure 8.3** Separation of the uterine artery

### 8.4.4 **Confirmation of the Cardinal Ligament** (Figure 8.4)

Another long L-shaped retractor is inserted into the pararectal space to push the rectum craniolateral side. The pararectal space is gradually expanded. Insertion of the L-retractor too deep into the pelvic floor risks the pelvic floor connective tissue being torn, resulting in bleeding which can be difficult to manage. Therefore, diligent placement of retractor tip in the pararectal space is important. The thick connective tissue bundle created between the paravesical space and pararectal space is a gross feature of the cardinal ligament (a two-directional arrow in Figure 8.4). The cardinal ligament is a thick connective tissue bundle formed between the internal iliac blood vessels and the sidewall of the uterus/upper vagina. The uterine artery and the superficial uterine vein run along the most ventral side of the cardinal ligament.

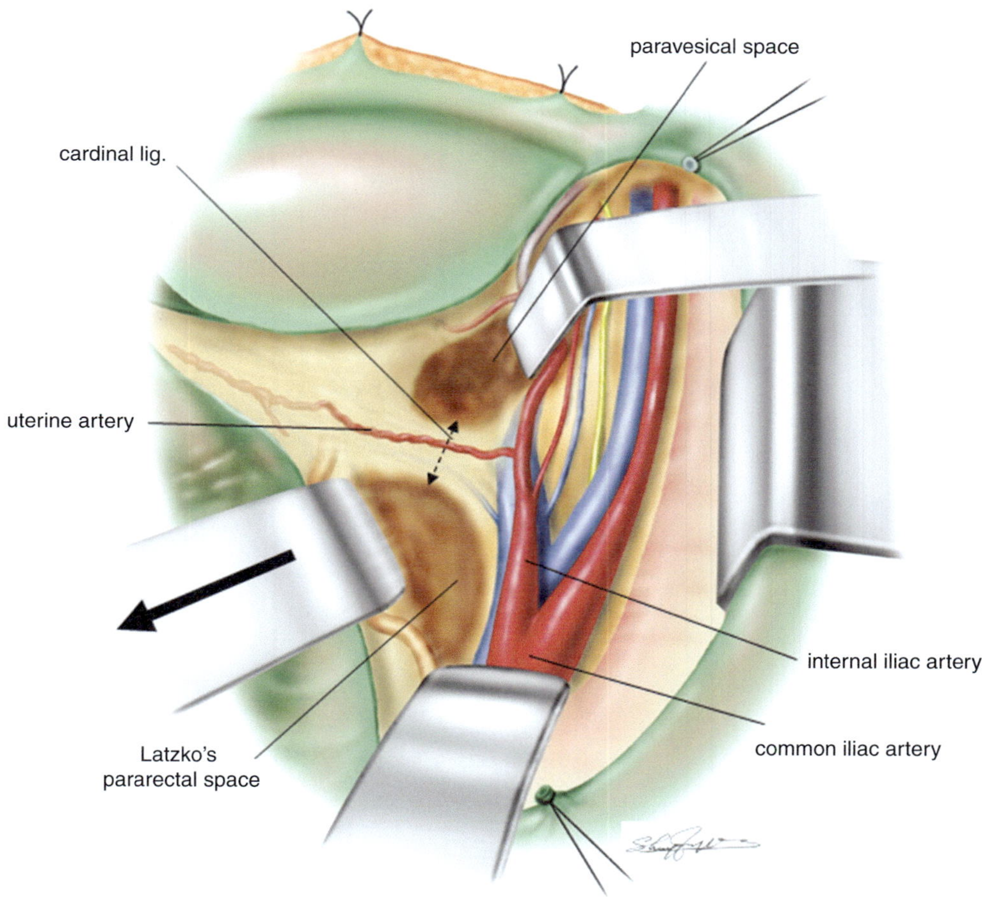


**Figure 8.4** Confirmation of the cardinal ligament. A two directional arrow is indicating the connective tissue bundle of the cardinal ligament surgically created between the pararectal space and paravesical space

### 8.4.5 Isolation and Division of the Uterine Artery (Figure 8.5)

The uterine artery originates from the internal iliac artery and passes into the sidewall of the uterus. The uterine artery is appreciated on the most ventral side of the cardinal ligament. The uterine artery is easily isolated, doubly clamped, and ligated. The uterine artery between the two ligatures is divided. The suture of the uterine side of the uterine artery is usually left as a longer piece to act as an anatomical landmark.

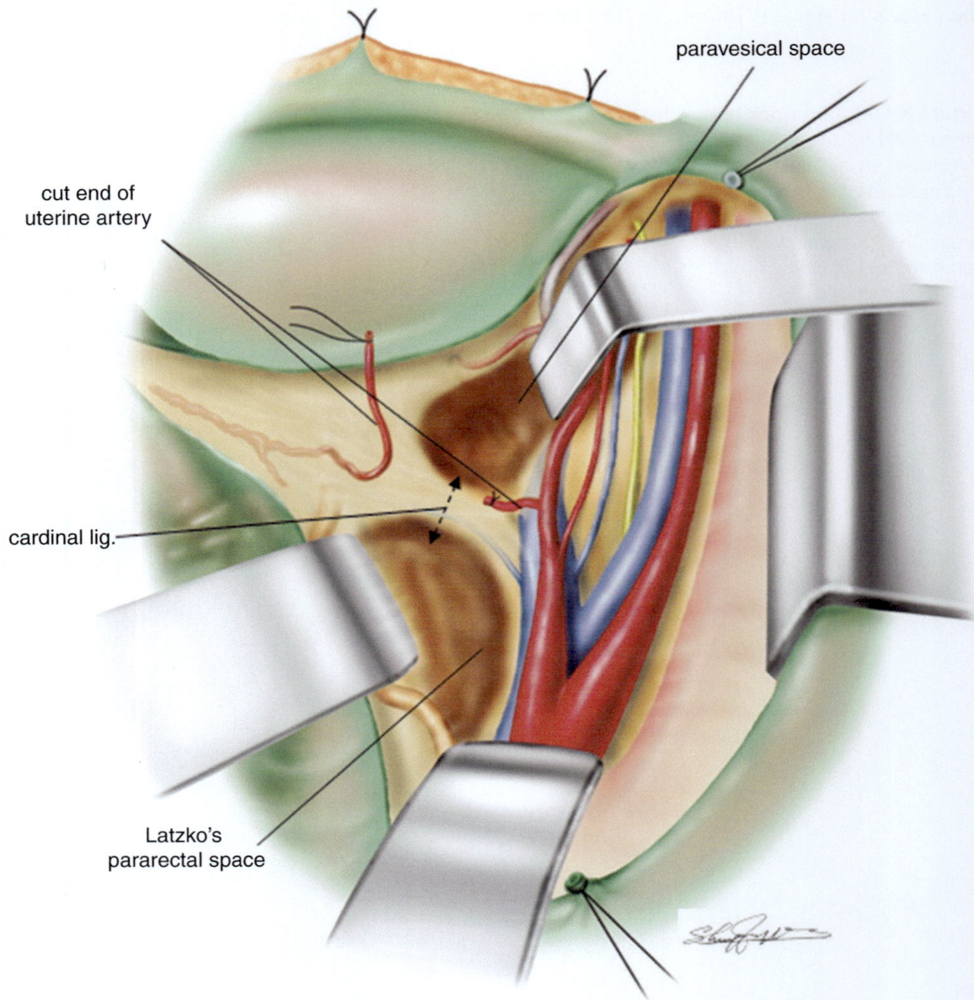


**Figure 8.5** Development of the paravesical space and confirmation of the uterine artery

### 8.4.6 Separation of the Superficial Uterine Vein (Figure 8.6)

Careful separation of the cut-end of uterine side of the uterine artery from the connective tissue of the cardinal ligament usually reveals the superficial uterine vein running parallel to the uterine artery. The superficial uterine vein is often fragile. Therefore, in order to isolate the superficial uterine vein, a careful approach is required. If the vessel is inadvertently damaged, monopolar or bipolar coagulation can be effective in achieving hemostasis. The superficial uterine vein does not always run parallel to the uterine artery. Rarely, it may run parallel to the ureter.

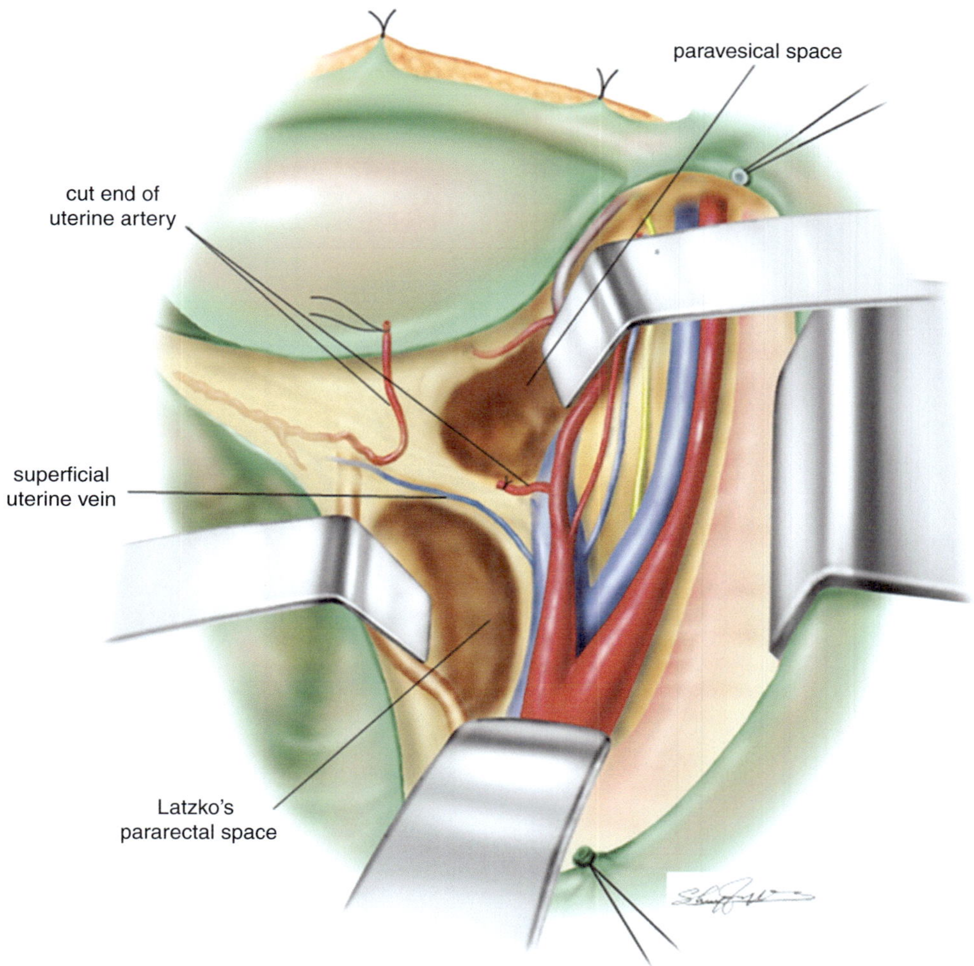


**Figure 8.6** Separation of the superficial uterine vein

### 8.4.7 Clamping and Division of the Superficial Uterine Vein (Figure 8.7)

The superficial uterine vein is isolated and doubly clamped by Pean forceps. Then the superficial uterine vein is divided between the two clamps. Each clamp is replaced by ligature. The connective tissue of the cardinal ligament is then separated toward the pelvic floor. In the cardinal ligament, a small vein or artery may be identified. In such cases, each small blood vessel should be sealed either by electrocautery or ligature. However, the deep uterine vein always resides in the dorsal part of the cardinal ligament. Careful separation of the connective tissue and lymph nodes in the cardinal ligament is required to identify the deep uterine vein.

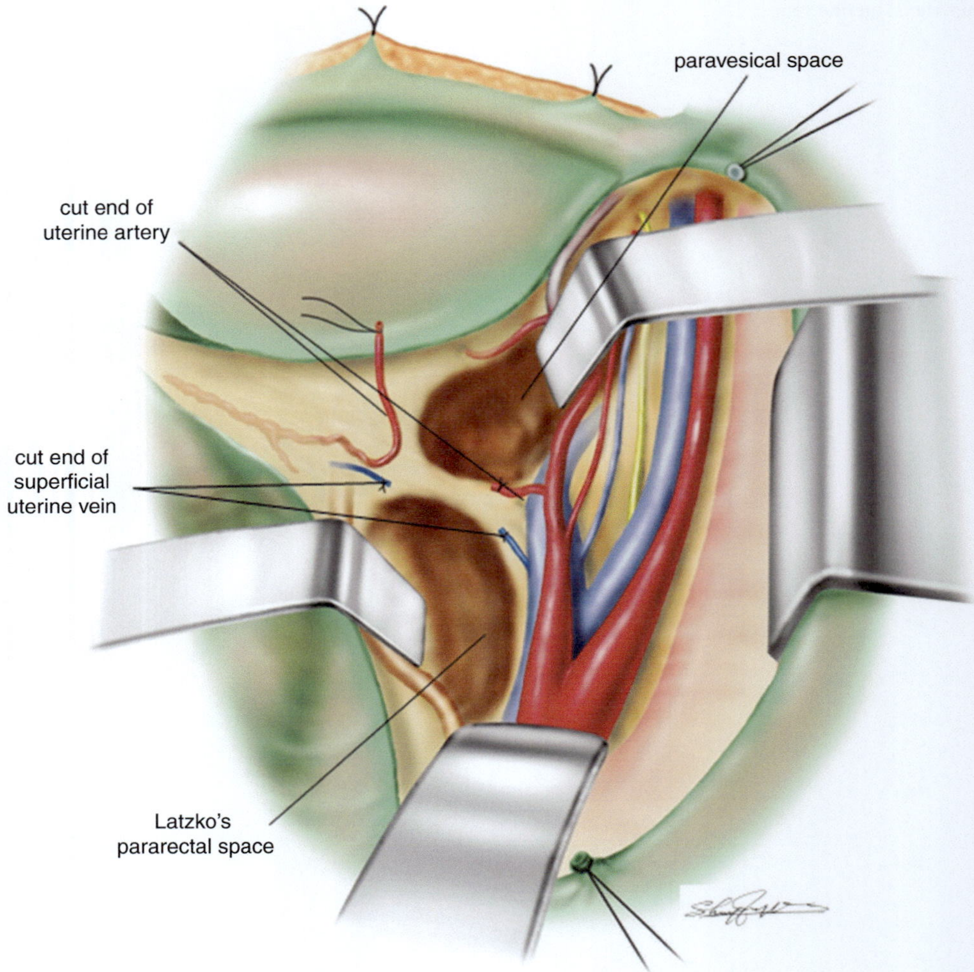


**Figure 8.7** Division of the superficial uterine vein

### 8.4.8 **Separation of the Deep Uterine Vein** (Figure 8.8)

Careful separation of the connective tissue and lymph nodes in the cardinal ligament can reveal a vein running from the uterine sidewall to the internal iliac vein (Figure 8.8a, b). This is the deep uterine vein. The connective tissue and adipose tissue surrounding the deep uterine vein should be cleaned as much as possible. Skeletonizing the dorsal side of the deep uterine vein is very important for the isolation of the deep uterine vein.

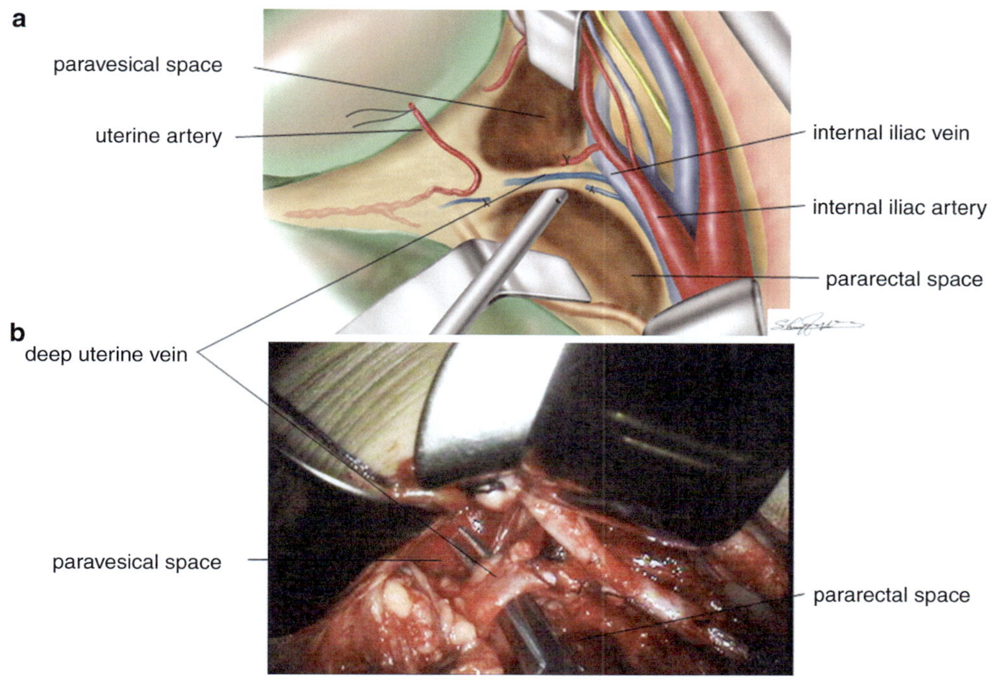


**Figure 8.8** Separation of the deep uterine vein. (**a**) is illustrating the deep uterine vein running between the uterine cervix and the internal iliac vein. (**b**) is a surgical photo of the deep uterine vein isolated between the uterine cervix and the internal iliac vein

### 8.4.9 Division of the Deep Uterine Vein Reveals the Pelvic Splanchnic Nerve (Figure 8.9)

In the dorsal part of the deep uterine vein, a white yellow bundle is usually running parallel to it. This is the pelvic splanchnic nerve. After isolation, the deep uterine vein is doubly clamped by Pean forceps. The deep uterine vein is then divided between the two clamps. Each clamp is replaced by ligature. There is a risk of heavy bleeding if the deep uterine vein is injured. However, hemostasis can be achieved effectively if the deep uterine vein has been clearly identified, and the damaged portion of the vessel can be detected. The skeletonization of the connective tissue and the adipose tissue in the base of the cardinal ligament (draining portion of the deep uterine vein into the internal iliac vein) is a very important step in performing safer nerve-sparing radical hysterectomy.

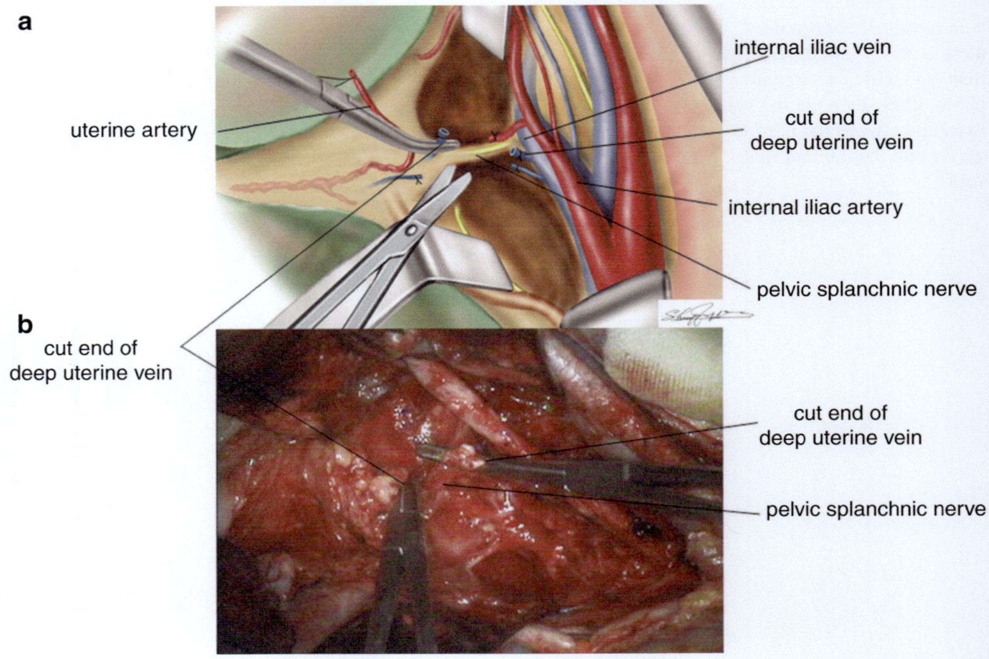


**Figure 8.9** Division of the deep uterine vein reveals the pelvic splanchnic nerve beneath the vein. (**a**) Relationship between the divided deep uterine vein and the pelvic splanchnic nerve. (**b**) A surgical photo of the divided deep uterine vein and the pelvic splanchnic nerve

## 8.5 Treatment of the Hypogastric Nerve

### 8.5.1 Isolation of the Hypogastric Nerve (Figure 8.10)

In the rectal sidewall of the pararectal space, 2–3 cm dorsal to the ureter, a white yellow bundle of the hypogastric nerve is appreciated. The hypogastric nerve is residing in the same connective tissue of the ureter. The hypogastric nerve is dissected and separated from the rectal sidewall.

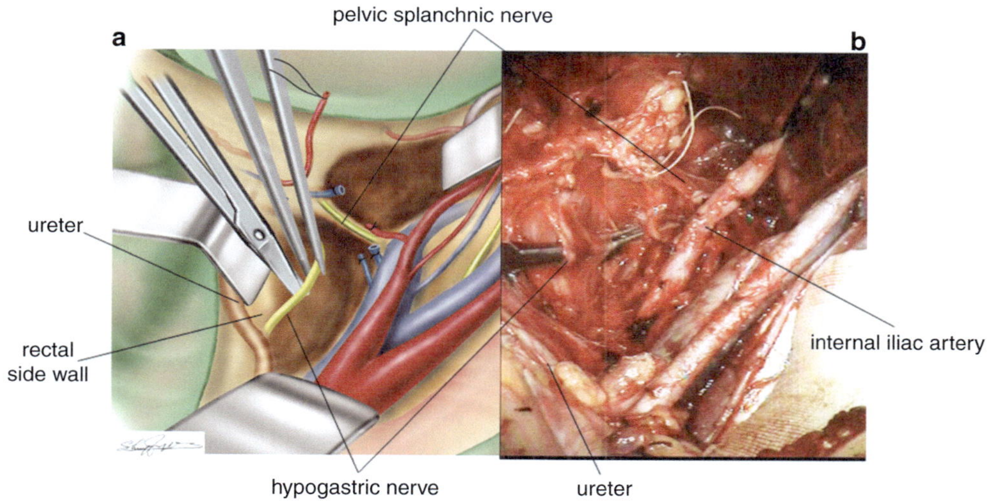


**Figure 8.10** Isolation of the hypogastric nerve. (**a**) An illustration of the separated hypogastric nerve from the lateral side wall of the rectum. (**b**) A surgical photo of the hypogastric nerve isolated from the lateral side wall of the rectum

### 8.5.2 Apply a Vessel Tape to the Isolated Hypogastric Nerve (Figure 8.11)

A vessel tape is applied for a marker of the isolated hypogastric nerve. The hypogastric nerve is better separated as close as possible to the uterine side of the pelvic splanchnic nerve.

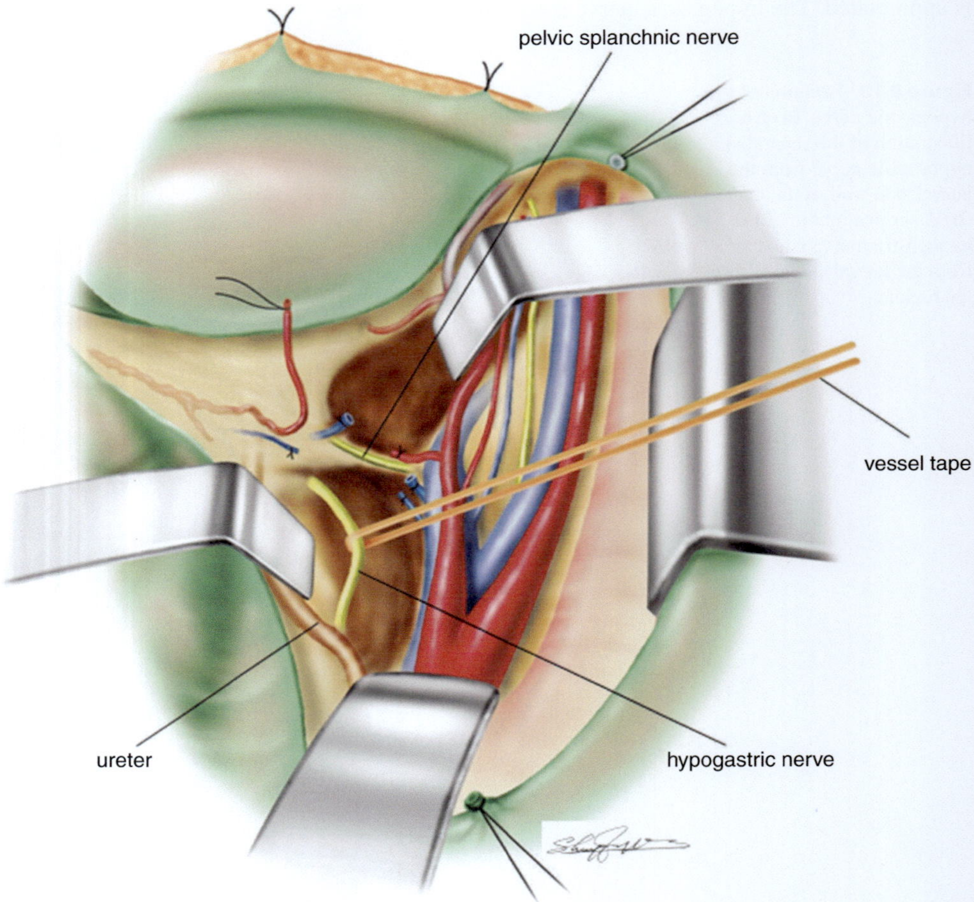


**Figure 8.11** Application of a vessel tape to the isolated hypogastric nerve

### 8.5.3 Separation of the Ureter from the Connective Tissue Plane and Application of a Vessel Tape to the Isolated Ureter (Figure 8.12)

The ureter can be identified on the ventral side of the hypogastric nerve. The ureter is isolated and a vessel tape is applied as a marker. The ureter is better separated as close as possible to the cut-end of the uterine side of the uterine artery.

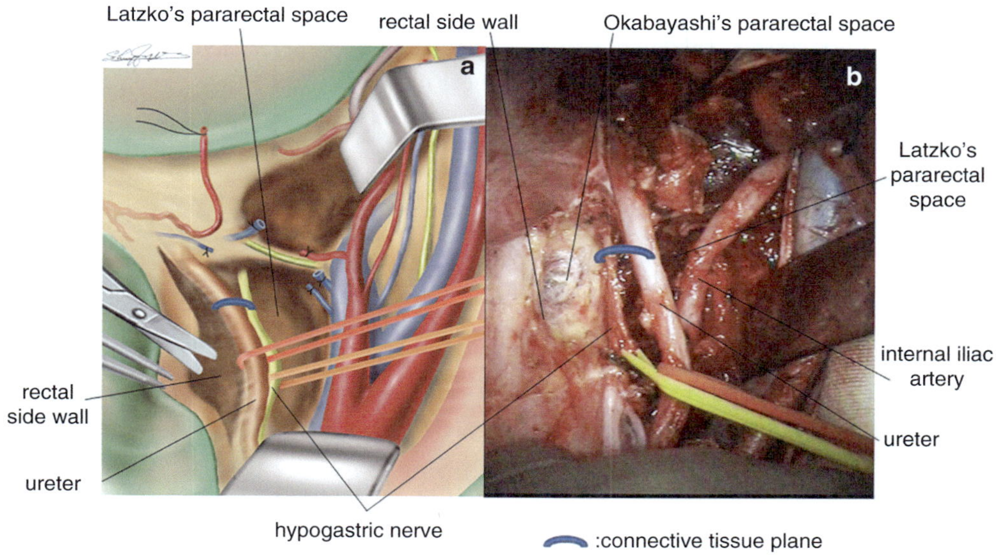


**Figure 8.12** Separation of the ureter from the connective tissue plane and application of a vessel tape to the isolated ureter. (**a**) A illustration of the isolated ureter and the hypogastric nerve with respective vessel tape. (**b**) A surgical photo of the isolated ureter and the hypogastric nerve with respective vessel tape

## 8.6 Development of the Rectovaginal Space and Division of the Uterosacral Ligament

### 8.6.1 Separation and Division of the Peritoneum of the Douglas' Pouch (Figure 8.13)

The uterus is drawn toward the pubic arch and the rectum with its peritoneal surface is stretched by hand toward the cranial side. The peritoneum between the uterus and the rectum is lifted from the base of the Pouch of Douglas. The incision is made on the elevated peritoneum and extended with scissors across the dorsal side (back) of the cervix. At the end of this step, both sides of the retroperitoneal space of the broad ligament are connected. The rectum is gently freed from the cervical/vaginal wall with scissors or with a finger. With the uterus held over to the pubic arch and the rectum stretched toward the cranial portion by hand, a loose connective tissue layer between the rectum and the cervix/vagina is appreciated. This is the landmark of the rectovaginal space.

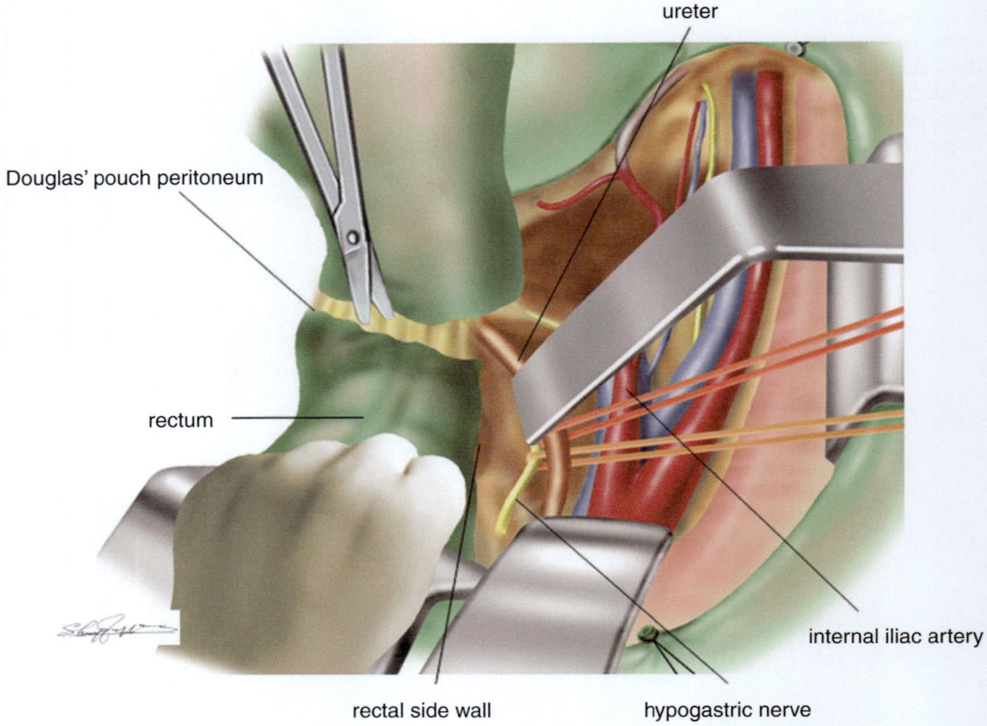


**Figure 8.13** Separation and division of the peritoneum of the Douglas' pouch

### 8.6.2 Development of the Rectovaginal Space (Figure 8.14)

If there are no dense adhesions or cancer invasion, the loose connective tissue layer between the rectum and the cervix/vagina is easily separated and the rectovaginal space can be developed. Pressing the tips of scissors against the cervical fascia, the rectum is bluntly detached from the cervix/upper part of the vagina. The separation should be carried out in the correct plane. The bilateral thick connective tissue bundles (the uterosacral ligament) can be identified between the rectovaginal space and the pararectal space.

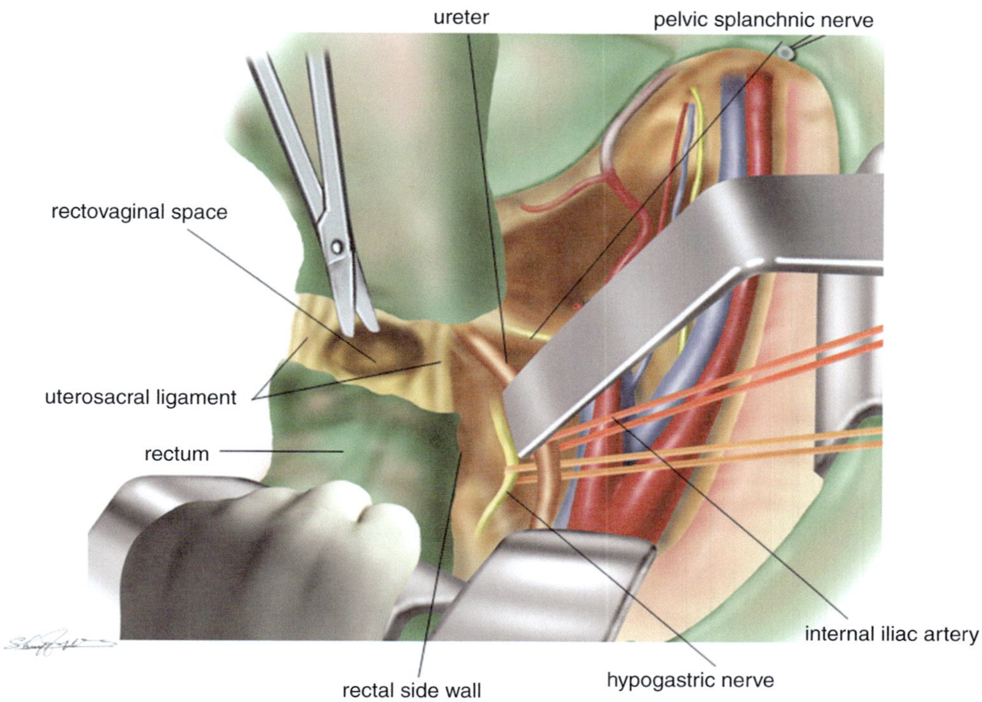


**Figure 8.14** Development of the rectovaginal space

### 8.6.3 Division of the Uterosacral Ligament (Figure 8.15)

The uterosacral ligament on either side is stretched forward and dissected at its base at the level of the rectal side wall. After confirmation/identification of the hypogastric nerve, the uterosacral ligament is isolated, and divided preserving the hypogastric nerve. If the uterosacral ligament is divided without confirmation of the hypogastric nerve, division of the hypogastric nerve can occur inadvertently during the division of the uterosacral ligament.

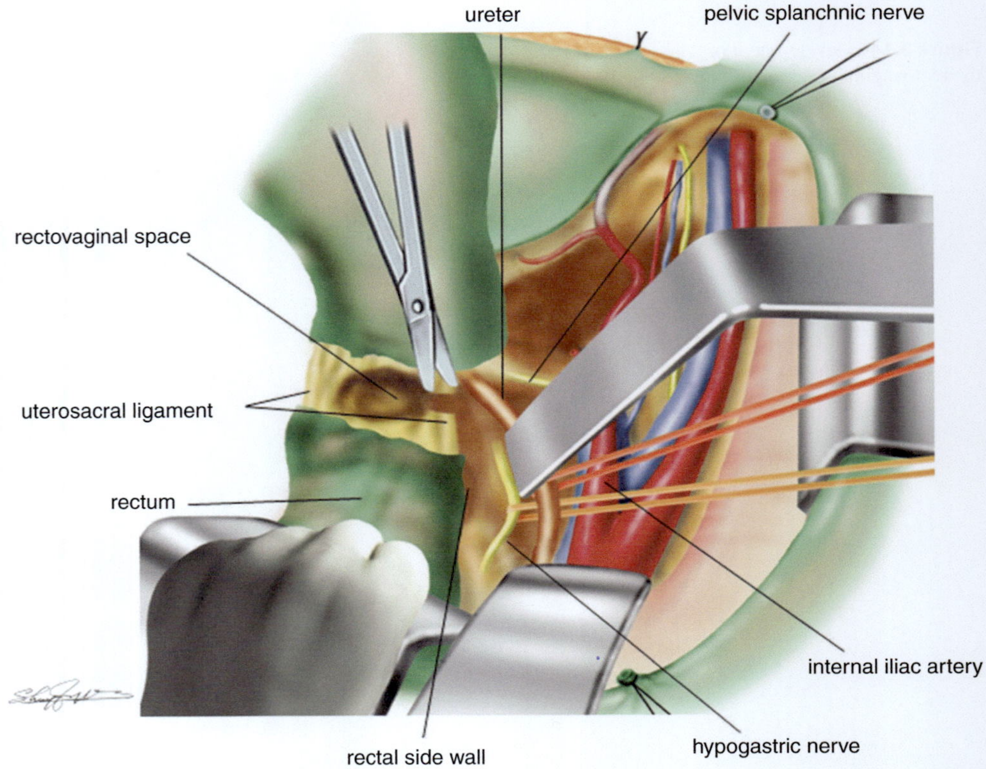


**Figure 8.15** Division of the uterosacral ligament

## 8.7 Separation of the Urinary Bladder and Anatomy of the Vesicouterine Ligament

### 8.7.1 Separation of the Urinary Bladder from the Cervical Fascia (Figure 8.16)

The peritoneum is divided across the ventral side of the cervix, just 1–2 cm below the vesicouterine fold where scissors can separate the peritoneum easily without any damage to the urinary bladder. The bladder is separated from the center of the cervical fascia at the level of the trigone of the urinary bladder. Connective tissue bundles are formed on the both sides of the cervix. The connective tissue bundle contains the ureter, the uterine artery, and several blood vessels. This is the vesicouterine ligament.

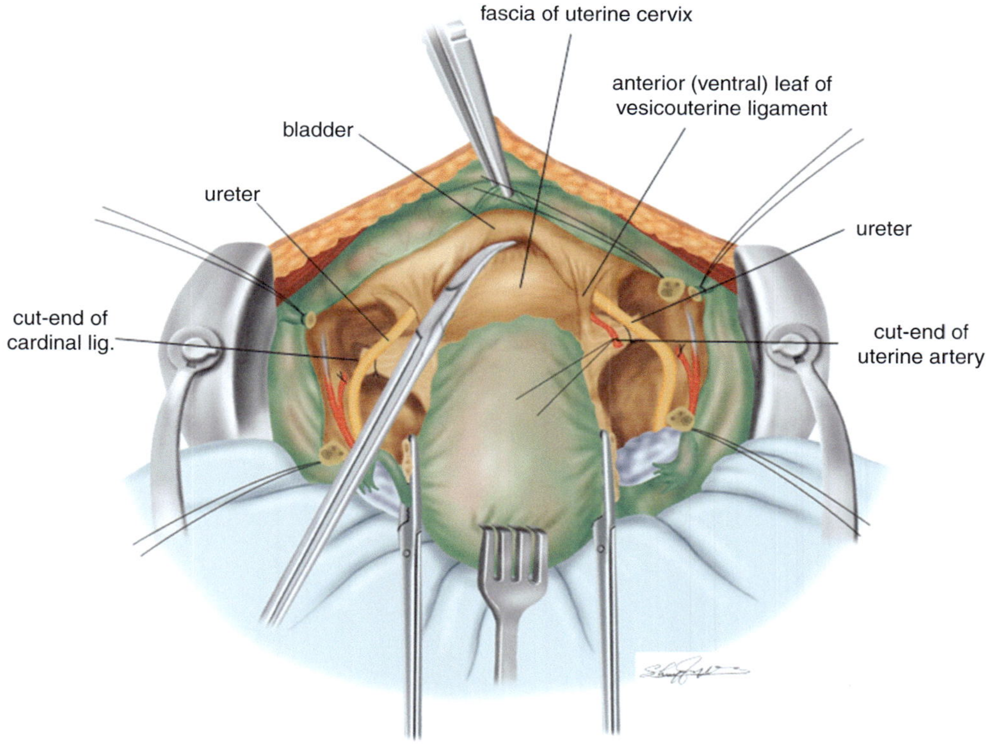


**Figure 8.16** Separation of the urinary bladder from the cervical fascia

### 8.7.2 Anatomy of the Vesicouterine Ligament (Figure 8.17)

Since the ureter is running in the vesicouterine ligament, separation of the connective tissue of the vesicouterine ligament is essential for radical hysterectomy. At first, the ventral part of the ureter should be unroofed. However, the detailed anatomy of the vesicouterine ligament was unclear for more than 100 years, until recently when it was clarified in 2007. Figure 8.17 (illustrated by Shingo Fujii) is showing a transparent view of the ureter and blood vessels in the vesicouterine ligament.

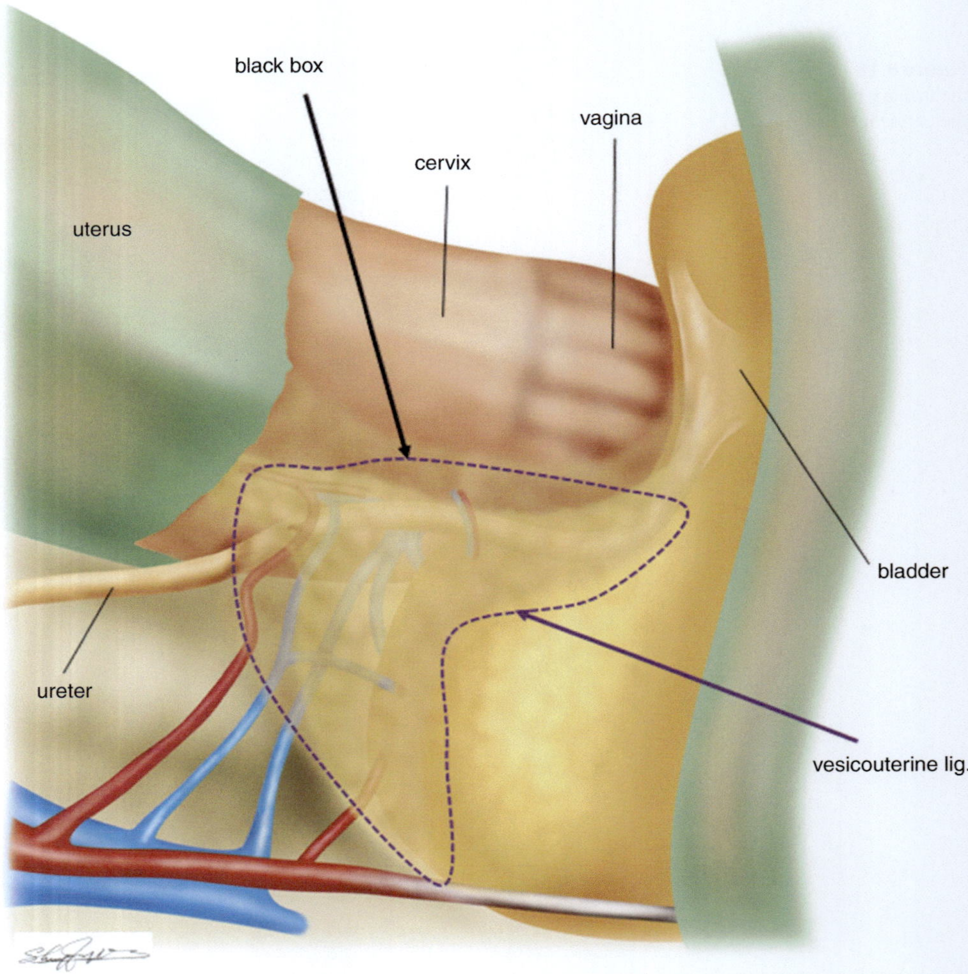


**Figure 8.17** Anatomy of the vesicouterine ligament. An area surrounded by a purple dotted line is a transparent view of the ureter and blood vessels in the vesicouterine ligament

### 8.7.3 Anatomy of the Anterior (Ventral) Leaf of the Vesicouterine Ligament (Figure 8.18)

Figure 8.18 illustrates the cut-ends of the blood vessels which reside in the anterior (ventral) leaf of the vesicouterine ligament and the blood vessels in the posterior (dorsal) leaf of the vesicouterine ligament (shown as a transparent view). After the separation of the anterior (ventral) leaf of the vesicouterine ligament, it is possible to roll the ureter laterally from the surface of the posterior (dorsal) leaf of the vesicouterine ligament.

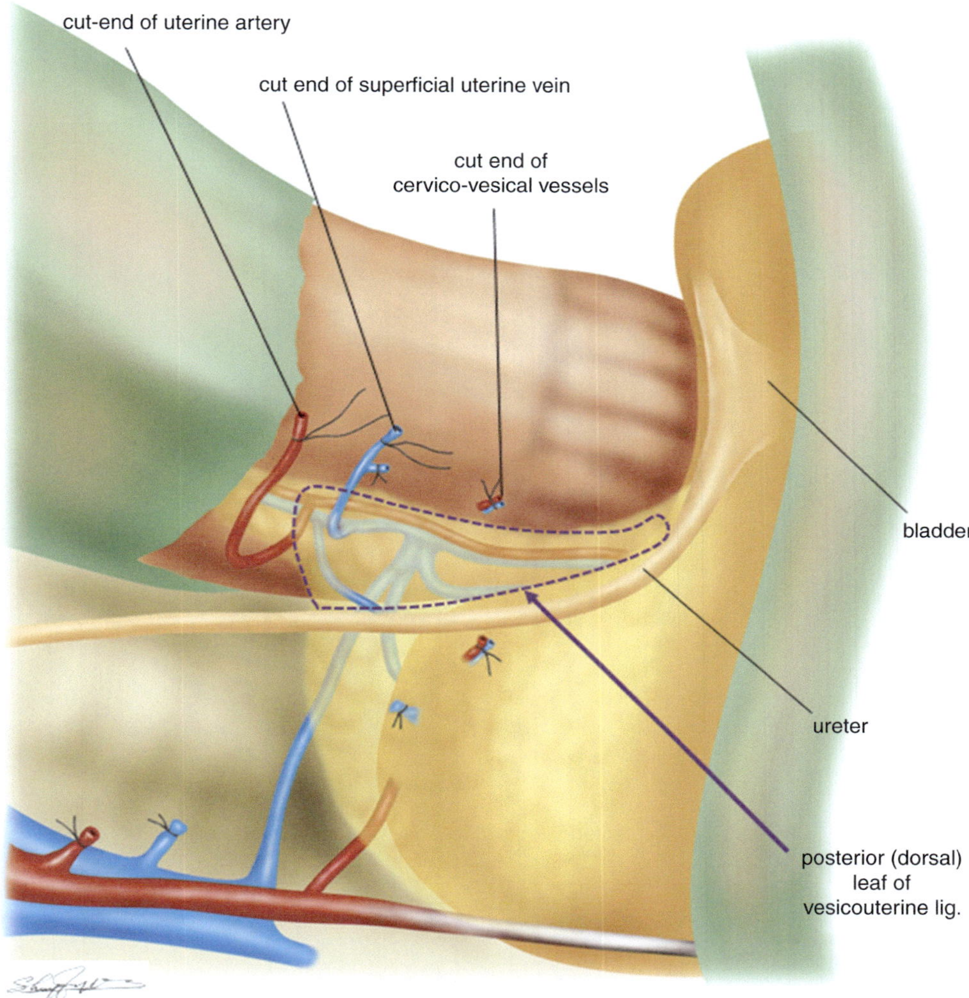


**Figure 8.18** The anatomy of the divided blood vessels in the anterior (ventral) leaf of the vesicouterine ligament with a transparent view of the blood vessels in the posterior (dorsal) leaf of the vesicouterine ligament (an area surrounded by a purple dotted line)

### 8.7.4 Anatomy of the Posterior (Dorsal) Leaf of the Vesicouterine Ligament (Figure 8.19)

By mobilizing the ureter toward the inguinal side, the surface of the posterior (dorsal) leaf of the vesicouterine ligament is exposed as the connective tissue triangle formed by the upper cervix/vagina and the ureter/the cranioventral side of the urinary bladder. Figure 8.19 shows a transparent view of the blood vessels in the posterior (dorsal) leaf of the vesicouterine ligament.

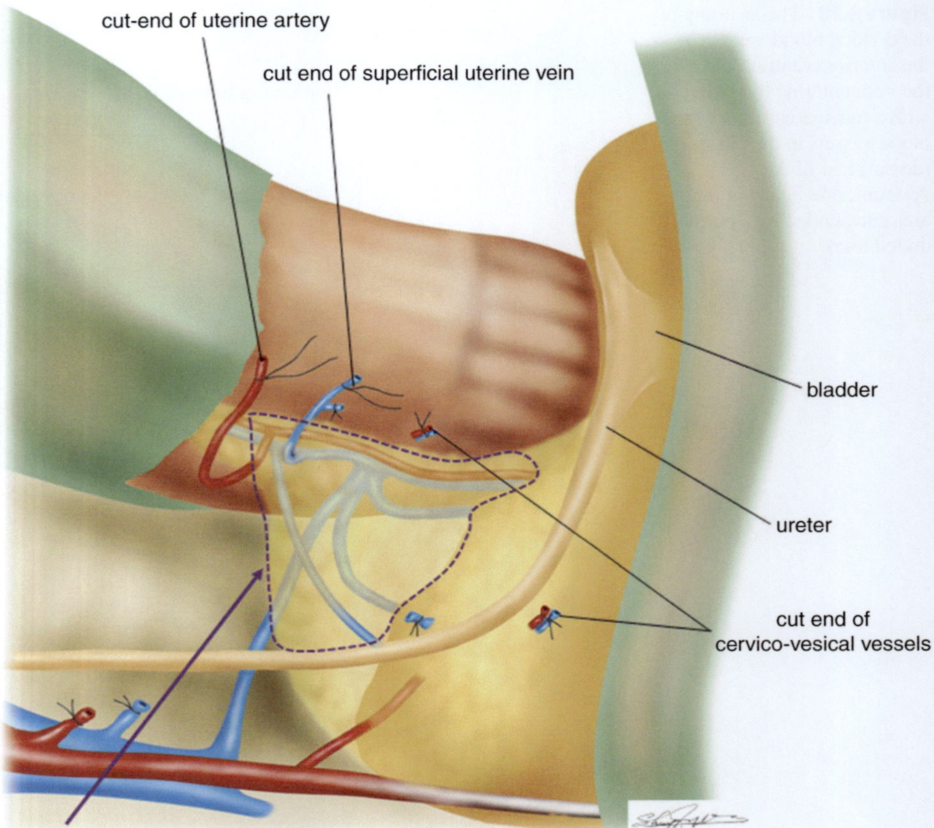


**Figure 8.19** Transparent view of the blood vessels in the posterior (dorsal) leaf of the vesicouterine ligament (an area surrounded by a purple dotted line)

### 8.7.5 Skeletonized View of the Blood Vessels and the Ureter in the Vesicouterine Ligament (Figure 8.20)

Figure 8.20 is a skeletonized view of the blood vessels and the ureter in the vesicouterine ligament. The inferior hypogastric plexus (IHP) between the blood vessels in the vesicouterine ligament and the uterus/cervix/vagina is also shown in Figure 8.20.

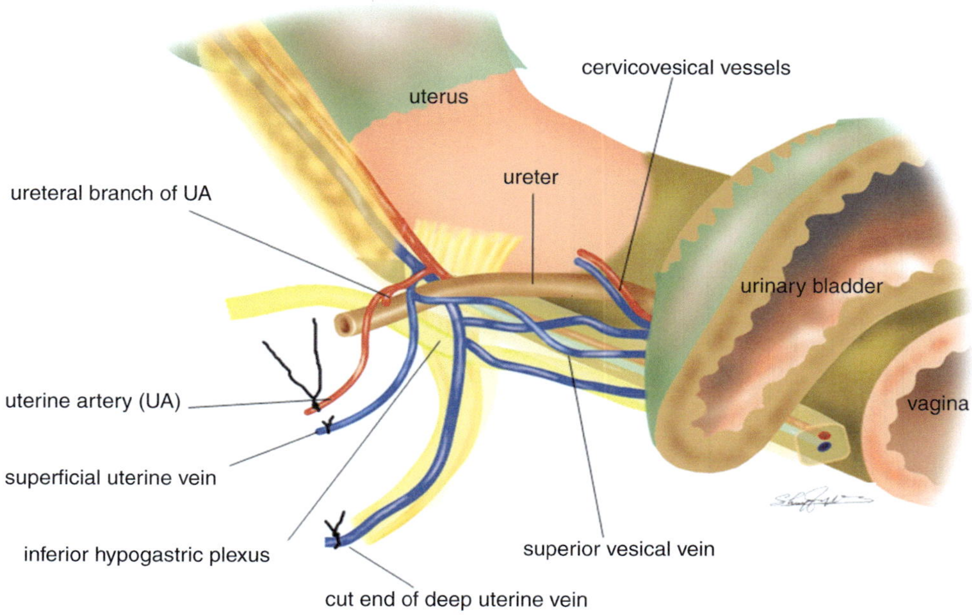


**Figure 8.20** Skeletonized view of the blood vessels and the ureter in the vesicouterine ligament from the symphysis side to the cranial side

## 8.8 Treatment of the Anterior(Ventral) Leaf of the Vesicouterine Ligament

### 8.8.1 Isolation of the Ureteral Branch of the Uterine Artery (Figure 8.21)

The cut-end of the uterine artery at the uterine side is lifted with forceps. The connective tissue between the ureter and the uterine artery is carefully divided. The ureteral branch of the uterine artery is often appreciated. It is usually clamped, cut, and ligated. However, if the ureteral branch of the uterine artery is not well developed, the vessel sealing system such as monopolar or bipolar device is enough to seal the ureteral branch.

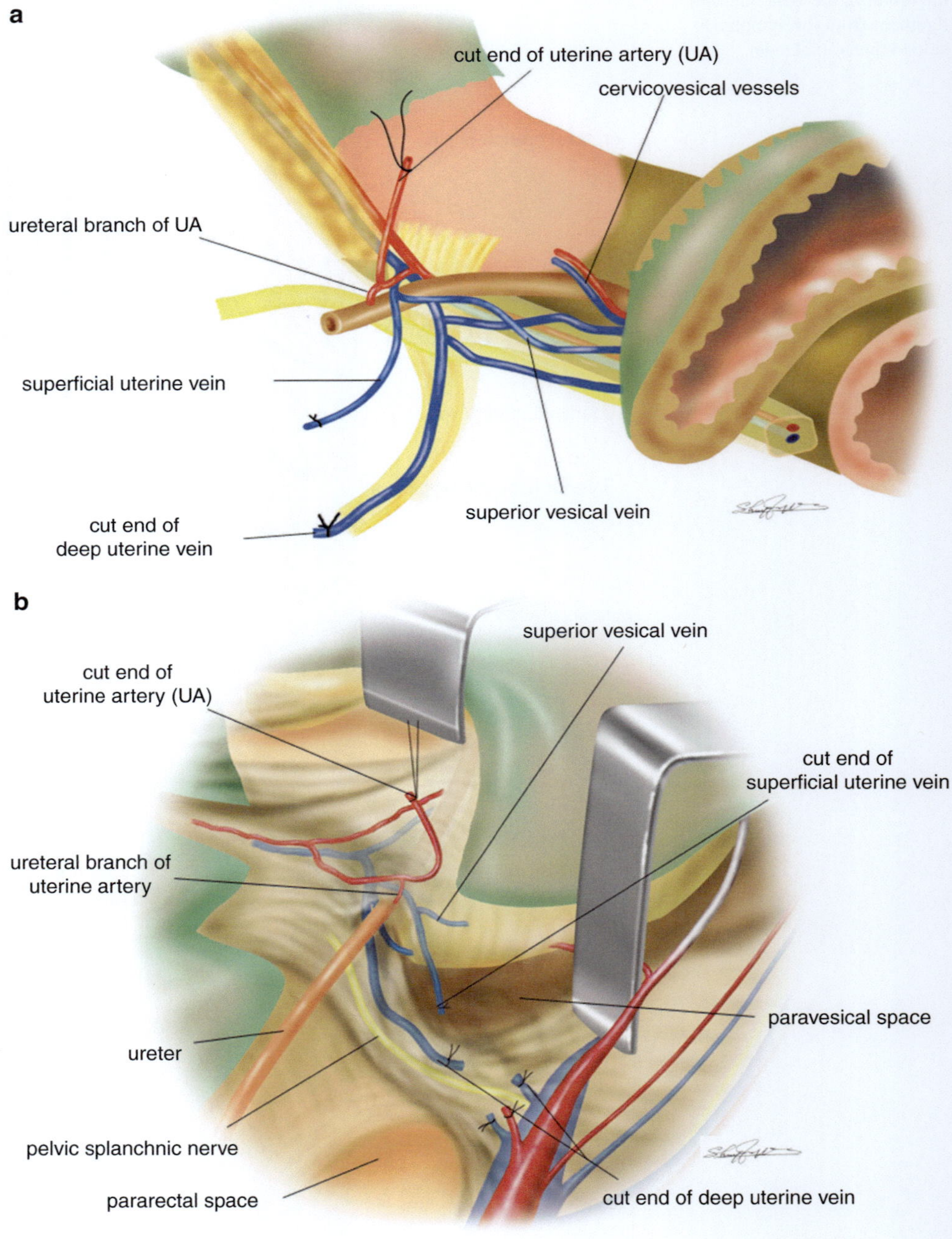


**Figure 8.21** Isolation of the ureteral branch of the uterine artery. (To provide more anatomical information of the paracervical area, two types of illustration are prepared for each surgical step). (**a**) Magnified skeletonized view of the paracervical area from the symphysis side to the cranial side. (**b**) Skeletonized view of the paracervical area and the pelvic cavity from the lateral side of the uterus

## 8.8.2 Division of the Ureteral Branch of the Uterine Artery (Figure 8.22)

The ureteral branch of the uterine artery is usually clamped, cut, and ligated. Following this step, the uterine artery is completely separated from the ventral side of the ureter.

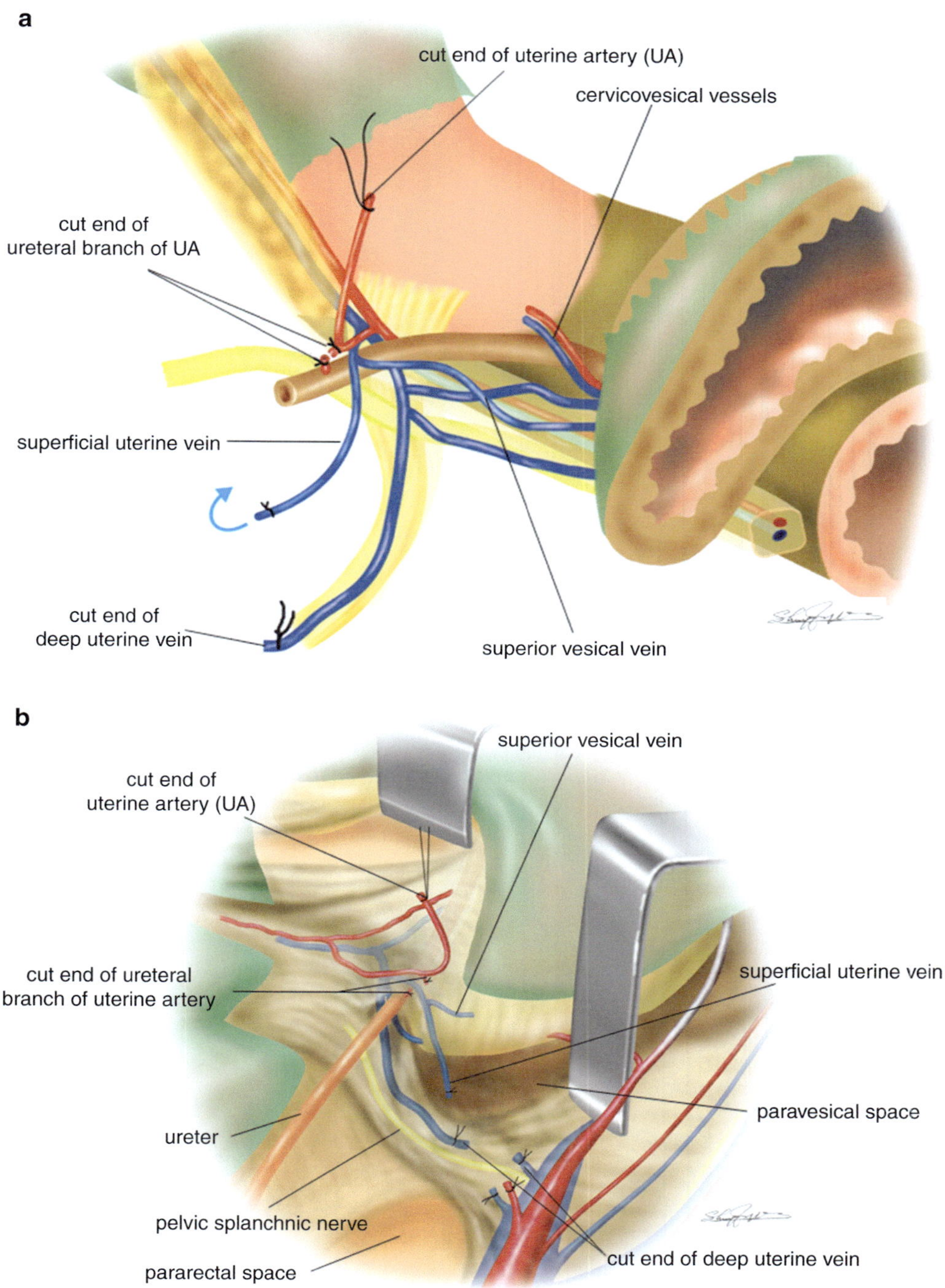


**Figure 8.22** Division of the ureteral branch of the uterine artery. (**a**) A view from the symphysis side to the cranial side. (**b**) A view from the lateral side of the uterus

### 8.8.3 Separation of the Superficial Uterine Vein from the Ureter and Isolation of the Superior Vesical Vein (Figure 8.23)

The superficial uterine vein usually runs parallel to the uterine artery. The cut-end of the superficial uterine vein is lifted gently with forceps and is carefully separated from the surface of the ureter. The separation of the connective tissue between the ureter and the urinary bladder exposes the vein draining from the urinary bladder into the superficial uterine vein. The vein is located in the most superior (ventral) portion of the urinary bladder and named the superior vesical vein. The superior vesical vein is carefully isolated.

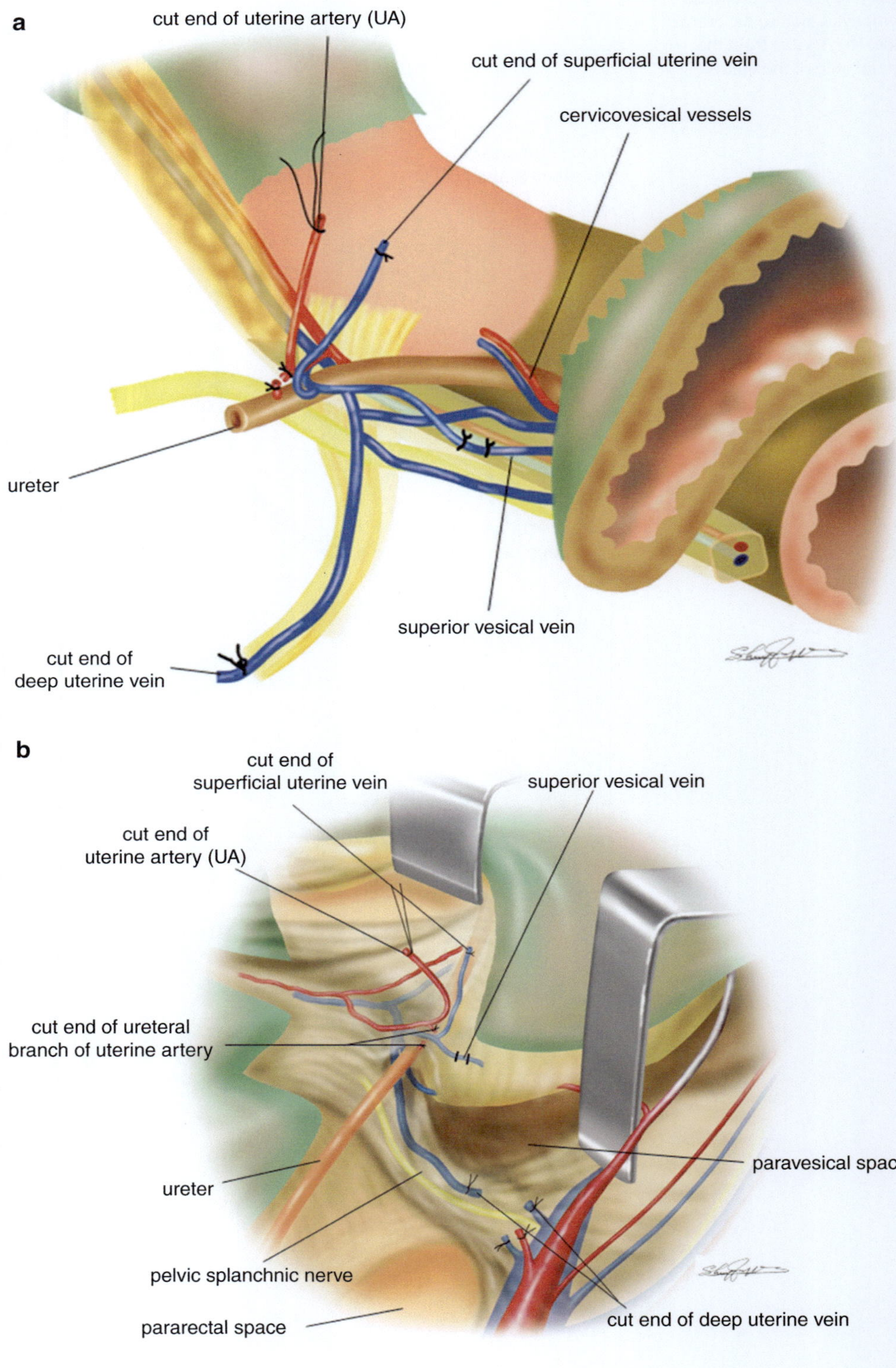


**Figure 8.23** Separation of the superficial uterine vein from the ureter and isolation of the superior vesical vein. (**a**) A view from the symphysis side to the cranial side. (**b**) A view from the lateral side of the uterus

### 8.8.4 Division of the Superior Vesical Vein (Figure 8.24)

The superior vesical vein is clamped, divided, and ligated.

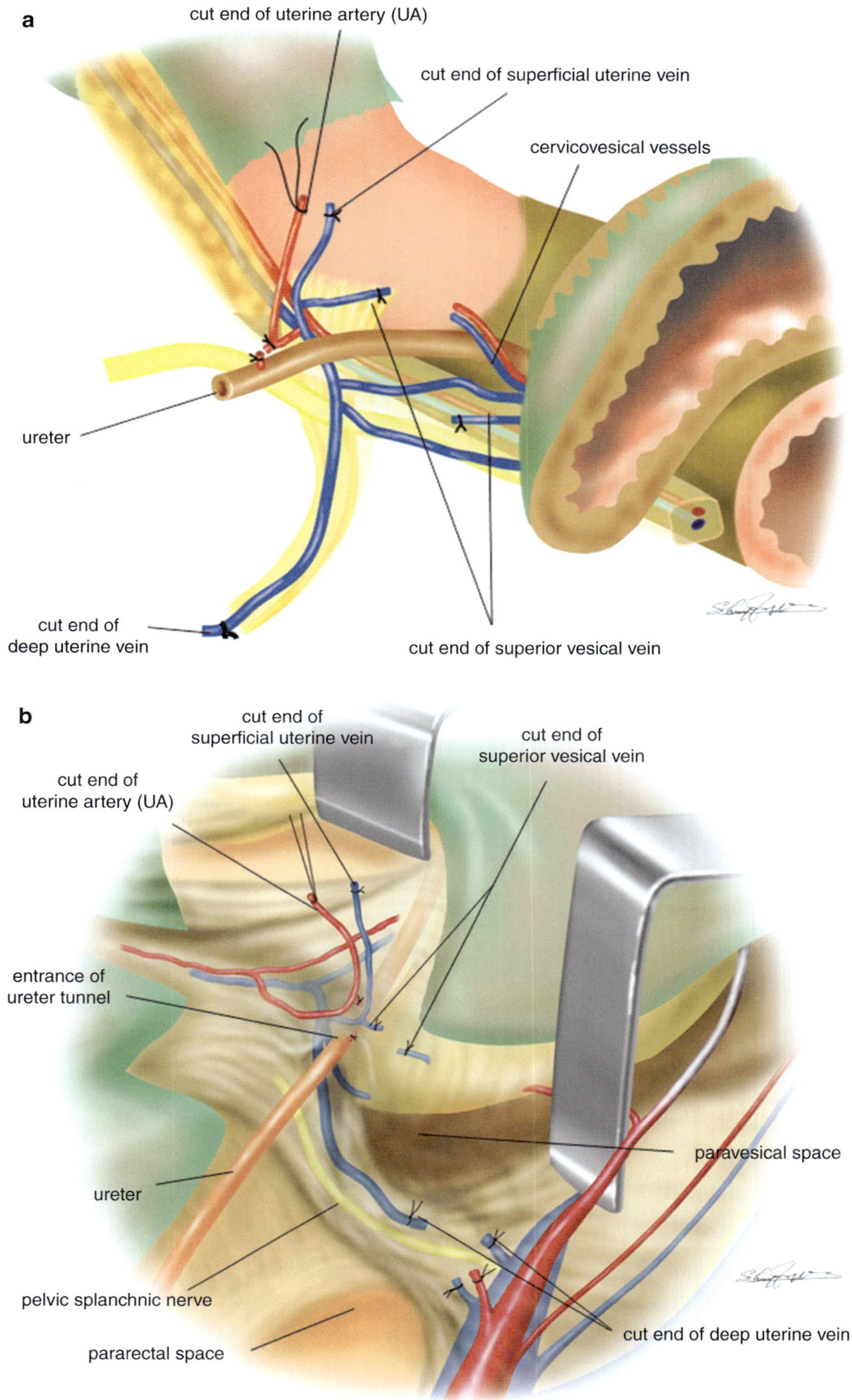


**Figure 8.24** Division of the superior vesical vein. (**a**) A view from the symphysis side to the cranial side. (**b**) A view from the lateral side of the uterus

### 8.8.5 Complete Separation of the Uterine Side of the Uterine Artery and the Superficial Uterine Vein from the Ventral Side of the Ureter (Figure 8.25)

The uterine side of the uterine artery with the superficial uterine vein is picked up and completely separated from the ventral side of the ureter. The connective tissue of the anterior (ventral) leaf of the vesicouterine ligament is exposed.

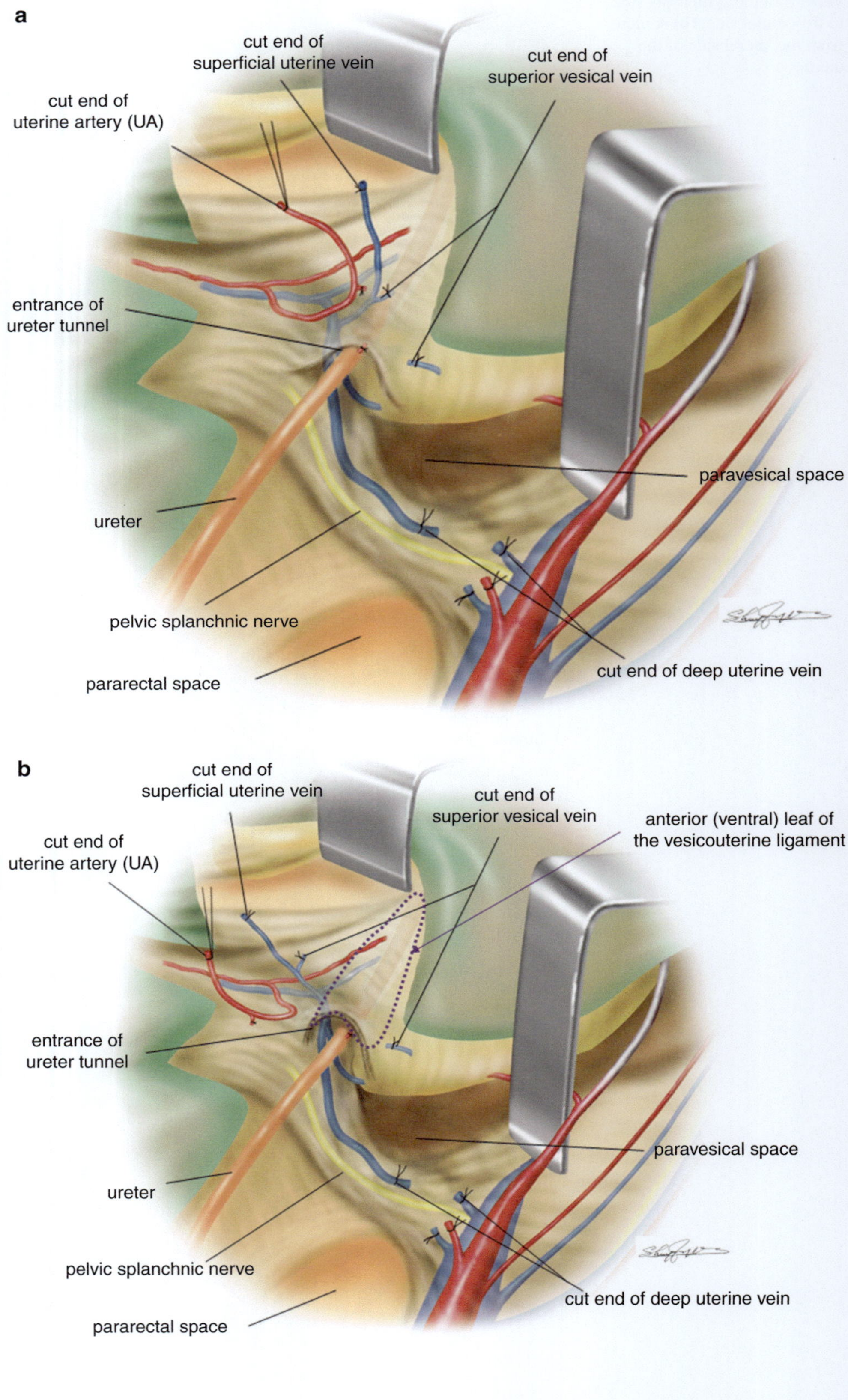


**Figure 8.25** Complete separation of the uterine side of the uterine artery and the superficial uterine vein from the ventral side of the ureter. (**a**) A figure just picking up the cut-ends of both the uterine artery and the superficial uterine vein. (**b**) After the division of the superior vesical vein, both cut-ends of the uterine artery and the superficial uterine vein are separated completely from the ureter and reveals the surface of the anterior (ventral) leaf of the vesicouterine ligament (an area surrounded by a purple dotted line)

### 8.8.6 Separation of the Anterior (Ventral) Leaf of the Vesicouterine Ligament (Figure 8.26)

Instead of developing the ureter tunnel, the connective tissue of the vesicouterine ligament is carefully separated by tracing the ureter from the entrance of the ureter tunnel. Usually, in the anterior (ventral) leaf of the vesicouterine ligament 1–1.5 cm apart from the entrance of the ureter tunnel, a pair of small blood vessels cross over the ureter from the bladder to the cervix, and are named as the cervicovesical vessels.

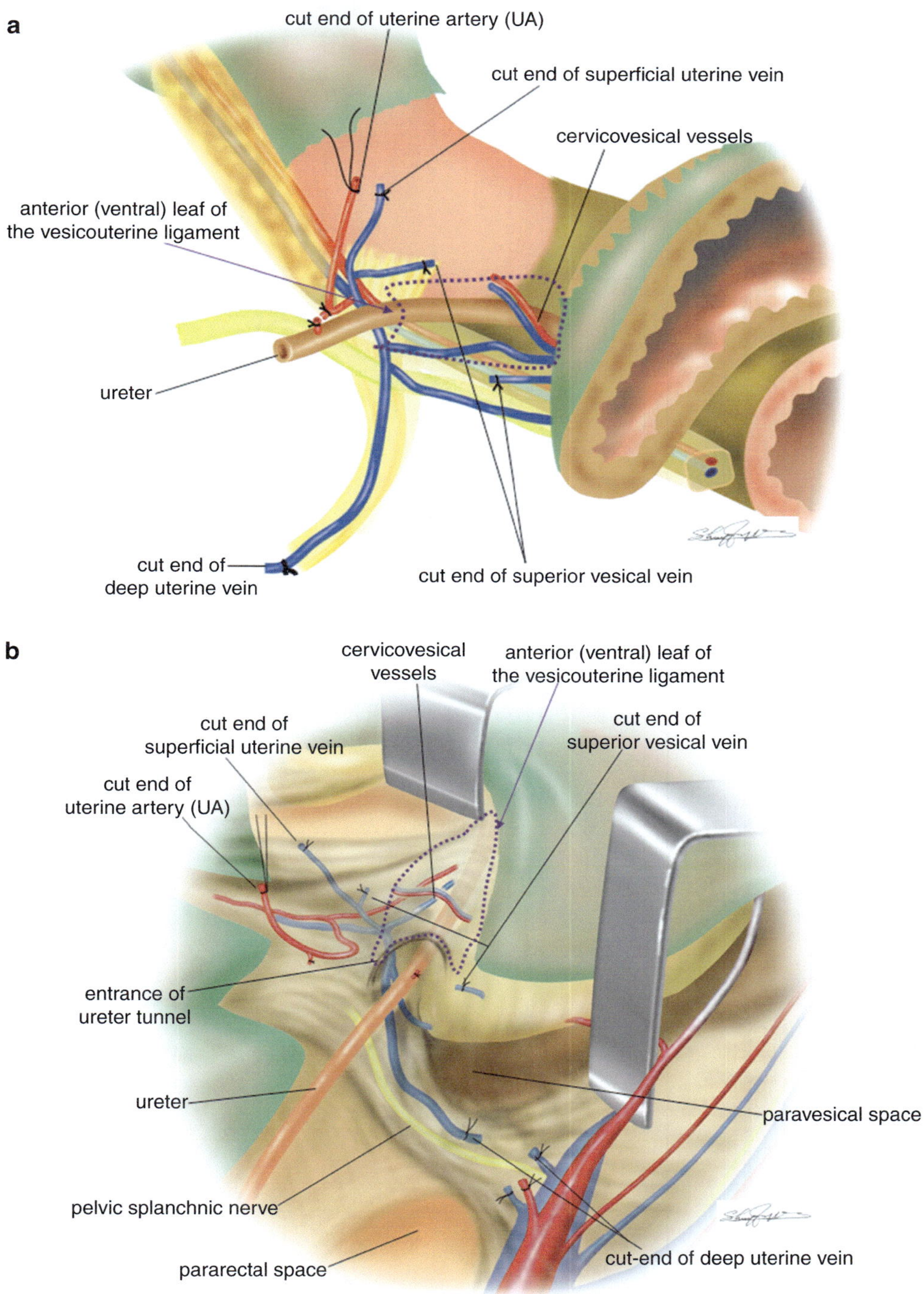


**Figure 8.26** Separation of the anterior (ventral) leaf of the vesicouterine ligament (an area surrounded by a purple dotted line) reveals the cervicovesical vessels. (**a**) A view from the symphysis side to the cranial side. (**b**) A view from the lateral side of the uterus

### 8.8.7 Isolation and Division of the Cervicovesical Vessels (Figure 8.27)

The cervicovesical vessels are isolated, doubly clamped, divided, and ligated. After the division of the cervicovesical vessels, the connective tissues surrounding the ureter are easily separated from the anterior (ventral) leaf of the vesicouterine ligament because other blood vessels are usually not identified in the anterior (ventral) leaf of the vesicouterine ligament. By dividing the connective tissues from the anterior (ventral) leaf of the vesicouterine ligament, the ureter is completely freed from its attachment to the posterior (dorsal) leaf of the vesicouterine ligament.

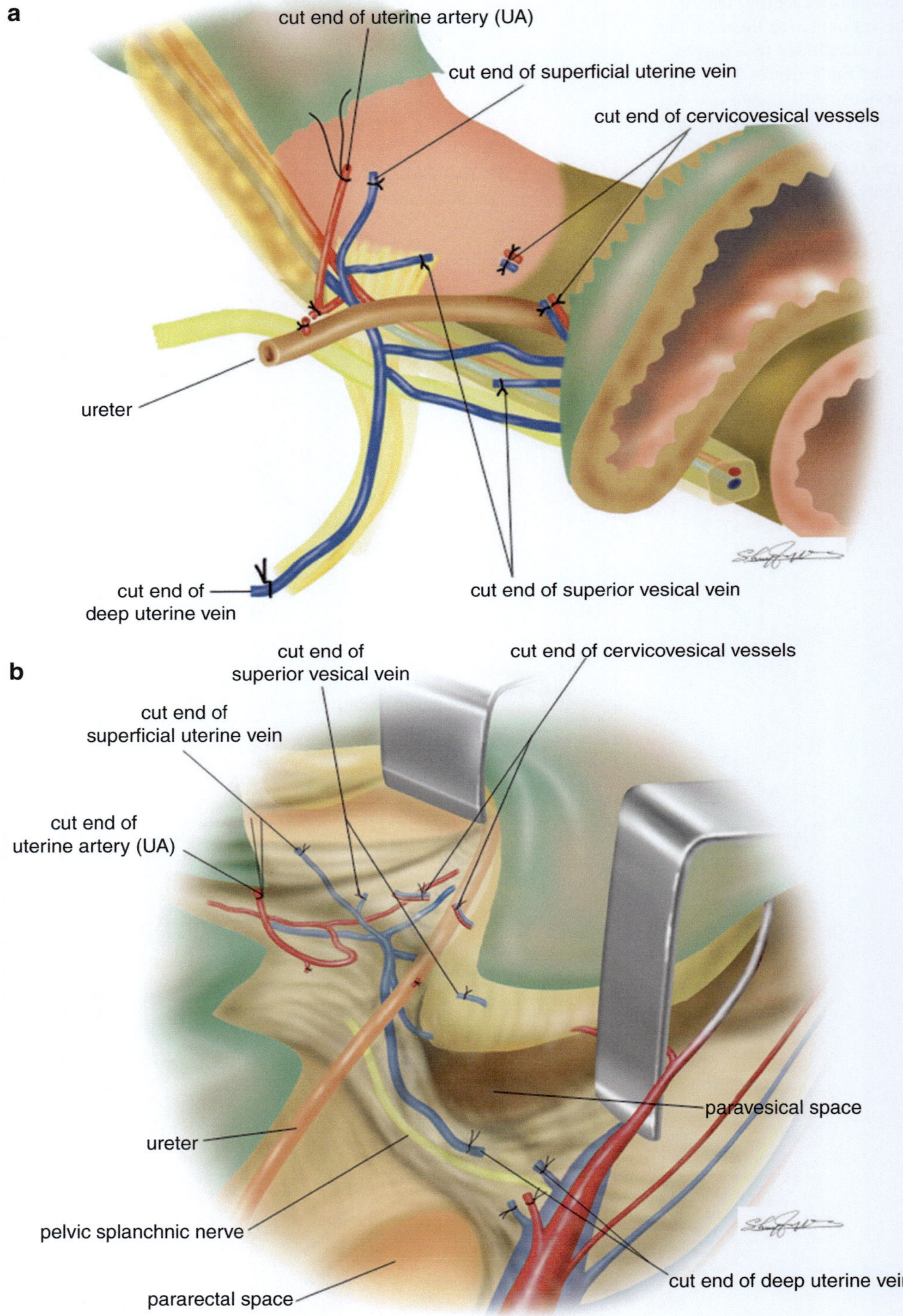


**Figure 8.27** Isolation and division of the cervicovesical vessels. (**a**) A view from the symphysis side to the cranial side. (**b**) A view from the lateral side of the uterus

## 8.9 Treatment of the Posterior (Dorsal) Leaf of the Vesicouterine Ligament

### 8.9.1 Mobilize the Ureter to the Symphysis Side and Confirm the Posterior (Dorsal) Leaf of the Vesicouterine Ligament (Figure 8.28)

Separate the connective tissue of the dorsal side of the ureter to detach the ureter from the ventral connective tissue of the posterior (dorsal) leaf of the vesicouterine ligament. Mobilize the ureter to the symphysis side to expose the posterior (dorsal) leaf of the vesicouterine ligament as wide as possible.

While mobilizing the ureter to the symphysis side, the connective tissue bundle between the ureter and the uterine cervix may give resistance, which is usually caused by a vein connecting the ureter with the cervix in the connective tissue bundle.

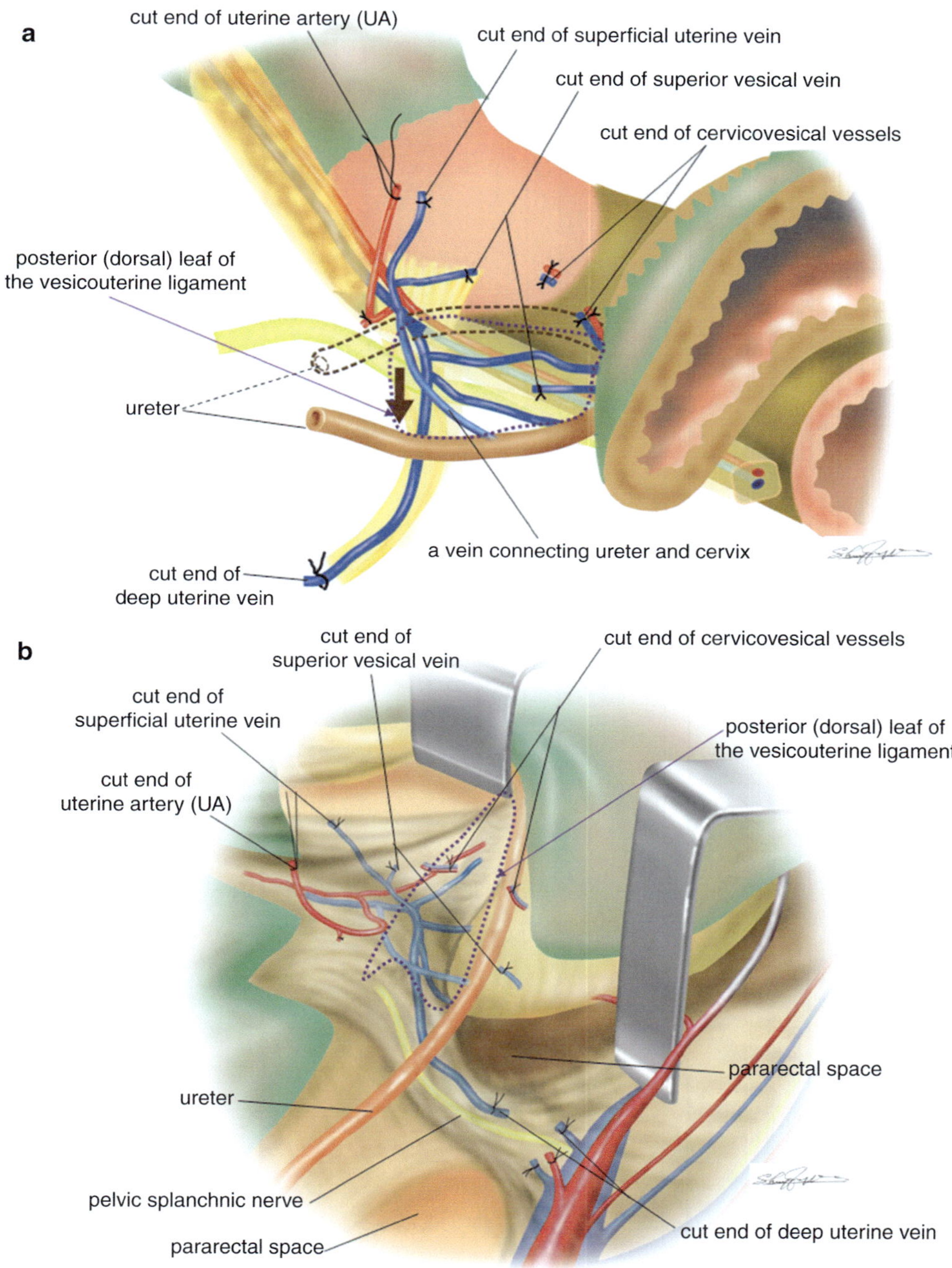


**Figure 8.28** Mobilizing the ureter to the symphysis side and confirm the posterior (dorsal) leaf of the vesicouterine ligament (an area surrounded by a purple dotted line). (**a**) A view from the symphysis side to the cranial side. (**b**) A view from the lateral side of the uterus

### 8.9.2 Isolation of a Vein Connecting the Ureter with the Cervix (Figure 8.29)

A vein connecting the ureter with the cervix is isolated.

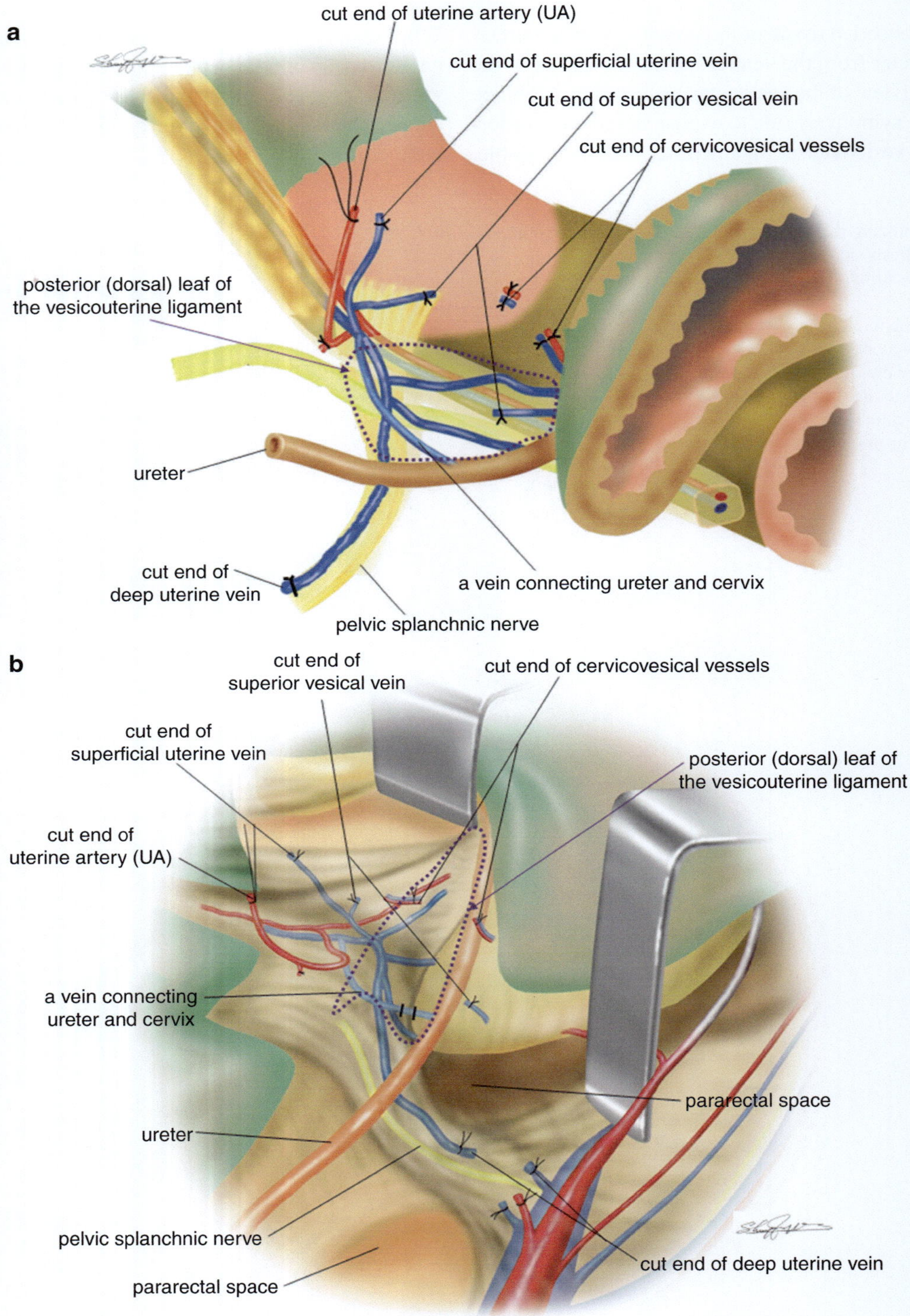


**Figure 8.29** Isolation of a vein connecting the ureter with the cervix from the cranial side of the posterior (dorsal) leaf of the vesicouterine ligament (an area surrounded by a purple dotted line). (**a**) A view from the symphysis side to the cranial side. (**b**) A view from the lateral side of the uterus. (**c**) A lateral side view of the isolated or divided blood vessels in the cardinal ligament and the posterior (dorsal) vesicouterine ligament (an area surrounded by a purple dotted line) with a transparent view of the hidden blood vessels and the nerve structure of the inferior hypogastric plexus

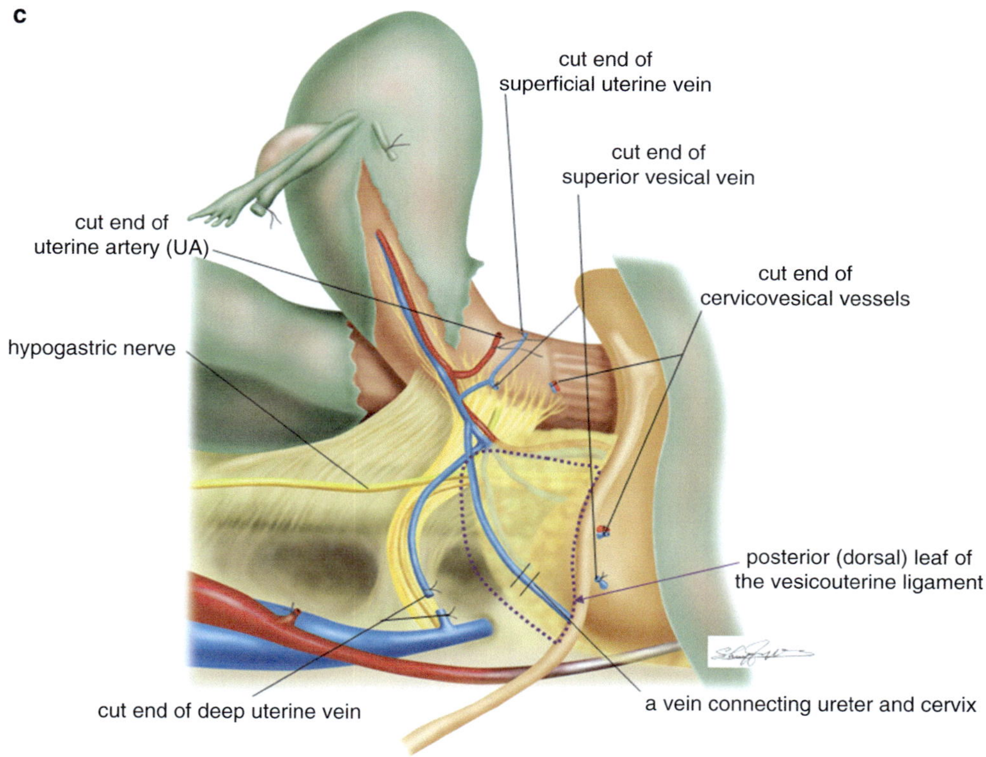


**Figure 8.29** (continued)

### 8.9.3 Division of a Vein Connecting the Ureter with the Cervix (Figure 8.30)

A vein connecting the ureter with the cervix is isolated, doubly clamped, divided, and ligated. Mobility of the ureter increases significantly following this step.

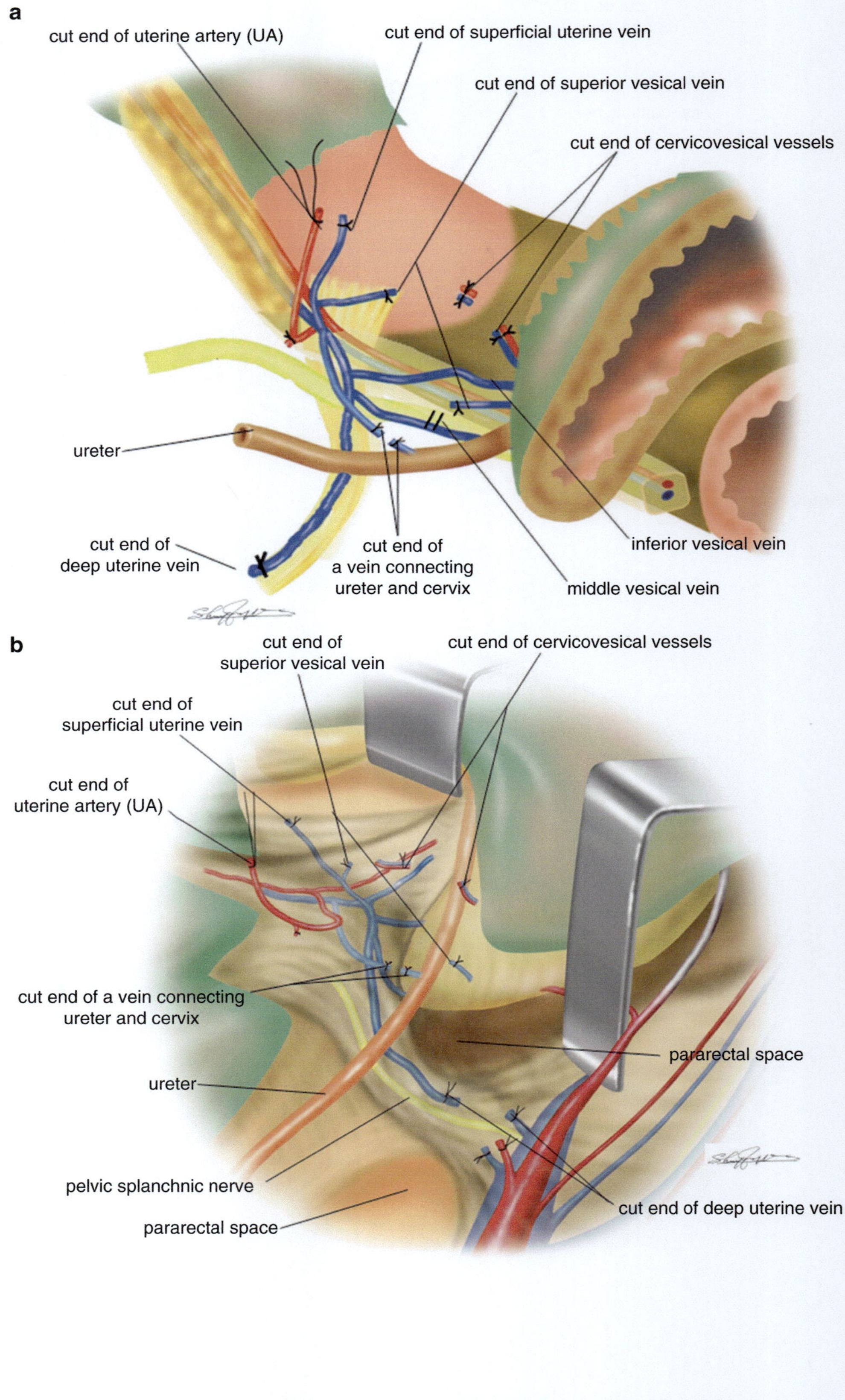


**Figure 8.30** Division of a vein connecting the ureter with the cervix. (**a**) A view from the symphysis side to the cranial side. (**b**) A view from the lateral side of the uterus. (**c**) A lateral side view of the isolated or divided blood vessels in the cardinal ligament and the posterior (dorsal) vesicouterine ligament (an area surrounded by a purple dotted line) with a transparent view of the hidden blood vessels and the nerve structure of the inferior hypogastric plexus

**Figure 8.30** (continued)

c

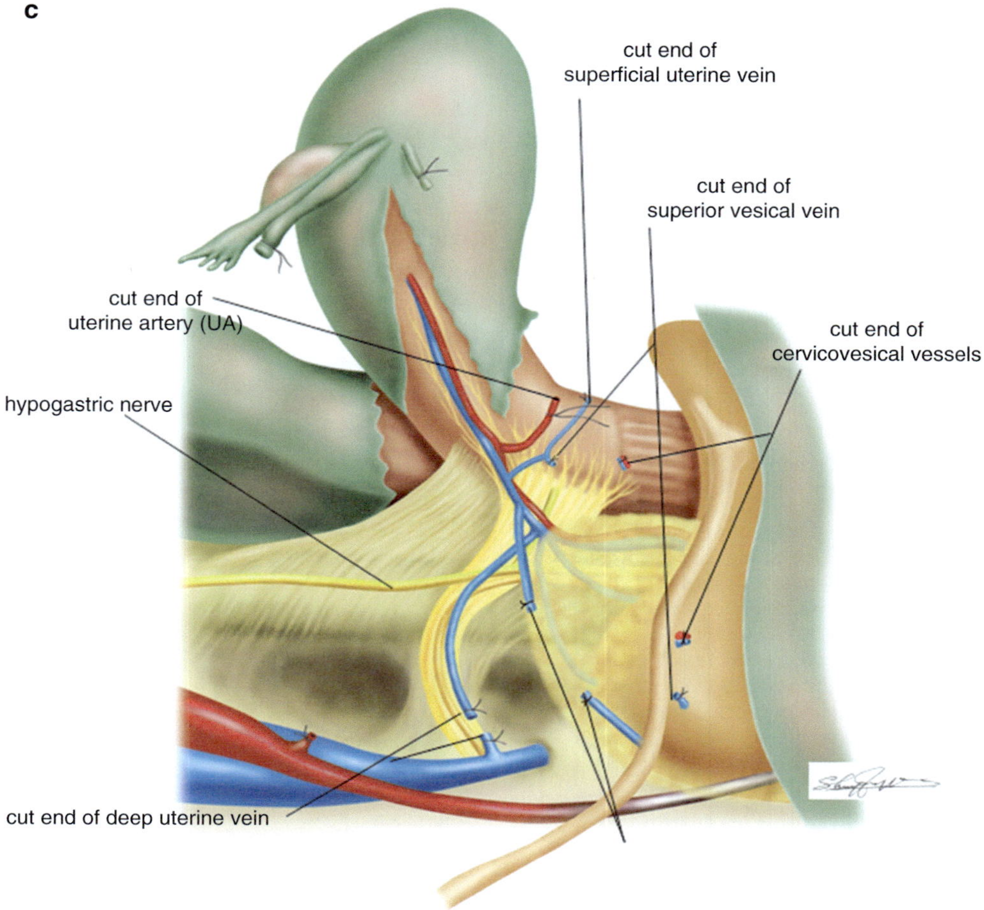

### 8.9.4 Separation of the Cut-End of the Deep Uterine Vein from the Pelvic Splanchnic Nerve (Figure 8.31)

Using two L-shaped forceps, the ureter and the urinary bladder are pulled toward the symphysis side as shown in Figure 8.31b. Then, the cut-end of the deep uterine vein is picked up and separated from the pelvic splanchnic nerve close to the sidewall of the rectum. Cranial traction of the cut-end of the deep uterine vein and the symphysis side traction of the ureter/the urinary bladder using L-shaped retractors gives tension to the posterior (dorsal) leaf of the vesicouterine ligament. This retraction exposes the structure of the connective tissues of the posterior (dorsal) leaf of the vesicouterine ligament between the bladder and the cut-end of the deep uterine vein.

**Notes:**
Giving tension between the cardinal ligament (the deep uterine vein) and the urinary bladder during the separation of the posterior (dorsal) leaf of the vesicouterine ligament will apply tension to the veins from the urinary bladder draining into the deep uterine vein. Separation of the connective tissue in the posterior (dorsal) leaf of the vesicouterine ligament will help expose and identify each vein from the bladder to the deep uterine vein.

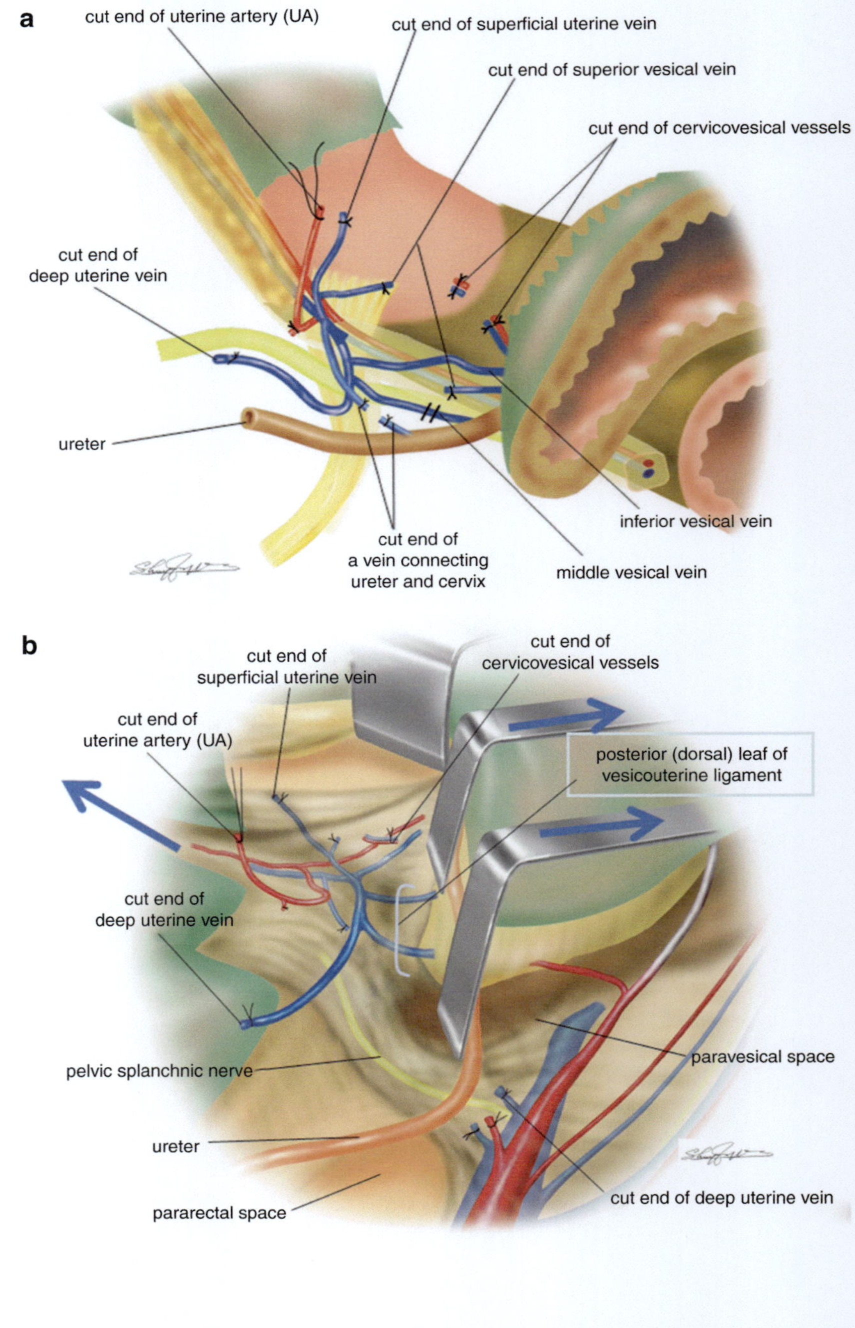


**Figure 8.31** Separation of the cut-end of the deep uterine vein from the pelvic splanchnic nerve. (**a**) A view from the symphysis side to the cranial side. (**b**) A view from the lateral side of the uterus. (**c**) A lateral side view of the isolated or divided blood vessels in the cardinal ligament and the posterior (dorsal) vesicouterine ligament with a transparent view of the hidden blood vessels and the nerve structure of the inferior hypogastric plexus

**Figure 8.31** (continued)

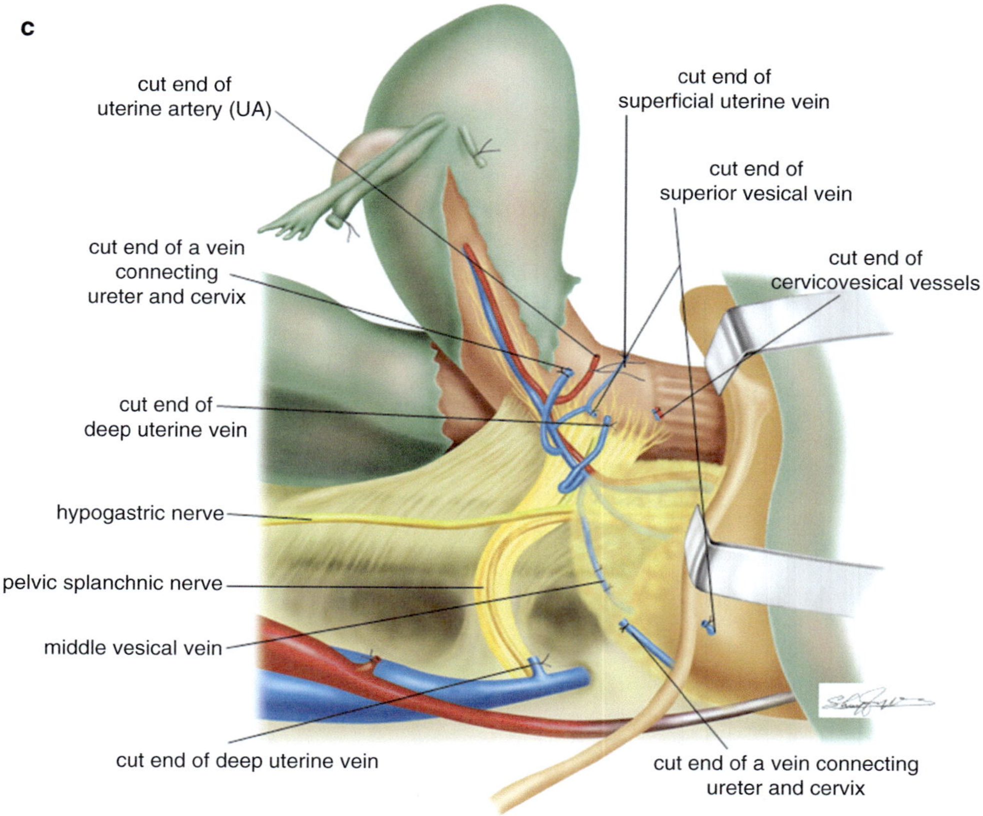

### 8.9.5 Importance of the Removal of the Adipose Tissues in the Posterior (Dorsal) Leaf of the Vesicouterine Ligament (Figure 8.32)

During the processes of the step-by-step nerve-sparing radical hysterectomy, the most important part is the separation of the posterior (dorsal) leaf of the vesicouterine ligament. Usually, adipose tissues are covering the rectal side of the vesicouterine ligament to the dorsal side of the urinary bladder as shown in the left side of Figure 8.32. Adipose tissues in the sidewall of the rectum and the dorsal side of the urinary bladder should be removed as much as possible as shown in the right side of Figure 8.32. The removal of adipose tissues is essential for an ideal nerve-sparing radical hysterectomy and enables the step-by-step separation of the posterior (dorsal) leaf of the vesicouterine ligament.

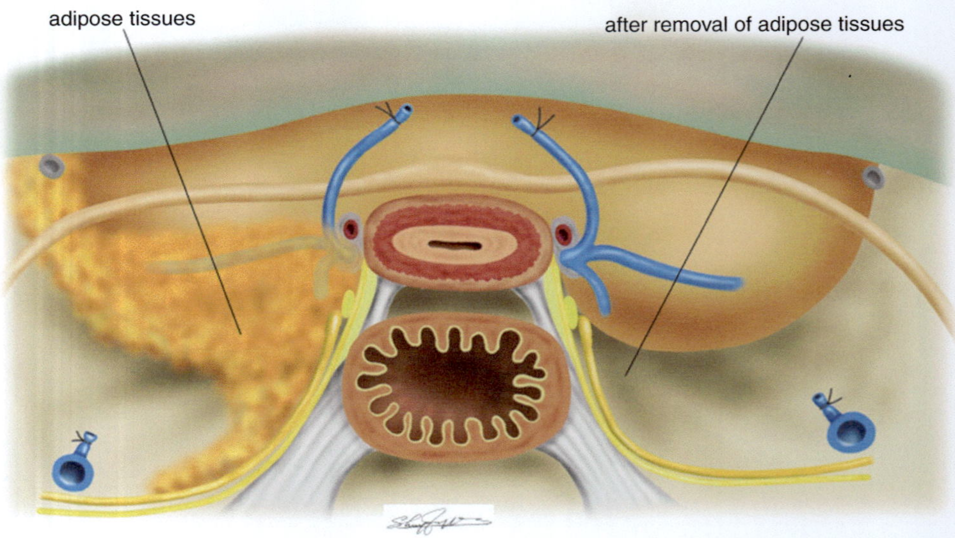


**Figure 8.32** Importance of the removal of the adipose tissues in the posterior (dorsal) leaf of the vesicouterine ligament. Adipose tissues in the side wall of the rectum/upper vagina and the dorsal side of the urinary bladder are illustrated in the left side of figure. Removal of the adipose tissues is illustrated in the right side

### 8.9.6 Clamp and Divide the Middle Vesical Vein (Figure 8.33)

The connective tissue in the posterior (dorsal) leaf of the vesicouterine ligament is carefully separated. In the cranial part of the posterior (dorsal) leaf of the vesicouterine ligament, a vein (the middle vesical vein) which runs from the urinary bladder to the deep uterine vein is visualized. The middle vesical vein is doubly clamped, divided and ligated.

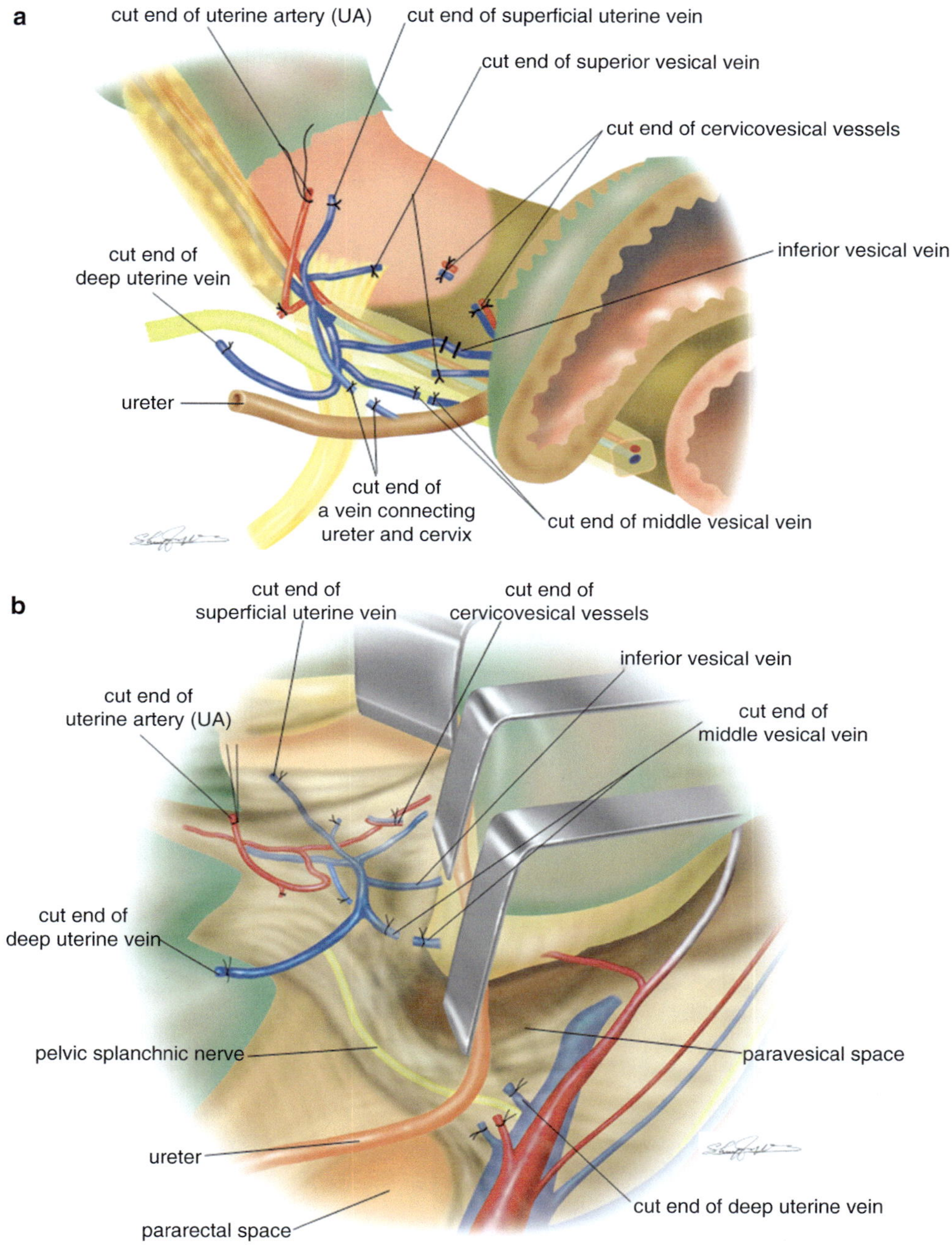


**Figure 8.33** Clamp and divide the middle vesical vein. (**a**) A view from the symphysis side to the cranial side. (**b**) A view from the lateral side of the uterus. (**c**) A lateral side view of the isolated or divided blood vessels in the cardinal ligament and the posterior (dorsal) vesicouterine ligament with a transparent view of the hidden blood vessels and the nerve structure of the inferior hypogastric plexus

**Figure 8.33** (continued)

c

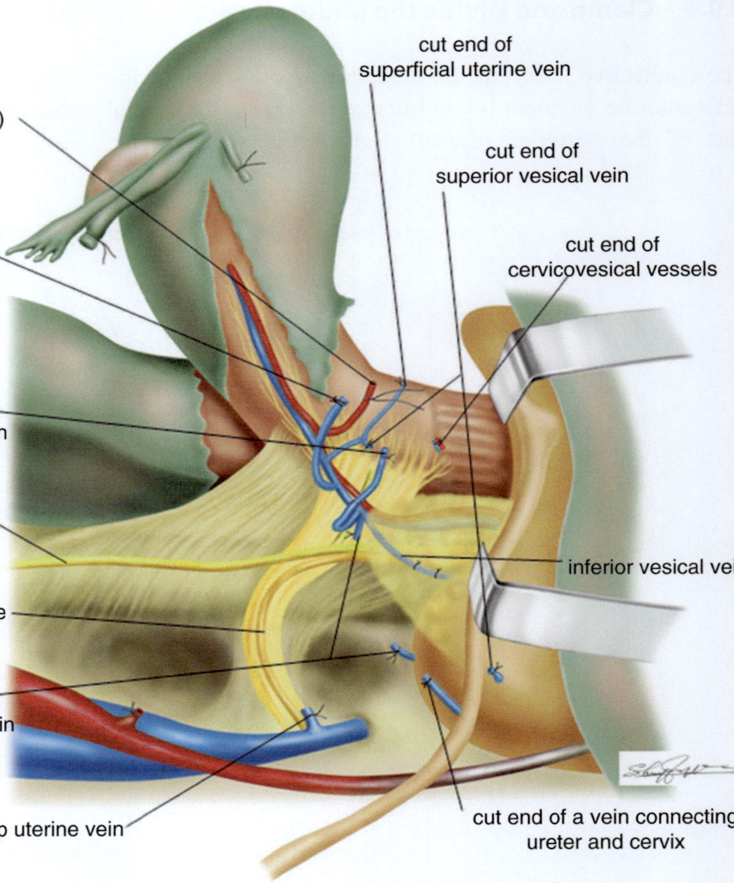

### 8.9.7 Clamp and Divide the Inferior Vesical Vein (Figure 8.34)

In addition, a vein (the inferior vesical vein) that runs parallel to the cervix from the posterior part of the urinary bladder, which also drains into the deep uterine vein, is also identified. The inferior vesical vein is doubly clamped, ligated, and divided. Usually, by the division of the inferior vesical vein, the urinary bladder with the ureter is completely separated from the lateral cervix and the upper vagina. Along the sidewall of the cervix and upper vagina, the blood vessels from the vagina can be identified. This is the paracolpium.

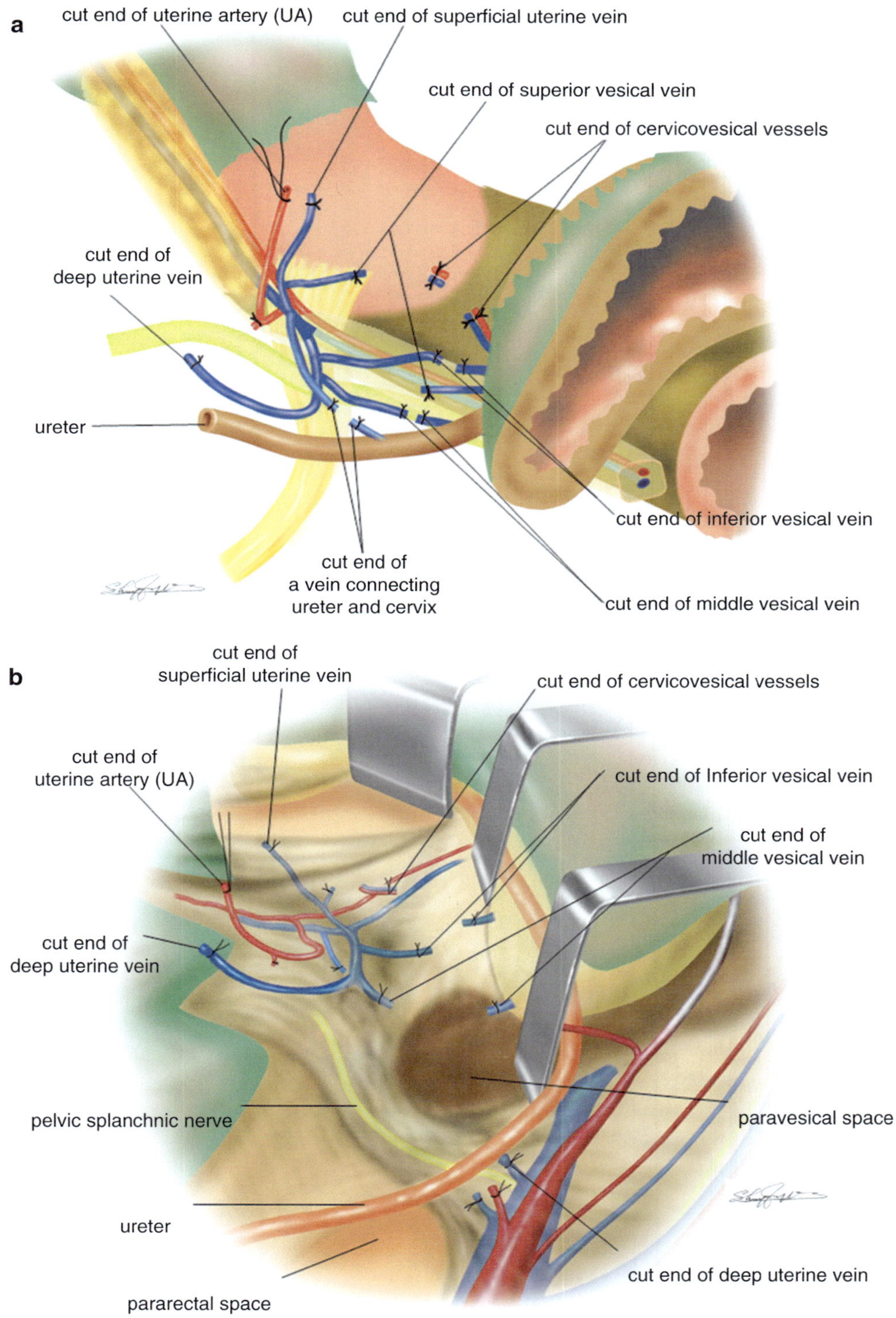


**Figure 8.34** Clamp and divide the inferior vesical vein. (**a**) A view from the symphysis side to the cranial side. (**b**) A view from the lateral side of the uterus. (**c**) A lateral side view of the isolated or divided blood vessels in the cardinal ligament and the posterior (dorsal) vesicouterine ligament with a transparent view of the hidden blood vessels and the nerve structure of the inferior hypogastric plexus

**Figure 8.34** (continued)

c

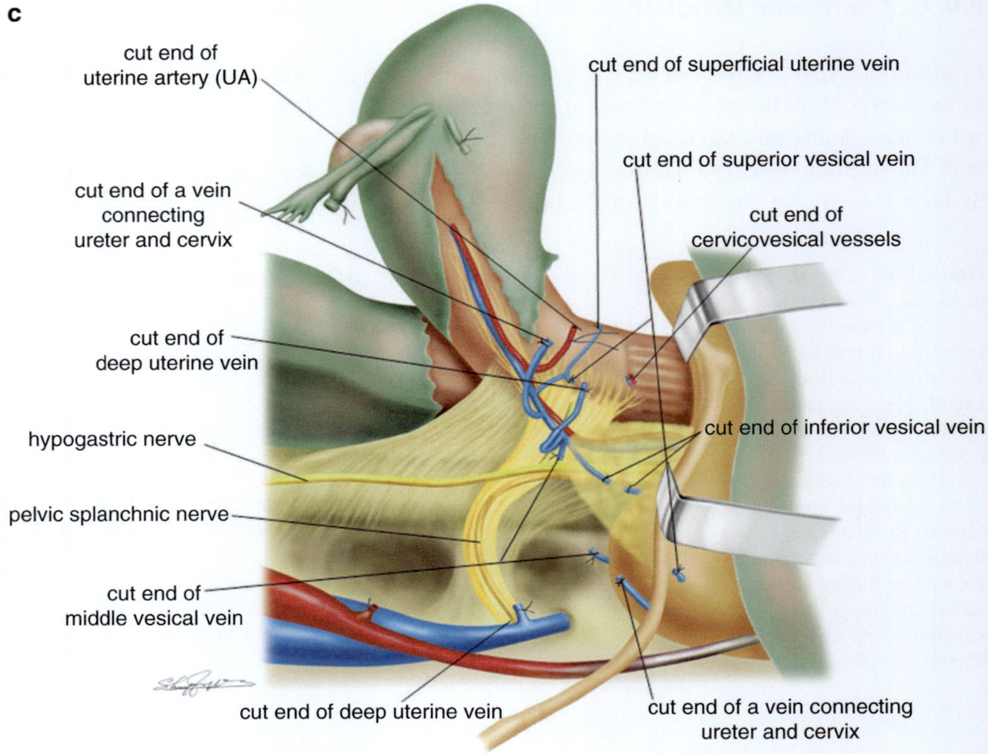

## 8.10 Confirmation of the Inferior Hypogastric Plexus (IHP) (Figure 8.35)

Following the removal of the adipose tissues residing between the dorsal part of the urinary bladder and the rectal sidewall, the pelvic splanchnic nerve is traced from the pelvic floor to the sidewall of the rectum. The hypogastric nerve can be followed from the cranial side of the rectum to the urinary bladder, up to the merging point of the hypogastric nerve to the pelvic splanchnic nerve (the IHP). From the IHP nerve bundles, the uterine branch and the bladder branch can be seen passing toward the uterus and the urinary bladder. The IHP formed by the hypogastric nerve, pelvic splanchnic nerve, uterine branch, and bladder branch can be seen as a shape of a cross at the plexus (Figure 8.35a–c).

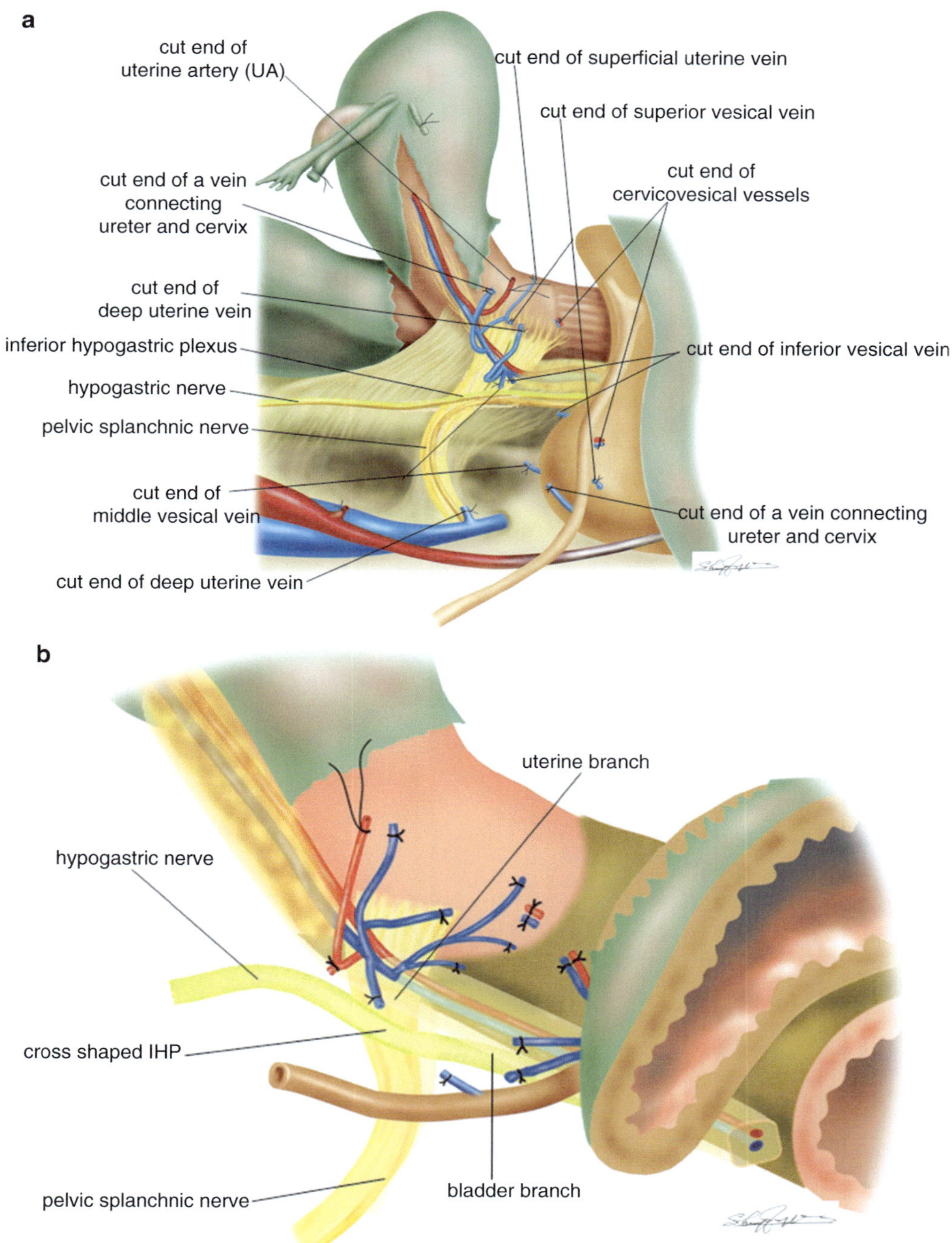


**Figure 8.35** Confirmation of the inferior hypogastric plexus (IHP). (**a**) A lateral side view of the nerve structure of the inferior hypogastric plexus (IHP). (**b**) A view from the symphysis side to the cranial side. (**c**) A surgical photo of the inferior hypogastric plexus (IHP)

**Figure 8.35** (continued)

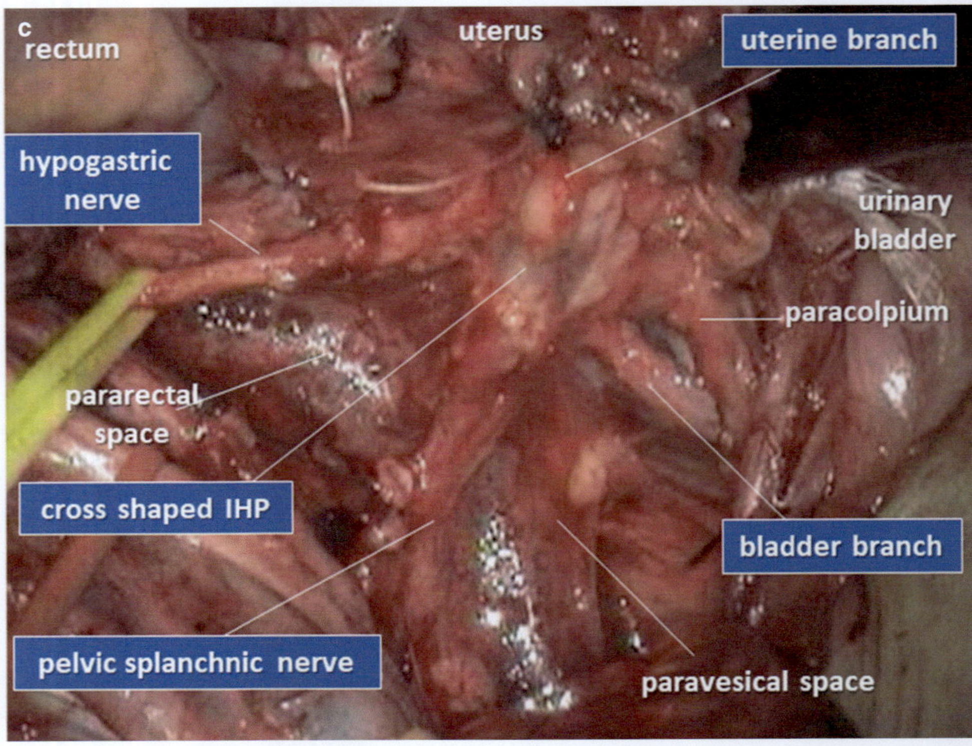

## 8.11 The Concept of the Pelvic Nerve Plane (Figure 8.36)

During the surgical processes of radical hysterectomy two spaces (such as the paravesical space and pararectal space) are developed, isolating the cardinal ligament between the two spaces. In the most dorsal part of the cardinal ligament, the pelvic splanchnic nerve runs from the pelvic wall to the sidewall of the rectum and merges with the hypogastric nerve. The merging point is the IHP with branches to the uterus and the urinary bladder. The IHP is formed by the hypogastric nerve, the pelvic splanchnic nerve, the bladder branch, and the uterine branch. Anatomically, all these nerves compose the IHP and can be identified in the same connective tissue plane between the lateral side of the uterosacral ligament and the rectal side of the two surgical spaces (paravesical and pararectal). Surgically, this connective tissue layer is separable from the rectum and the uterus/vagina without blood loss. In the ventral side of the same connective tissue layer, the ureter runs parallel to the hypogastric nerve. The connective tissue surrounding the ureter is called as the *mesoureter*. However, the dorsal side of the connective tissue layer from the hypogastric nerve including all the components of the IHP can be called as the *pelvic nerve plane*. An appropriate separation of the pelvic nerve plane is necessary for nerve-sparing radical hysterectomy.

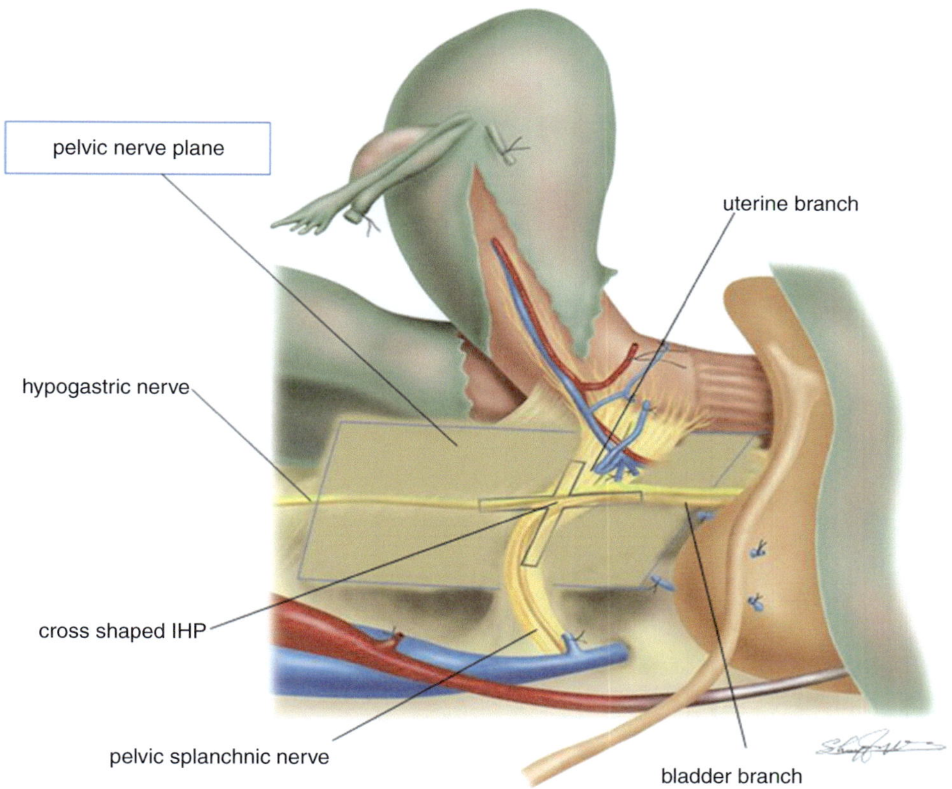


**Figure 8.36** Pelvic nerve plane that includes the whole structure of the inferior hypogastric plexus is illustrated using a square sheet surrounded by a blue line

## 8.12 Separation of the Rectovaginal Ligament (Figure 8.37)

Pushing the rectum up separates the lateral side of the connective tissue layer between the rectum and the cervix/vagina. After the division of the uterosacral ligament, the rectovaginal ligament is appreciated between the rectum and the vagina.

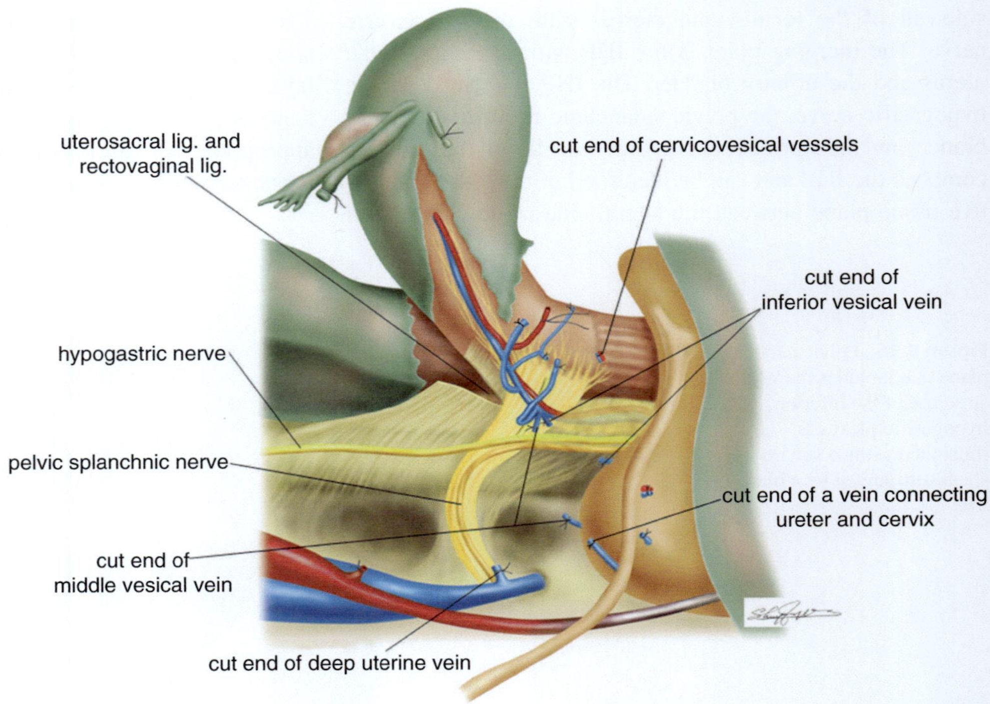


**Figure 8.37** Separation of the rectovaginal ligament

## 8.13 Separation of the Bladder Branch from the Paracolpium (Figure 8.38)

In order to perform nerve-sparing radical hysterectomy, isolation of the uterine branch from the IHP is necessary. Before the isolation of the uterine branch, separation of the bladder branch from the vaginal blood vessels (paracolpium) is required. During the separation of the bladder branch from the paracolpium, at the ventral side of the bladder branch close to the IHP, a loose connective tissue depression (v-shaped depression) is appreciated.

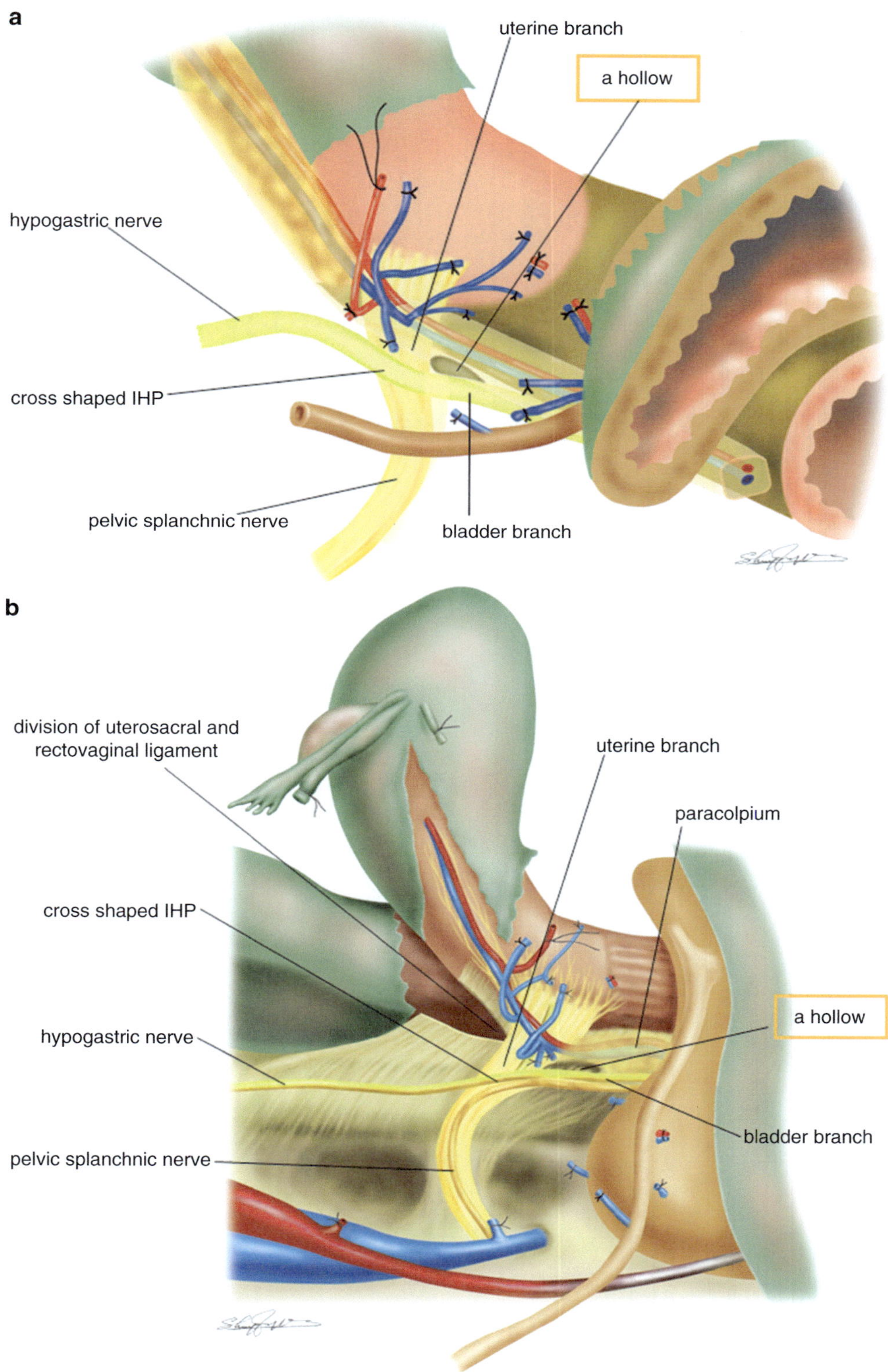


**Figure 8.38** Separation of the bladder branch from the paracolpium. At the cranial side of the bladder branch, a hollow is created between the bladder branch and the paracolpium. (**a**) A view from the symphysis side to the cranial side. (**b**) A lateral side view of the nerve structure of the inferior hypogastric plexus. (**c**) A surgical photo of the inferior hypogastric plexus

**Figure 8.38** (continued)

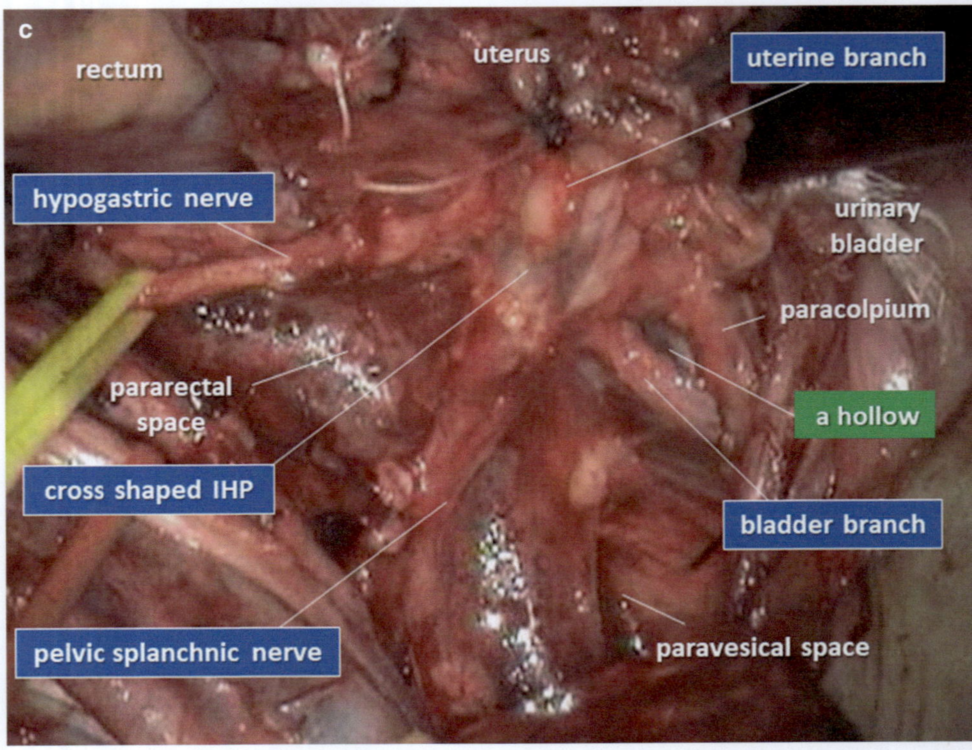

## 8.14 Separation of the Uterine Branch from the IHP (Figure 8.39)

From the ventral level of the v-shaped depression created between the bladder branch and the paracolpium, Pean forceps is insinuated towards the ventral level of the hypogastric nerve. Pean forceps can isolate the uterine branch of the IHP from the cervix/vagina.

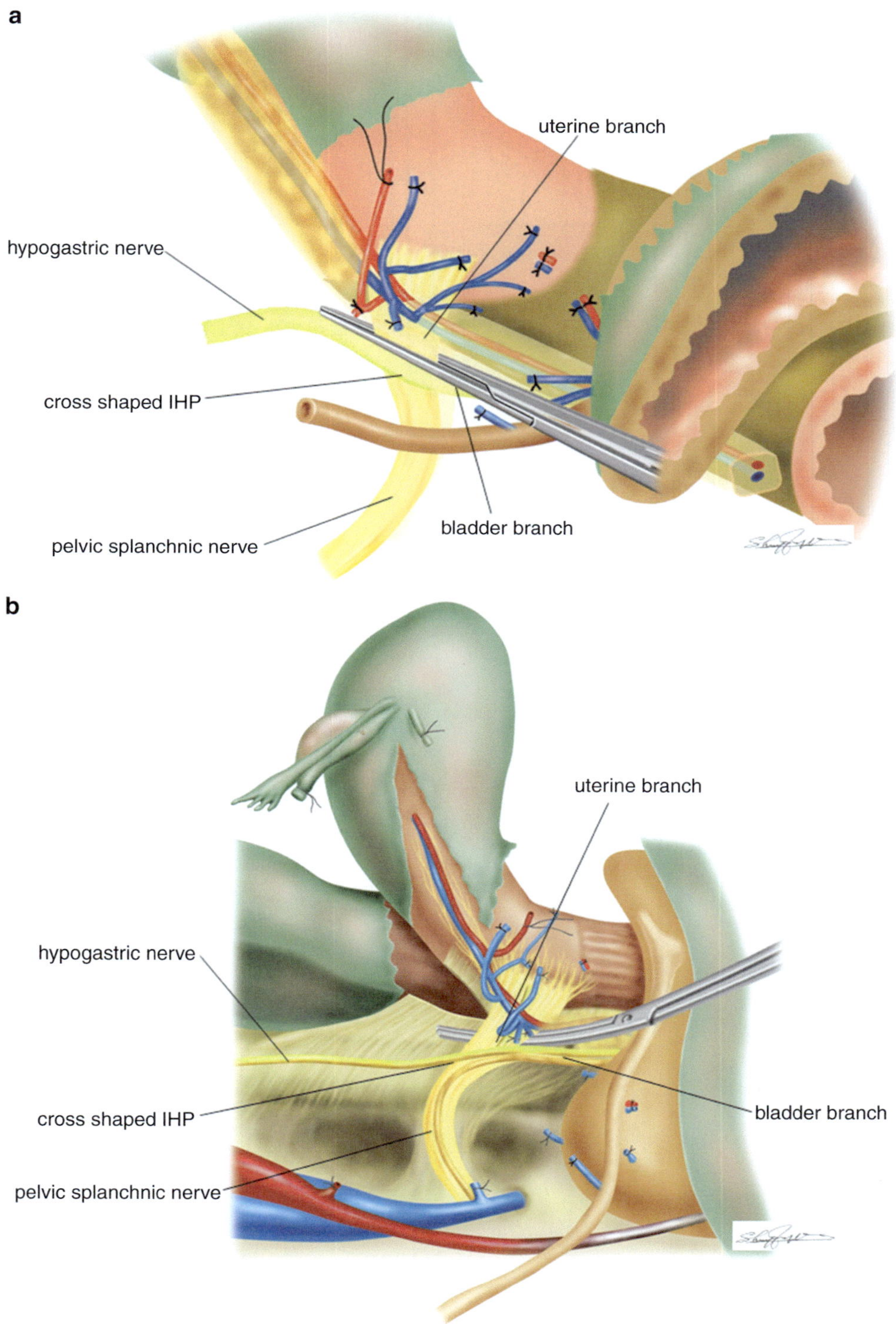


**Figure 8.39** Separation of the uterine branch from the inferior hypogastric plexus. (**a**) A view from the symphysis side to the cranial side. (**b**) A lateral side view of the nerve structure of the inferior hypogastric plexus. (**c**) A surgical photo of the inferior hypogastric plexus

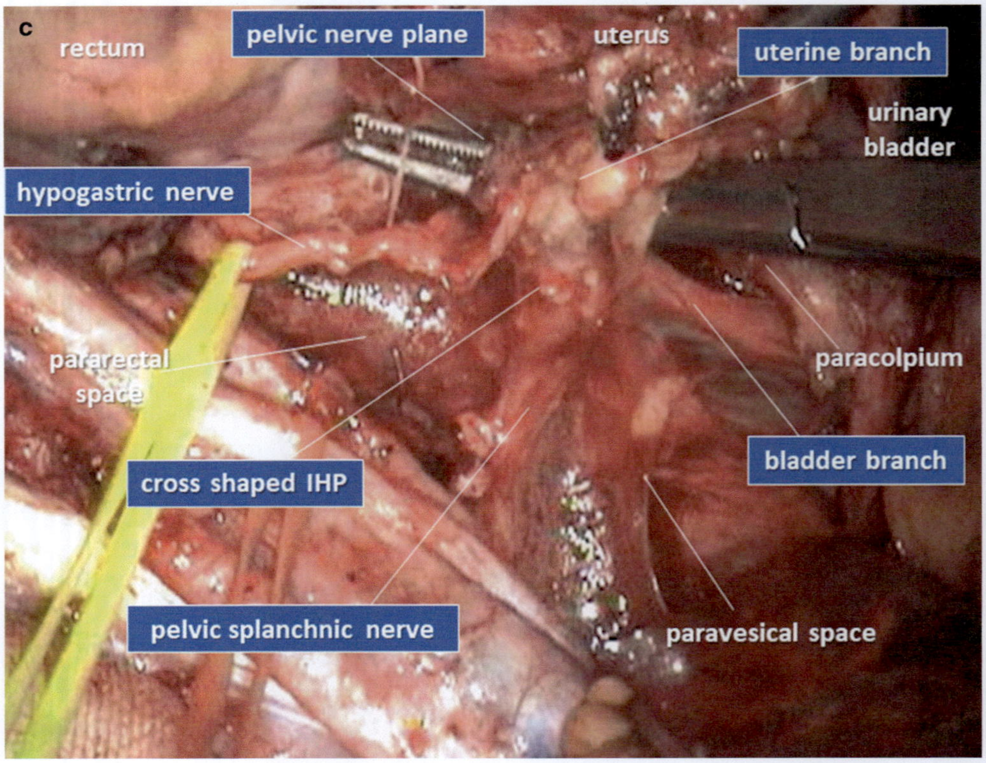


**Figure 8.39** (continued)

## 8.15 **Division of the Uterine Branch** (Figure 8.40)

Two Pean forceps are applied to the separated uterine branch. One is applied parallel to the hypogastric nerve/the bladder branch, and another is applied to the cervical side. The reason why two Pean forceps are applied to the uterine branch is to avoid bleeding from the small vessel running parallel to the uterine branch. The uterine branch between the two forceps is divided with scissors. When the uterine branch is divided, the surgeon will experience a sensation similar to that of a stretched string breaking with a snap. Each forceps is replaced by ligature. Electrocautery is not recommended for the division of the uterine branch, in case of inadvertent damage to the remaining nerves.

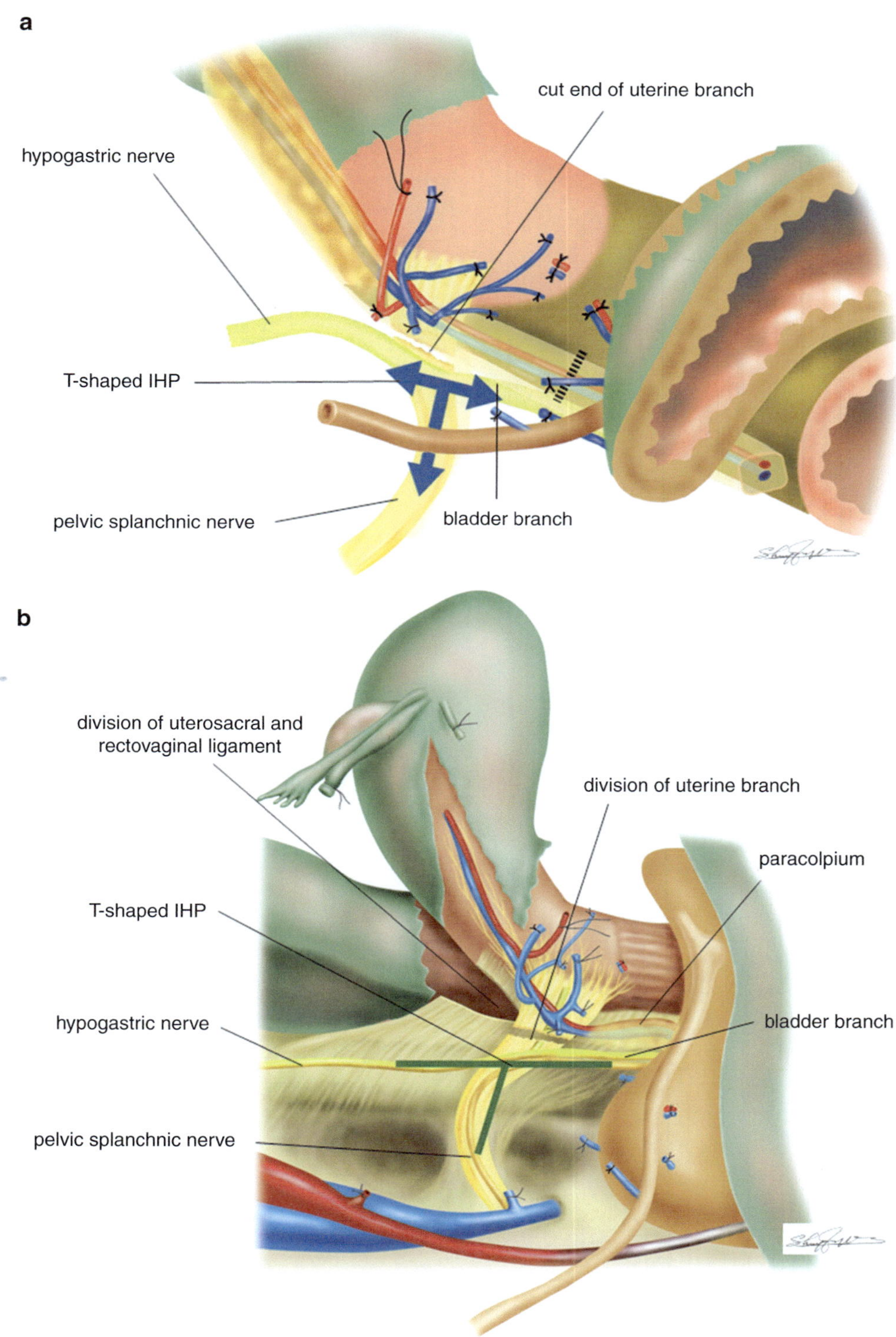


**Figure 8.40** Division of the uterine branch. (**a**) A view from the symphysis side to the cranial side (T-shaped IHP). (**b**) A lateral side view of T-shaped inferior hypogastric plexus. (**c**) A surgical photo of T-shaped inferior hypogastric plexus

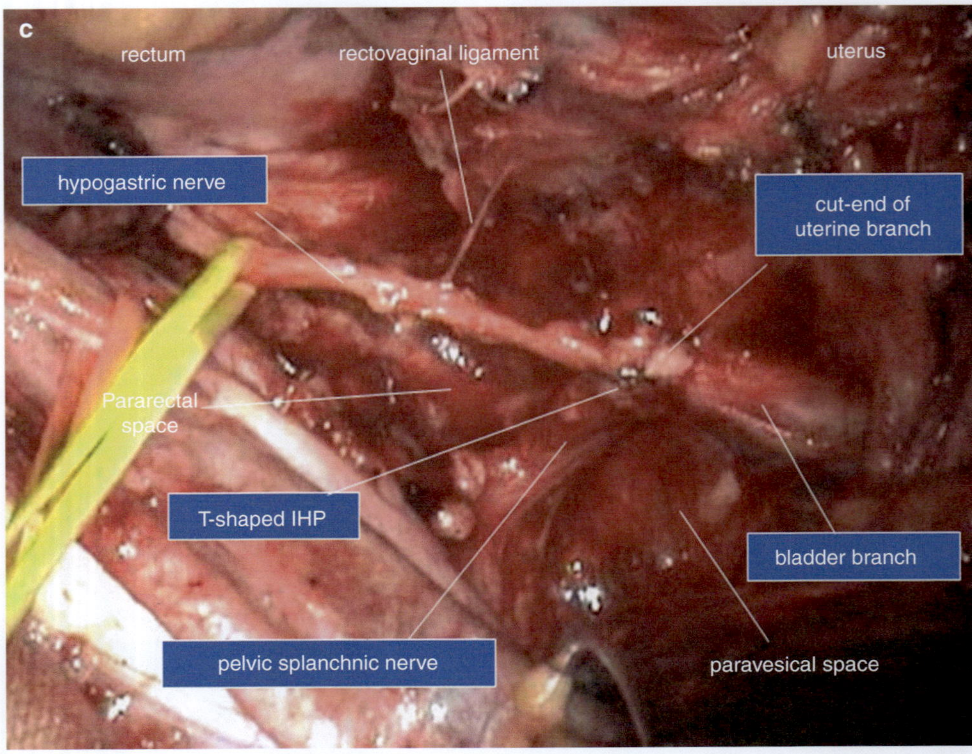


**Figure 8.40** (continued)

## 8.16 Separation of the Rectovaginal Ligament Preserving T-Shaped Nerve Plane (Figure 8.41)

After the division of the uterine branch from the IHP, the rectovaginal ligament is divided toward the vaginal wall. The bladder branch is gradually separated from the blood vessels of the paracolpium. By pushing the rectum up, the rectovaginal ligament between the rectum and the vagina is divided using bipolar scissors toward the upper vagina excluding the T-shaped IHP. The separation can extend caudally to obtain a vaginal length that is deemed appropriate by the extent of cervical disease.

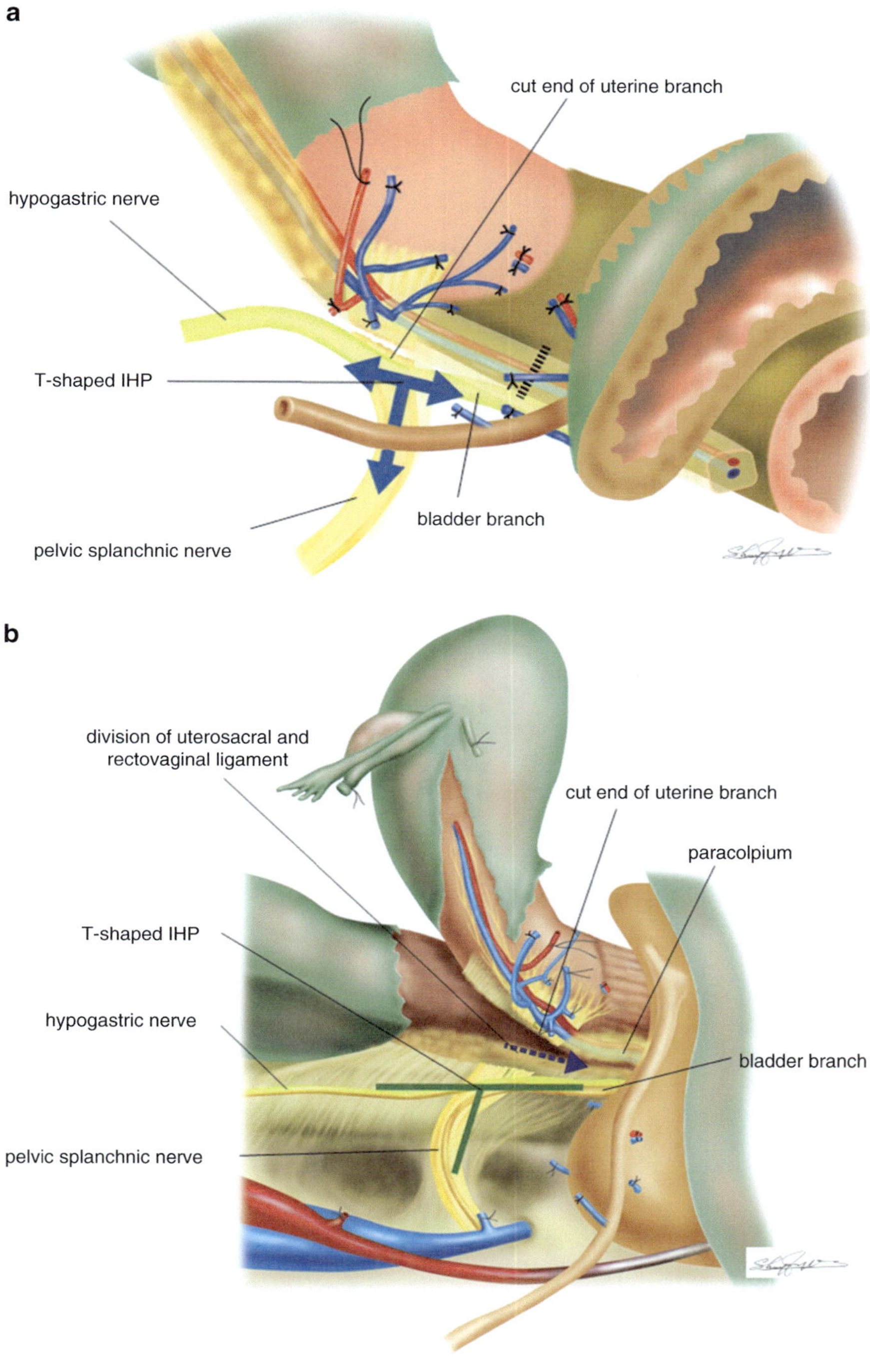


**Figure 8.41** Separation of the rectovaginal ligament preserving T-shaped nerve plane. (**a**) A view from the symphysis side to the cranial side. (**b**) A lateral side view of the T-shaped inferior hypogastric plexus. (**c**) A surgical photo of the T-shaped inferior hypogastric plexus and rectovaginal ligament

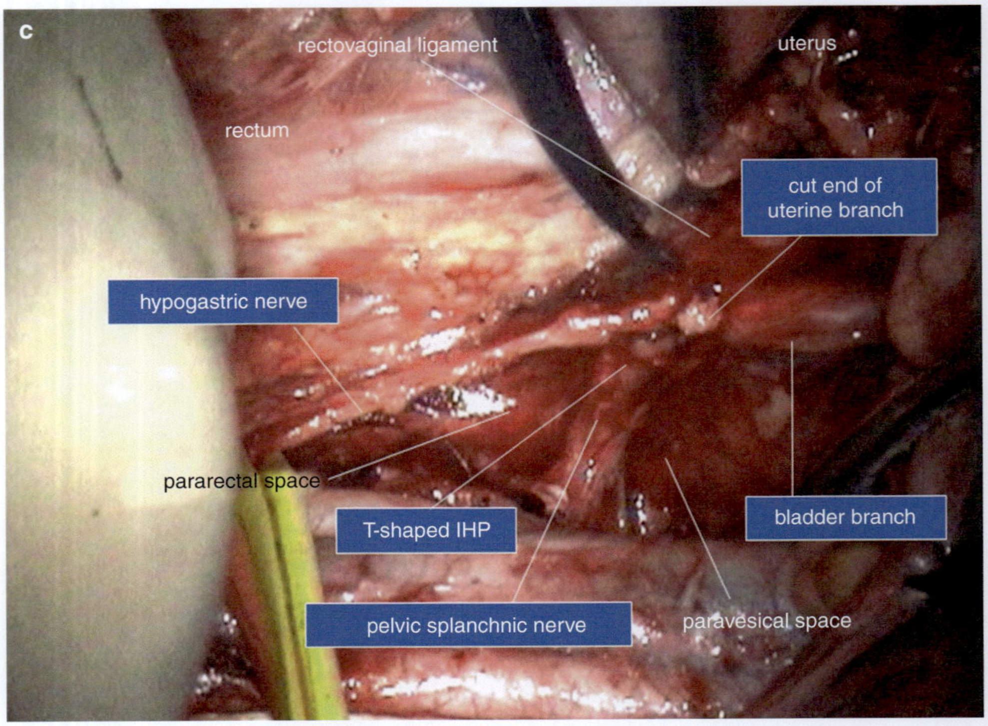


**Figure 8.41** (continued)

## 8.17 Clamp of the Paracolpium (Figure 8.42)

At the appropriate level, the blood vessels of the paracolpium are doubly clamped.

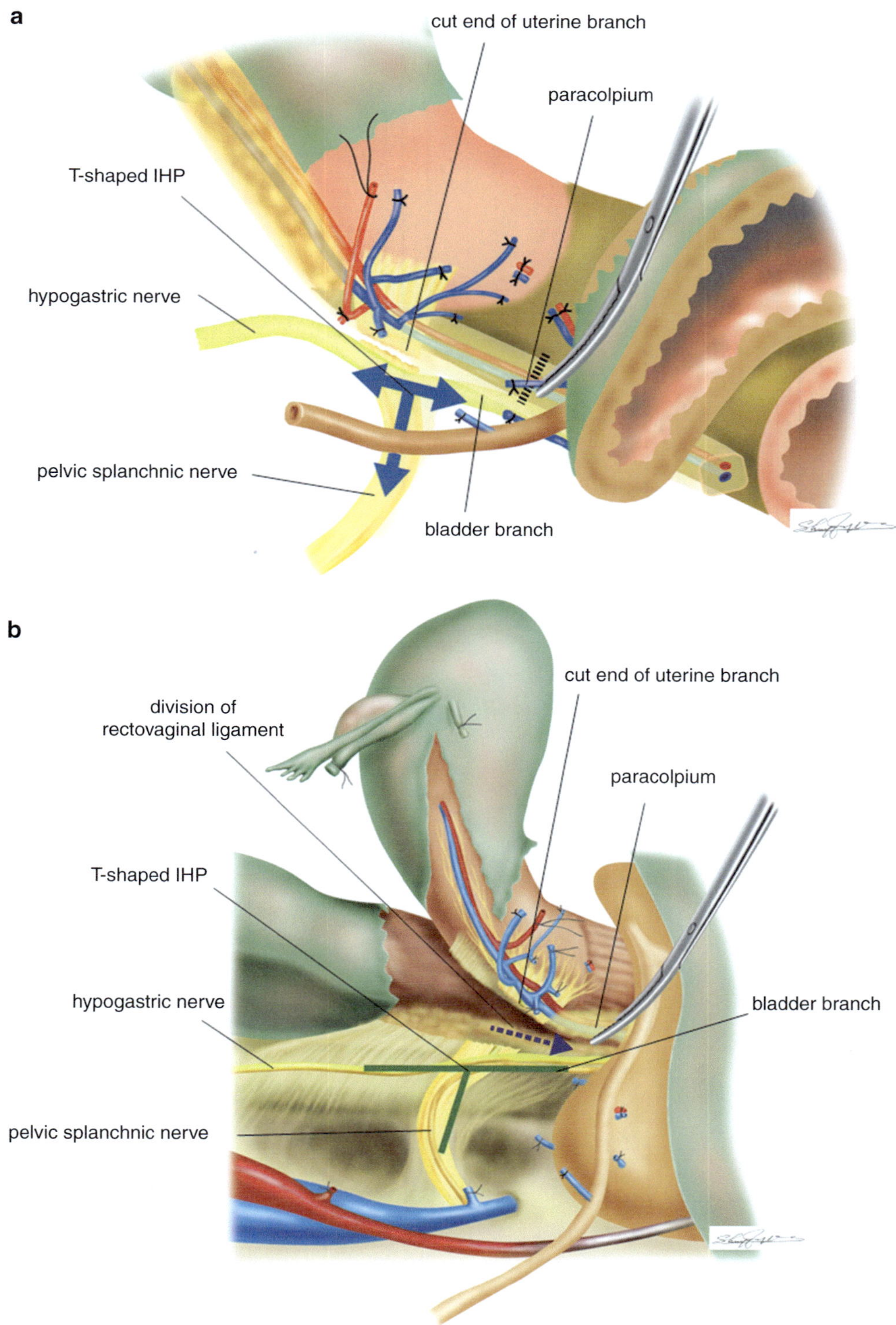


**Figure 8.42** Clamp the paracolpium. (**a**) A view from the symphysis side to the cranial side. (**b**) A lateral side view of the paracolpium. (**c**) A surgical photo of the paracolpium

**Figure 8.42** (continued)

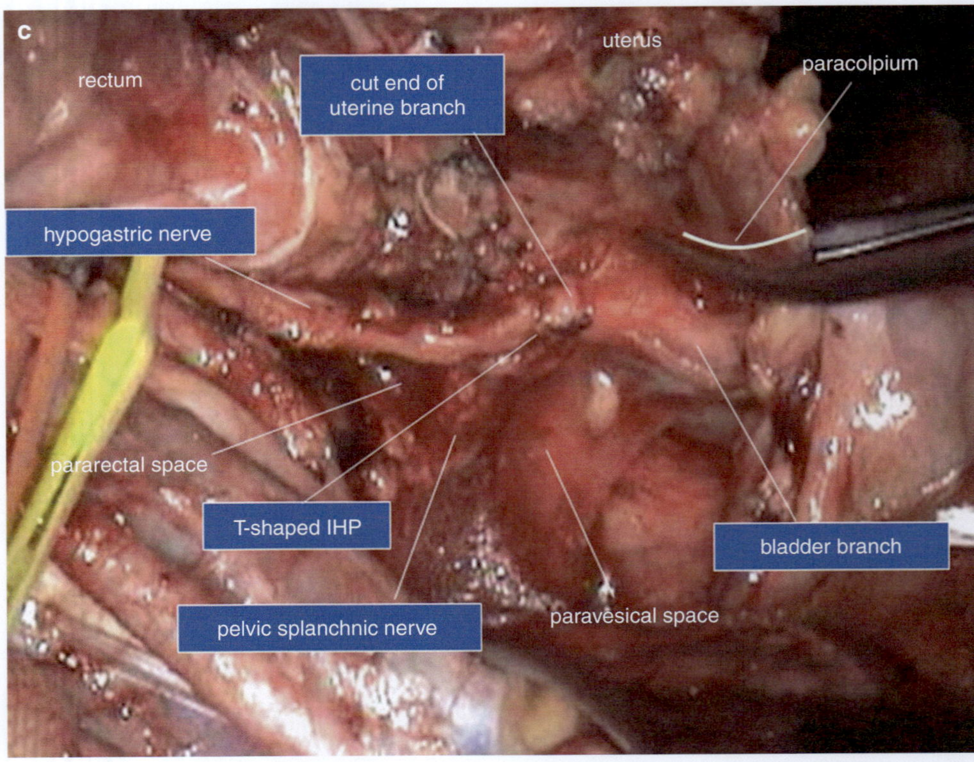

## 8.18 Ligation and Division of the Paracolpium (Figure 8.43)

Between the two forceps, the paracolpium is divided. The forceps are replaced by the ligature. The T-shaped nerve plane formed by the hypogastric nerve, the pelvic splanchnic nerve, and the bladder branch from the IHP is completely preserved. The uterus is left connected only with the vagina. After the same step is completed on the opposite side, the length of the vaginal cuff that needs to be excised is confirmed.

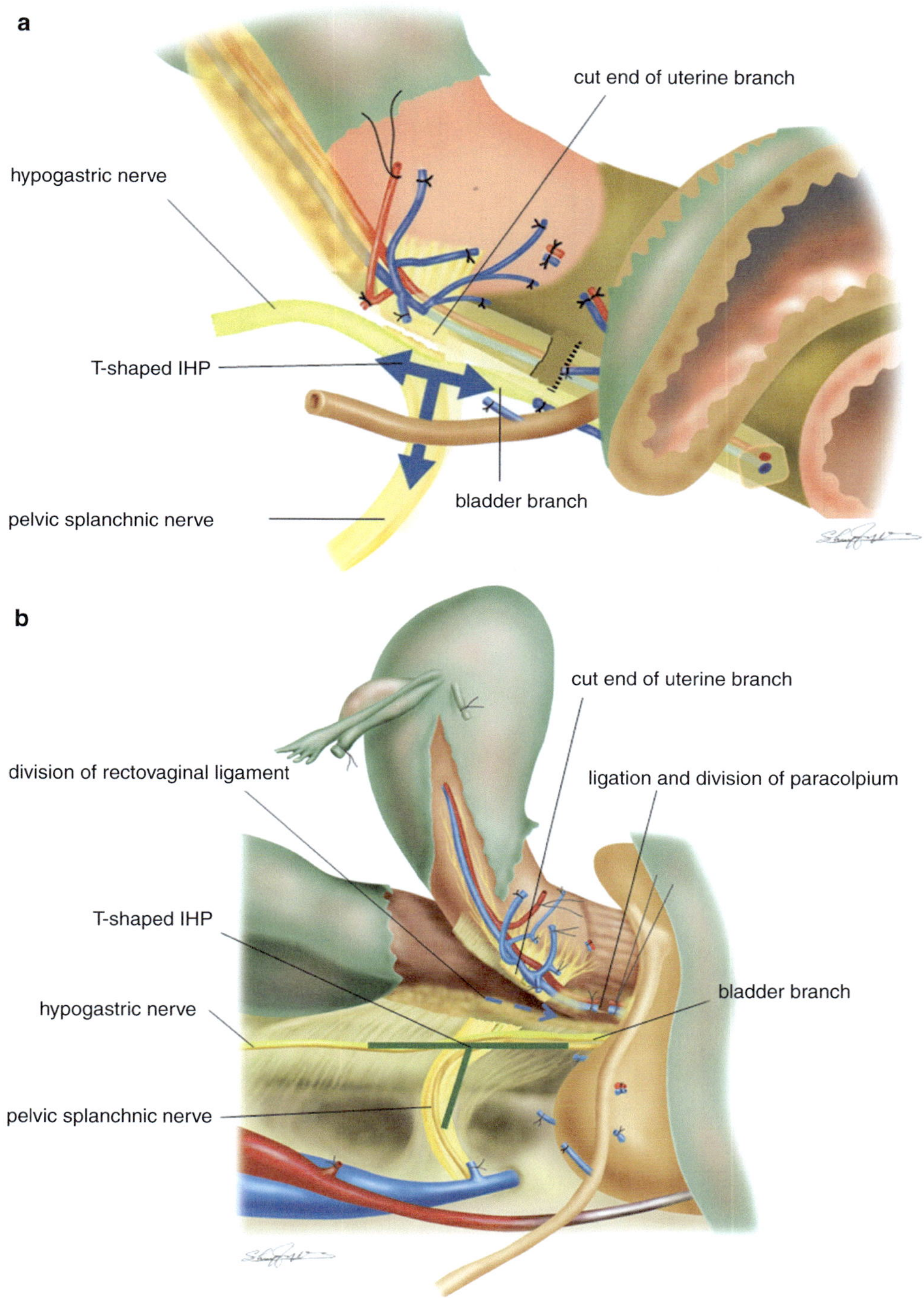


**Figure 8.43** Ligation and division of the paracolpium. (**a**) A view from the symphysis side to the cranial side. (**b**) A lateral side view of the paracolpium. (**c**) A surgical photo of the paracolpium

**Figure 8.43** (continued)

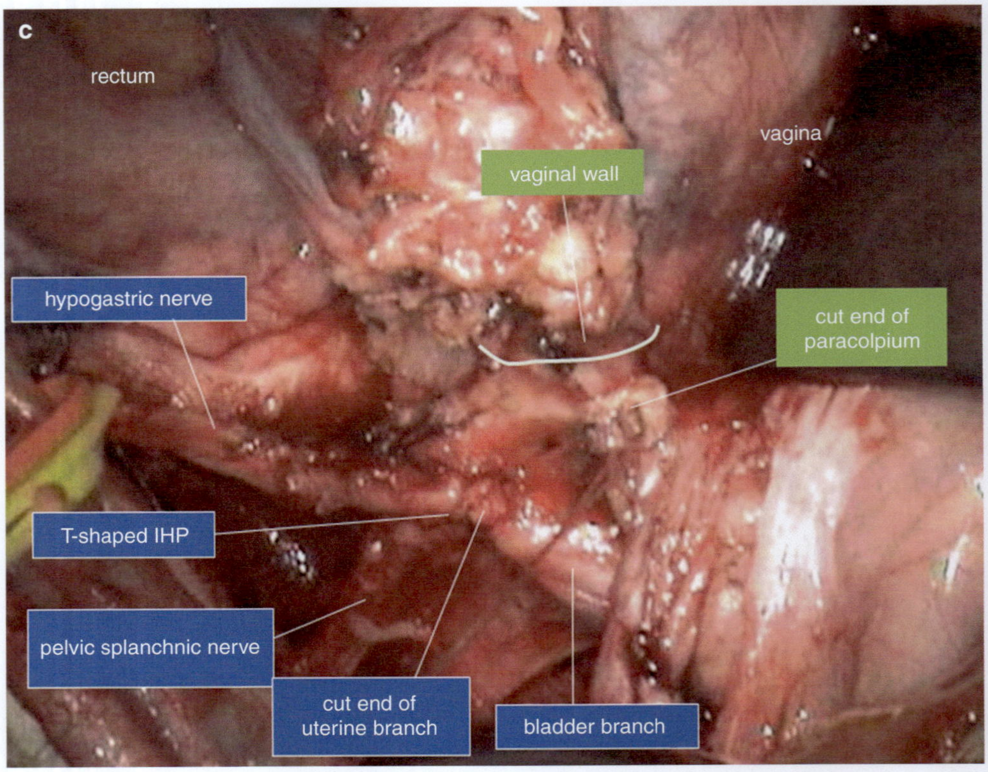

## 8.19 Incise the Vaginal Wall for Amputation of the Vagina (Figure 8.44)

An incision is made on the vagina and the uterus along with the vaginal cuff is amputated from the vagina.

**Figure 8.44** Incision of the vaginal wall for amputation of the vagina

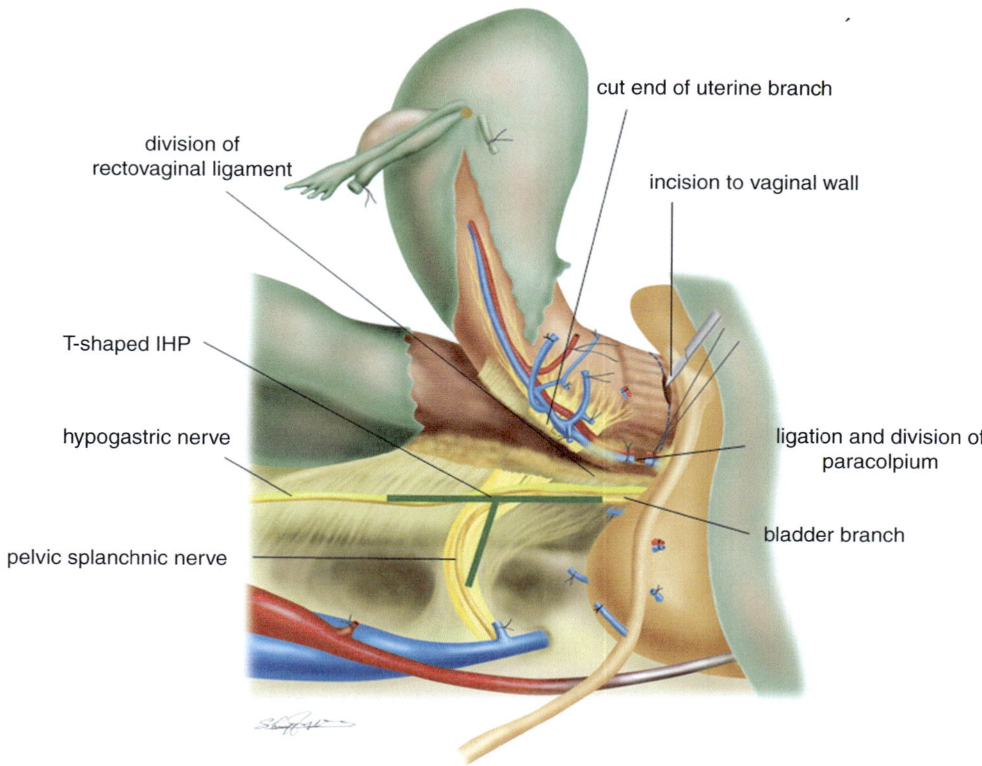

## 8.20 Removal of the Uterus Preserving T-Shaped Nerve Plane (Figure 8.45)

After the removal of the uterus, T-shaped IHP is preserved. The goal of nerve-sparing radical hysterectomy is achieved. The urinary functions after surgery are complete voiding, a good feeling of bladder fullness, and a satisfactory feeling of micturition.

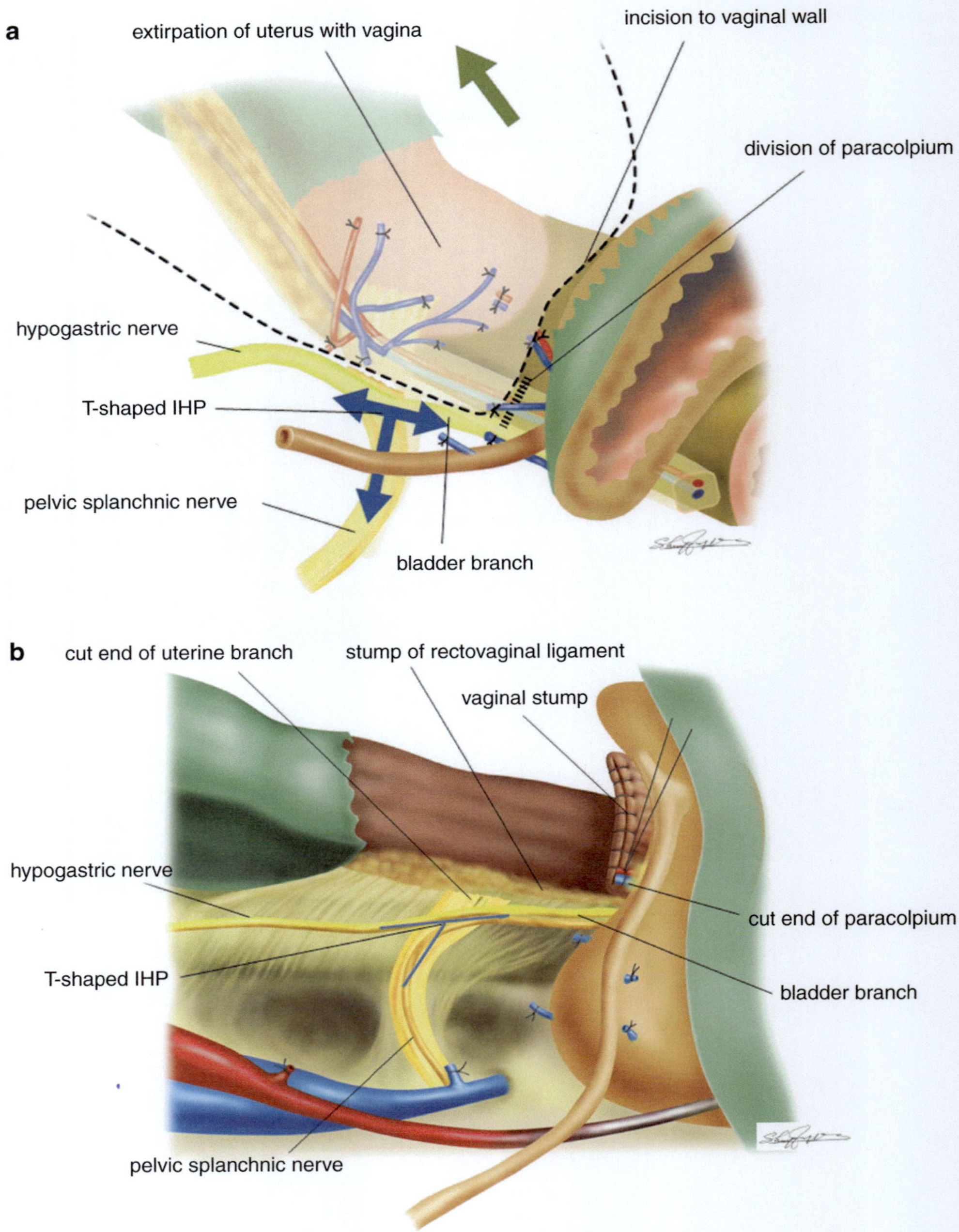


**Figure 8.45** Removal of the uterus preserving T-shaped nerve plane. (**a**) A view from the symphysis to the cranial side. (**b**) A lateral side view of vaginal stump and the preserved T-shaped nerve plane

## 8.21 Closure of the Vaginal Cuff

At the division of the vaginal wall, long Kocher forceps is applied to the foot side of the divided vaginal wall. After extirpation of the uterus, each long Kocher forceps is replaced by ligature. Two to three stitches are taken from the ventral vaginal edge to the dorsal vaginal edge and the vaginal cuff is closed by ligature.

## 8.22 Partial Suture to the Pelvic Peritoneum and Insertion of Drains into the Retroperitoneal Space

Careful observation of the pelvic cavity is undertaken to identify bleeding and ensure hemostasis. The pelvic cavity is then washed with saline water. Partial closure of the visceral peritoneum is undertaken between the peritoneum of the cranial side of the urinary bladder and the peritoneum of the Pouch of Douglas. The peritoneum of the ventral side of the pararectal space is not closed in order to facilitate absorption of lymph fluid by the surface of the peritoneum secondary to lymphadenectomy. Pelvic drains are inserted transabdominally into the retroperitoneal space bilaterally. The drainage tubes are usually removed if bleeding is not observed for 2 days.

## 8.23 Closure of the Abdominal Cavity

After the suture of the ventral abdominal peritoneum and the fascia, interrupted skin suture is undertaken with cosmetic suture being popular. Using a vaginal speculum, the packed gauze is removed from the vagina and the vaginal stump suture is checked. The surgery is now finished.

## 8.24 Management After Nerve-Sparing Radical Hysterectomy

Postoperatively, bladder function is objectively measured by assessing the time to obtain a postvoid residual volume (PVR) of less than 50 mL. Subjective measures of self-reported sensation of bladder fullness and satisfaction of micturition are evaluated after draining the bladder for 4 days using a Foley catheter. The Foley catheter is clamped and the urinary bladder is filled with urine. If the patient feels a good sensation of bladder fullness, the catheter is removed. If the patient does not feel a good sensation of bladder fullness, the Foley catheter is not removed by postoperative day (POD) 7. If surgery could preserve complete T-shaped nerve plane on either side of the rectum/upper vagina, the patient should retain good sensation of bladder fullness within 7 days after the surgery. Spontaneous voiding with a postvoid residual urine volume (PVR) less than 50 mL is usually achieved within a couple of days after the removal of the Foley catheter. Satisfaction of micturition is typically obtained within 7 days after removal of the Foley catheter. If the uterine branch from the IHP is divided using electrocautery, recovery of the urinary function can be delayed.

# Correction to: Precise Neurovascular Anatomy for Radical Hysterectomy

**Correction to:**
**S. Fujii, K. Sekiyama, *Precise Neurovascular Anatomy for Radical Hysterectomy*, https://doi.org/10.1007/978-981-13-8098-3**

This book was inadvertently published without giving credit to the original publication in the copyright statement. This has now been amended in the copyright page.

The updated original version of the book can be found at https://doi.org/10.1007/978-981-13-8098-3


S. Fujii, K. Sekiyama, *Precise Neurovascular Anatomy for Radical Hysterectomy*,
https://doi.org/10.1007/978-981-13-8098-3_9

MIX
Papier aus verantwortungsvollen Quellen
Paper from responsible sources
FSC® C105338

If you have any concerns about our products,
you can contact us on
**ProductSafety@springernature.com**

In case Publisher is established outside the EU,
the EU authorized representative is:
**Springer Nature Customer Service Center GmbH**
**Europaplatz 3, 69115 Heidelberg, Germany**

Printed by Libri Plureos GmbH
in Hamburg, Germany